THE CONSTRUCTION OF THE SELF

The Construction of the Self

Developmental and Sociocultural Foundations

second edition

Susan Harter

Foreword by William M. Bukowski

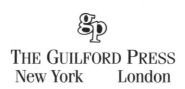

THE GUILFORD PRESS
New York   London

Library of Congress Cataloging-in-Publication Data

Harter, Susan, 1939–
 The construction of the self : developmental and sociocultural foundations /
Susan Harter. — 2nd ed.
    p. cm.
 Includes bibliographical references and index.
 ISBN 978-1-4625-0297-4 (hardcover : alk. paper)
 1. Self in children.   2. Self in adolescence.   I. Title.
 BF723.S24H37 2012
 155.2—dc23

                                                    2011045275

To my daughter, Karen

She has, with enthusiasm and courage, embraced
and carried on the generational childhood educational mission
that my mother began. In only her fourth year in the classroom,
Karen received a coveted accolade as the most talented
elementary school teacher in our large Colorado county.
How proud I am of my mother (to whom I dedicated the first
edition) and now my daughter. Each has had a profound impact
on my understanding of children.

About the Author

Susan Harter, PhD, is Professor Emerita of Psychology at the University of Denver. Her research focusing on self-esteem, the construction of multiple selves, false-self behavior, classroom motivation, and emotional development has been funded by the National Institute of Child Health and Human Development and the W. T. Grant Foundation. Her interests and research also include the study of gender issues across the lifespan. Most recently, she has turned her attention to school violence and the role of the self system in provoking both depressive and violent ideation. A new theme, emanating from the experience of the high-profile school shooters, is the role of humiliation—its causal roots, correlates, and behavioral reactions such as revenge.

Dr. Harter's research has resulted in the development of a battery of assessment instruments that are in widespread use in the United States and elsewhere. She has published numerous scholarly articles and chapters; has served on National Institute of Mental Health study sections, including chairing the committee on Cognition, Emotion, and Personality; and is a member of the editorial boards of journals including *Developmental Psychology, Child Development, Psychological Review, Psychological Bulletin, Development and Psychopathology,* and the *American Educational Research Journal.* In addition, she has given numerous invited colloquium talks worldwide.

Dr. Harter is the recipient of two major faculty awards from the University of Denver for national and international recognition in one's chosen field of research: the University Lecturer of the Year in 1990 and the John Evans Professorship Award in 1993. The latter is the highest scholarly honor the University can bestow upon a faculty member. In two separate publications, Dr. Harter was named one of the world's top 50 developmental psychologists.

Foreword

The "self" is not an easy concept. It is hard to define, it has no easily observable properties, and it can be difficult to measure. Even when one has measures of "it," it is often difficult to know exactly what the measure means. To make matters more challenging, the self is believed to have a vast array of features and characteristics and to be implicated in a wide variety of processes and experiences. Although there is little agreement about exactly what and where the self is, there is nearly universal agreement that the self is real and that it exists within each of us.

In this second edition of *The Construction of the Self*, Susan Harter makes the reality of the self very clear. She does this by situating it within a rich set of ideas, perspectives, and findings drawn from different scholarly domains, including philosophy, psychology, cultural studies, and history. Each of these areas brings a different perspective to the topic of what the self is, how it is formed, and how it functions. The book covers the vast territory of the empirical literature regarding the components that make up the self and how variations in these components affect adaptation and well-being. Perhaps the most important territory of this volume is the extensive presence of basic questions about how the self fits into human life. Beyond her careful and comprehensive description of the vast breadth of the empirical literature related to aspects of the self, Harter provides a deep and reflective consideration of the self's fundamental pertinence to our understanding of the experience of being a person at a particular time in a particular place. Insofar as the self is essentially a meaning-laden construct, then a book about the self needs to consider what it means and how it achieves a place of functional meaning in a person's life. These considerations are the centerpiece of this book.

Harter begins by discussing historical changes in the self. She shows how the prevailing social and cultural structures at specific moments of history colluded to define the basic features of the self. During the periods of 18th- and 19th-century romanticism, the self was comprised of considerations of love, interpersonal loyalty and passion, the power of nature, and morality. In contrast, during the rationalist period of 21st-century modernism, the self became dependent on the concepts of self-direction, individuality, self-reliance, autonomy, and individual strength. The focus also shifted to rationality and the need to scientifically verify claims about the self. These changes revealed how views of the self reflect the prevailing cultural and political zeitgeist. Contemporary formulations focus on the implications of postmodern thought, where a more contextualized perspective, revealed in the construction of multiple selves, leads to a potential cause for concern.

Harter also situates the self within a developmental perspective. Just as the self has changed across history, it also changes over the course of a person's life, at least in part for some of the same reasons. Harter argues persuasively that the self is not the direct result of experience but is instead the result of several constructive processes that are dependent on a person's cognitive abilities and their intersection with experience and developmental history. The self-concept of young children is often very narrow due to limitations in their cognitive skills. They typically think of themselves according to simple and easily observable features such as physical appearance or basic physical skills ("I can run fast!"). They also have trouble creating a comprehensive impression of their overall worth as a person (i.e., their global self-esteem or self-worth). Creating this type of general self-representation requires a higher-order integration of impressions from specific domains of functioning. For young children, specific domains of functioning are not clearly distinguished from each other and therefore defy integration. Older children, however, whose cognitive skills include a facility with articulation, are able to make careful distinctions between domains of experience and integrate them in nuanced ways. They are also better able to compare themselves to/with others and understand the features and dynamics of the broader social and cultural context. As a result, they can construct a richer and more complex self that is comprised of their own likes and dislikes and their similarities to and differences from others. Just as important, their increased ability to create personal narratives allows them to construct a view of themselves that has a past, a present, and a future.

Older children are also better able to compare themselves to others and to understand the implications of the similarities and differences they observe. Social comparison skills can, paradoxically, lead to more negative perceptions of the self, *if* one concludes that one is lower on the evaluative hierarchy. This example highlights a major contribution of Harter's developmental analysis. At each level of childhood and adolescence, she points to the *normative liabilities* of self-development. She distinguishes these often transitory liabilities from more stable pathological manifestations of the self at each level.

If there are periods of the lifespan to which the self has been most strongly connected, they are adolescence and "emerging" adulthood. Several changes occur during these periods, including the ability to engage in abstract thinking and self reflection, an increased level of intimacy in interpersonal relations, and a wider range of contexts in which persons spend their days. These pressures, in turn, lead to changes in several fundamental aspects of the self, including one's chosen goals, sense of vulnerability to risk, ability to project oneself into the future, and sense of connection to others. These periods of the lifespan take on both the passionate features of the historical period of romanticism and the rational features of modernism. Harter's present description of the self-related dynamics of emerging adulthood (Chapter 4) is the best explication I have ever read of this developmental period.

Many questions about the self ultimately lead back to questions about what it is. One persistent self-related question has to do with authenticity; another has to do with accuracy. Harter grapples with these challenging aspects of the self in her concluding chapter. It would be easy to write off these questions as irrelevant. Why should one be concerned with the self's authenticity and accuracy? Presumably the self is the self, and that's all that matters. It turns out, however, that authenticity and accuracy *do* matter. The importance of authenticity appears to be strongest in the present postmodernist era, when guidance about what the self should be is, for most persons, no longer available from traditional sources such as religion and powerful cultural forces. Moreover, as persons tend to function in a more diverse set of circumstances and take on a broader set of roles, the self necessarily becomes more differentiated. This level of differentiation makes integration and authenticity more difficult. Considering that having a sense of authenticity is positively associated with well-being, this postmodernist lack of an integrated and authentic self may be a malaise of the postmodern world. Having an inaccurate self (i.e., one that differs from objective indicators) may be a form of malaise also. Persons whose distortion is positive (i.e., they think they are better than they really are) appear to be at risk for anger, hostility, and aggression; those whose distortion is negative are at risk for depressed affect. Harter's rich discussion of these issues touches upon not only the basic features of the self but also the question of what kind of self is the "best."

Two chapters that are new to this revised volume offer other perspectives on how the self intersects with contextual factors. Chapter 8 provides a thorough discussion of cultural variations in the self, especially as they are related to contextual differences in the importance of individualism and collectivism. This chapter shows clearly that the self is deeply rooted in daily cultural practices that regulate many of our thoughts, emotions, and expectations of others, and give meaning to our experiences. Although there have been some claims that the concepts of individualism and collectivism have been overused to the point of becoming clichés, this chapter shows their fundamental relevance to our sense of who we are and what we do. This emphasis on "what we do" is seen also in Chapter 7's discussion of how several fundamental self-related processes affect achievement motivations and outcomes. Harter does not shy away from describing the complex nature of the multilevel processes in which the self is implicated in academic achievement.

Given that the "self" is of interest to many audiences, this book will appeal to a broad set of readers, including *developmental psychologists* who wish to understand the origins and ontogenetic changes in the self, *philosophers* who wish to enhance their understanding of how conceptual formulations stand up to empirical scrutiny, *social psychologists* who are interested in a developmental perspective on the structure and functional dynamics of the self, *clinical psychologists* and other *mental health professionals* who are concerned with how self-processes relate to forms of psychopathology such as depression and aggression, *educators* interested in how the self is related to classroom motivation, and *cross-cultural psychologists* interested in refining previous conceptualizations. This multilayered and scholarly volume offers much to each of these groups; it speaks to all audiences.

Perhaps the most impressive aspect of the book has to do with how it speaks. This book has a voice, and for me this voice comes directly from its author. As I read this book I could hear Susan Harter speaking to me. I truly felt as if she were in the room with me, kindly providing a gentle and scholarly lecture about the self and all the fascinating components and processes related to it. In this way, this book is a manifestation of a part of Susan's learned and reflective self that has developed over a rich and productive career of research on what the self is and how it fits into development.

WILLIAM M. BUKOWSKI, PHD
Department of Psychology
Concordia University
Montreal, Quebec, Canada

Preface

During its long history, the self has continued to evolve in its definition as well as its determinants, correlates, and consequences. Since the publication of this book's first edition in 1999, the years have witnessed shifting and expanding conceptualizations of the self, on several fronts: (1) theoretical approaches to the self, (2) the identification of new developmental stages such as "emerging adulthood" (Arnett, 2000), (3) methodological innovations to capture the nature of self-processes, (4) a sociocultural appreciation for how one's inner self (self-esteem) is intimately related to one's outer self (perceptions of physical appearance or attractiveness), (5) clinical attention to implications of self-dynamics that bear upon our understanding of psychopathology, (6) the educational relevance of self-constructs as they play out in the classroom, and (7) an appreciation for cross-cultural differences in the conceptualization of the self.

This second edition addresses these themes. Five new chapters cover self-processes during emerging adulthood, the inextricable link between self-esteem and perceived appearance, self-processes and motivation in the classroom, cross-cultural and multicultural considerations, and a reconsideration of the self that focuses on authenticity. Three other chapters, on self-processes during childhood, self-processes during adolescence, and self-conscious emotions, have undergone significant revision.

Throughout the second edition, a recurring theme is concern with Americans' *preoccupation* with the self. This excessive focus on the self can be observed in adult displays of self-enhancement strategies, self-serving biases, narcissistic tendencies, and false-self behavior. The revised chapters on childhood and adolescence examine the developmental precursors of the motives and skills necessary to engage in these behaviors, which are argued to compromise the display of the authentic self.

Following the introductory chapter, the next three chapters delineate critical developmental issues for childhood (Chapter 2), adolescence (Chapter 3), and emerging adulthood (Chapter 4). Three substages (early, middle, and late) of both childhood and adolescence are discussed in Chapters 2 and 3, respectively. Such an approach deviates from many common treatments of the self that merely compare childhood to adolescence as two monolithic developmental stages. Moreover, since Arnett (2000) first identified a distinct period of "emerging adulthood," it becomes critical to distinguish the self-representations of older adolescents from those of young, emerging adults (ages 18 to 25).

The chapters on the development of the self during childhood, adolescence, and emerging adulthood address three separate themes: (1) normative descriptive features of the self, (2) normative *liabilities* of self-development, and (3) *pathological* manifestations of self-development that reflect individual differences within a given substage. It is important to make the distinction between normative liabilities, more transient in nature, and pathological processes, which are likely to be more enduring and severe.

The content of Chapters 2 and 3 has been expanded and organized to address developmental changes in seven different self-processes that will be explored across the three substages of childhood and three substages of adolescence: (1) self-awareness (including self-agency, self-continuity, and self-coherence), (2) egocentrism, (3) the accuracy of self-appraisals, (4) global self-esteem, (5) narcissism, (6) true-self versus false-self behavior, and (7) self-enhancement strategies.

Chapter 4, new to this edition, fleshes out those dimensions of *emerging adulthood* that are particularly relevant to the self. This stage is most likely to be normative for those middle-class youth who have the luxury of exploring various dimensions of their identity prior to making strong commitments. Thus, they experiment with occupational possibilities, with social and intimate relationships, and with belief systems (e.g., religious, moral, and political identification). Differences associated with social class as well as culture cast doubt on the universality of this new stage of development, suggesting the need for refinements in the conceptualization of emerging adulthood.

Chapter 5, also new to this edition, tackles the inextricable link between *perceived appearance* and *global self-esteem*. Our own research reveals that across the entire lifespan (young children to senior adults), there is a strong, positive relationship between perceived appearance and self-esteem, with correlations ranging from .55 to .80, consistent with the findings of others. The major contributor to this robust relationship between perceptions of one's outer and inner selves can be found in the cultural icons who represent the gold standard of attractiveness, as broadcast in the media. Movies, television, the Internet, and magazine advertising all tout the importance of adherence to unattainable societal standards of attractiveness. Failure to measure up to these standards can be psychologically crippling. Historically, women have been the targets of these cultural messages, but more recently the bar of attractiveness has been raised for men. Those who acknowledge that they base their self-esteem on perceptions of their appearance are more likely to experience negative outcomes such as low self-esteem, depression, and eating-disordered behavior.

Chapter 6, on *self-conscious emotions*, has been considerably broadened since the first edition. In addition to shame and guilt, the second edition adds *embarrassment* and *humiliation* to the list. Humiliation, in particular, has received virtually no attention in the empirical emotion literature, despite the fact that every day in schools and neighborhoods, children are being bullied and harassed, leading to humiliation. My own interest in this topic was spurred by an examination of the media reports of 12 high-profile school shooting cases. The histories of the all-male, white, middle-class school shooters reveal that they not only suffered from chronic bullying and harassment, but also experienced the self-conscious emotion of humiliation at the hands of the perpetrators. Humiliation, in turn, provoked acts of revenge and retaliation. I contrast the four negative self-conscious emotions—shame, guilt, embarrassment, and humiliation—across six defining and differentiating dimensions: (1) the *causes* of each emotion, (2) implications for the *self*, (3) the role of *others*, (4) *emotional correlates*, (5) *behaviors and reactions*, and (6) *adaptive functions*. The literature points to the sociocultural conclusion that we require negative self-conscious emotions to curb our tendencies to violate self- and societal norms.

Chapter 7, also new to this edition, delves into the role of self-processes in the *classroom* and their links to student *motivation*. Findings consistently reveal that those with negative perceptions of their scholastic ability invariably report lower levels of academic motivation and/or types of motivation that can be debilitating—for example, an extrinsic orientation to external rewards and sanctions within the classroom. Those more intrinsically motivated by curiosity, exploration, and the joy of mastery are much more likely to report more positive perceptions of their ability. The educational system itself has been indicted for encouraging the more debilitating extrinsic orientation, beginning with the transition to middle and junior high schools. Educational practices such as an emphasis on *ability* rather than *effort*, bolstered by the focus on grades and test scores and exacerbated by public social comparison (posting of grades, honor roll lists, and so forth), are commonplace. They conspire with the normative self-consciousness of adolescence, diminishing the motivation of all but those students at the top of the academic totem pole.

Chapter 8, another addition to this second edition, addresses *cross-cultural* and *multicultural* approaches to the self. It begins with distinctions by previous scholars in the field that contrast *individualistic* and *collectivistic* cultures. In so doing, this chapter differentiates or disentangles the *value systems* of each cultural orientation from its respective *self-appraisals*—an *independent* versus an *interdependent* construal of the self. Most contemporary cross-cultural scholars acknowledge that the lines between these distinctions have been too sharply drawn. This chapter provides a critique that addresses these issues from theoretical, methodological, and empirical perspectives. That said, there are cross-cultural distinctions that remain robust, for example, the *self-enhancing* strategies that dominate in Western individualistic cultures, in contrast to the more self-effacing tendencies of Eastern, collectivistic, cultures.

Multiculturalism speaks to the adaptation of those who have moved from their country of origin to a different culture (typically to the United States), in which they are in the minority. Acculturation issues, such as acceptance versus rejection by the dominant culture, loom large. The consequences of different acculturation styles vary in terms of their adaptiveness and implications for the self. Chapter 8 highlights how American values and self-construals can produce unrealistic self-enhancement strategies and self-serving biases. These not only preclude authentic connectedness to others but eventually backfire, with negative consequences for the self.

A new concluding Chapter 9, "Reconsidering the Self: In Search of Authenticity," builds upon the previous chapters. It suggests that the contemporary self is clearly cause for concern. The fact that the majority of the material reviewed in the first chapters addressing self-development during childhood, adolescence, and emerging adulthood is consumed with negative implications for the self (liabilities and pathological manifestations) is one clue. Another is the observation that the self has actually become a curse (see Leary, 2004). Rampant preoccupation with the self, self-enhancing strategies that unrealistically promote the self through self-aggrandizement, self-serving biases, and narcissism are all on the rise. There are also pluralistic demands for the individual to create multiple social selves whose voices are no longer compatible. Intrapsychic distress, conflict, chaos, and confusion represent the postmodernist's characterization of the 21st-century self. In addition, the "self-esteem movement," claiming that enhancing the self-esteem of the citizenry and our students would cure many societal ills, floundered badly and has come under severe criticism. In large part, the failure of these efforts stemmed from the fact that they sought to *unrealistically* inflate the self-evaluations of individuals, with negative consequences for the self. These efforts also promoted an even greater use of the very self-enhancement strategies and self-serving biases that have come to define the curse of the self (Leary, 2004).

Fortunately, there are those who have countered postmodernism pessimism with a vision of hope for the self. Paramount are pleas that the self rediscover its authenticity. Realistic self-appraisals are urged as one pathway to the true self. The positive psychology movement has also contributed to a more optimistic vision of the self. Topics such as compassion for others as well as the self, mindfulness, gratitude, hopefulness, authenticity, and a quiet ego have emerged in the consciousness of the field. It remains to be seen how these more encouraging themes will play out. It is an exciting time to study the self (and be oneself, in the process).

Acknowledgments

Many collaborative efforts brought this volume to fruition. Over several decades, graduate students and postdoctoral trainees at the University of Denver have constituted the backbone of our research program. Financial backing from granting agencies has made this body of work possible. The cooperation of numerous schools has been vital. Several colleagues have provided welcome encouragement and support. Finally, the completion of the book was facilitated through the devoted efforts of those at The Guilford Press.

Numerous talented graduate students and several undergraduate honors students have contributed their insights and energies, culminating in groundbreaking theses that have formed the basis for the research presented in this volume. Because their invaluable efforts cannot be prioritized, I am listing them in alphabetical order: Kauser Ahmed, Lisa Badanes, Natasha Bolling, Heather Bouchey, Shelly Bresnick, Bonnie Buddin, Cris Chandler, Chris Chao, Jim Connell, Barbara Danis, Jackie Dougherty, Kay Freyer, Maria Elena Guzman, Jane Haltiwanger, Brad Jackson, Crystal Johnson, Don Johnson, Eric Johnson, Lori Junkin, Diana Kastelic, Lisa Kiang, Patty Kowalski, Kevin Lancelotta, Peggy Lane, Sabina Low, Donna Marold, Wanda Mayberry, Kendall McCarley, Tara Mehta, Bonnie Messer, Ann Monsour, Jennifer Neemann, Rosanna Ng, Diana Nikkari, Lisa Pettitt, Robin Pike, Danielle Pulham, Mari Jo Renick, Andrew Renouf, Shauna Rienks, Nancy Robinson, Valerie Simon, Ayelet Talmi, Robert Thompson, Amanda Volenec, Nancy Whitesell, and Nancy Winfrey.

Two students who contributed extensively to our research program deserve special mention. Nancy Whitesell continued as a primary colleague after obtaining her PhD and for many years was central to our research program. Nancy contributed her many talents in terms of research design, her insights into self-processes, her knowledge of the increasingly sophisticated statistical techniques that emerged, and her clarity in shaping the final presentation of our findings to the professional community. Donna Marold, a trained clinician at the time of her graduate training, continued to contribute her expertise in the areas of depression, suicide, and the effects of early abuse on the functioning of children and adolescents. This collaborative research received support from the W. T. Grant Foundation, leading to the publication of several articles and chapters.

Complementing these efforts have been the contributions of a coterie of gifted postdoctoral trainees who have represented junior colleagues. They have brought their own talents, unique ideas, and expertise, enriching the studies that ensued. At their particular period of training, they rounded out a vibrant research team, also serving as mentors to graduate students. I am indebted to Kym Baum, Paula Bealle, Jeff Elison, Jennifer Kofkin, Kristin Neff, Clare Stocker, and Tricia Waters. Elison, Neff, and Waters continued to collaborate after they moved on to accept tenure-track faculty positions in highly reputable institutions.

Over the years, we have been grateful for the generous financial support from several agencies. The National Institute of Child Health and Human Development supported our research for several decades. The National Institute of Mental Health provided two decades of support for our Post-Doctoral Research Training Program in Developmental Psychology at the University of Denver. The W. T. Grant Foundation provided funds for the studies that I conducted with Donna Marold on the links between the self system and depressive reactions displayed by adolescents. More recently, the W. T. Grant Foundation supported our seminal research on the role of humiliation.

The research we have conducted over the years would not have been possible without the cooperation of numerous schools whose student participants enhanced our understanding of childhood and adolescence. I am particularly indebted to Principal Steven Cohen of Flood Middle School in Englewood, Colorado, for his continued support over the years. Part of our success stemmed from his insights into the need to bring together a collaboration of our own research team with his teachers and the students' parents. I would also like to thank other school administrators and their students at Arapahoe High School, Bear Creek High School, Cherry Creek High School, Rangeview High School, Smoky Hill High School, St. Mary's High School, Hamilton Middle School, Indian Hills Elementary School, Laredo Middle School, Merrill Middle School, and Steele Street Elementary School.

Several close colleagues have provided continued encouragement as I crafted this volume. They were particularly helpful as I sought to bring my research program to bear upon more applied issues, for example, within the classroom and within our multicultural world, and as our research addressed clinical issues such as depression and more outward displays of aggression toward others. So thank you, Catherine Cooper, Barbara McCombs, and Stephen Shirk.

Special gratitude goes to Kendall McCarley, a 2009 PhD, who was an integral part of our most recent research team. Kendall worked tirelessly on this volume. She researched numerous topics and tracked down relevant publications and made them available, all of which allowed me to cover the literature during the past decade. As the chapters of the book evolved, she critiqued them thoughtfully. Moreover, her eagle editorial eye helped immensely in shaping the manuscript. Finally, she came to understand the ultimate, somewhat controversial message that I chose to deliver, helping me to craft the chapters toward a compelling conclusion.

Finally, no such volume could have come to fruition without the guidance of those at The Guilford Press. Seymour Weingarten, Editor-in-Chief, shared my belief that a second edition would illuminate the many new self issues that continue to emerge in our rapidly changing world. Editor Kristal Hawkins provided the day-to-day support, guiding me through the process. Barbara Watkins was a most conscientious developmental editor, whose thoughtful suggestions were immensely helpful in clarifying the points I wished to express and in ensuring that my grammar led to the most forceful conclusions.

I am most grateful to the many people who have collectively constituted "Team Susan Harter." Everyone brought their A-game throughout the entire process and I will forever be indebted.

Particular thanks go to Bill Bukowski for providing a thoughtful and extensive review of the manuscript. His suggestions were invaluable in allowing me to make more nuanced arguments. He also supported my speaking in my own voice. I am also very appreciative of the laudatory endorsements of Jacque Eccles, Mark Leary, and Rich Ryan, all scholars of great renown, each of whom have made major contributions to our understanding of self-development.

Contents

Chapter 1

Introduction

A Contemporary Approach
to Self-Development

The goal of this book is to explore the *development* of the self and those cognitive-developmental as well as sociocultural influences that shape its formation. I will focus on the antecedents that contribute to self-development as well as on the functional consequences of the self. With regard to antecedents, it will become evident that the self is both a *cognitive* and a *social* construction, two major themes around which the developmental material will be organized. Cognitive determinants illuminate normative *developmental* features of self-development. Social antecedents (child-rearing practices, cultural factors) are more likely to produce *individual differences* in how the self is crafted.

From a cognitive perspective, the construction of the self is inevitable. Those self-theorists devoted to the study of adults (e.g., Epstein, 1991; Greenwald, 1980; G. A. Kelly, 1955; Leary & Tangney, 2003; Markus, 1980; Sarbin, 1962) have forcefully argued that our species has been designed to actively create *theories* about our world, including the construction of a theory of *self* in order to make meaning of our experiences. Cognitive-developmental theorists, particularly neo-Piagetians (e.g., Case, 1992; Fischer, 1980) have concurred, pointing to the changing cognitive structures that determine the nature of the self-theory that children construct at different periods of development. As cognitive processes undergo normative-developmental change, so will the very structure and organization of the self undergo alterations. Thus, the particular cognitive limitations and advances at each developmental period will dictate the emerging features of the self-portrait that can be crafted. The very unity of the self

1

can be compromised as adolescents develop the ability to construct multiple selves that may not always speak with a singular voice. As a result, a pressing concern may arise: Just which is my "true self"?

The self is clearly also a *social* construction. Socialization experiences, initially within the crucible of interpersonal relationships with family, will dictate the *content* and *valence* of the self, resulting in a balance of positive and negative self-evaluations. As will become evident, the evaluative-content self is largely defined by the valence of the reflected appraisals of how significant others treat the self. These appraisals become internalized as children come to appreciate the perspective of others toward the self. The scope of those who offer evaluations of the self broadens as children develop, as various peer groups, teachers, and other adults cast their evaluative gaze upon the self. Other sociocultural factors become increasingly critical. For example, the school becomes a microcosm of society that can profoundly impact the developing self. Broader cross-cultural influences have a powerful impact on the dimensions that shape the self.

A major theme throughout the book focuses on the contemporary self as a cause for *concern*. Adult social psychologists have identified numerous self-enhancement strategies, self-serving biases, unrealistic self-perceptions, and narcissistic tendencies, all of which can dilute the quality of interpersonal relationships and compromise the authenticity of the self. From a developmental perspective, Chapters 2 and 3 on childhood and adolescence and their substages, respectively, address the extent to which the *motives* as well as the *skills* to engage in these strategies exist. At what point in development do they emerge? My analysis suggests that they emerge when these various self-enhancing strategies become available and potentially carried into adulthood. The concluding chapter focuses on how the authenticity of the self can become compromised, beginning with experiences in childhood and continuing into adolescence. I offer suggestions for how the authentic self might be resurrected, although the barriers in our culture are legion. Many of these themes have their roots in historical conceptualizations of the self, to which I now turn.

Shifting Conceptualizations of the Self in Historical Perspective

The self has never represented a static construct. Philosophers of past historical periods, later to be displaced by more academic and scientific intellects, offered their own perspectives on the self (see Baumeister, 1987; Gergen, 1991; Harter, 1997, for reviews). During the 18th- and 19th-century period of *romanticism*, the psychological interior and unobservable qualities of the self were accentuated, including intrinsic worth, morality, creative inspiration, passion, spirituality, and the soul. The subsequent period of *modernism* was ushered in by the scientific and technological advances of the 20th century. The emerging values of reason, objective evidence, and rationality were incompatible with the romanticist perspective. Paradigms for scientific inquiry were predicated on the belief that there were absolute universal truths that could be revealed through the pursuit of science and reason (see L. Hoffman, Stewart, Warren, & Meek, 2009). These principles led to a reconceptualization of the self, where *rationality* and reason became the essence of humanity. The self was cast as a material reality (Norman, 2006) that obeyed the laws of science and became self-directing, consistent over situations and time, coherent in its organization, unwavering, principled, and authentic (see Gergen, 1991; Vitz, 2006). Modern man made conscious and intelligent inferences about behaviors, attributes, and strengths that were *observable*.

Modernism has, in recent years, given rise to our current period of *postmodernism*. As Vitz (2006) describes, from a scientific perspective, truths were no longer believed to be universal; that is, they became relative ("Your truth, my truth"). As such, the values espoused during the era of modernism, objective reality and scientific reasoning, lost their luster. In their place, the limitations of reason and science were highlighted as erroneous and misleading pursuits, in what Vitz characterizes as a rather nihilistic movement. Thus, postmodernism became a critique of the previously entrenched assumptions of modernism, a reaction against the assumptions of universality and strict rationalism (Norman, 2006). As Hoffman et al. (2009) observe, radical arbitrariness and anarchistic relativism came to define the parameters of postmodernism. Pluralism, contextualism, and the multiplicity of perspectives became watchwords.

These shifting philosophical conceptualizations of the self were paralleled by trends within the *academic* discipline of psychology that emerged at the end of the 19th century. During the early period of *introspection*, a remnant of the era of romanticism, legitimate inquiry into topics concerning the self and psyche flourished. William James (1890, 1892) contributed to this zeitgeist. Of paramount importance was his introduction of the distinction between the I-self and the Me-self. James (1890) defined the I-self as the actor or *knower*, whereas the Me-self was identified as the object of one's knowledge, "an empirical aggregate of things objectively known" (p. 197). The Me-self, as a product, was most clearly reflected in the conscious construction of one's self-esteem. The distinction between the I-self and the Me-self has proven to be amazingly viable over the decades, and is a recurrent theme in many theoretical treatments of the self (see Dickstein, 1977; Harter, 1983; M. Lewis, 1994; M. Lewis & Brooks-Gunn, 1979; Wylie, 1979). Until recently, major empirical attention has been devoted to the Me-self as an object of one's evaluation, as evidenced by myriad studies on self-concept and self-esteem that began to emerge in the 1970s (see Harter, 1983, 2006a; Montemayor & Eisen, 1977; Wylie, 1979, 1989).

It was also James's (1890) contention that the individual creates *multiple Me-selves*, paralleling the different social roles that one must perform. He thoughtfully observed that these multiple selves may not always speak with the same voice. This conscious "conflict of the different Me's" arose because of the incompatibility of the multiple social roles that one must negotiate. However, there were countertrends to this introspective conceptualization of self-processes.

With the emergence of radical behaviorism in the 1920s and 1930s, James's (1890) subjective, mentalistic constructs were excised from the scientific vocabularies of many theorists. The principles of modernism came to dominate conceptualizations of the self. Thus, the writings of James and likeminded scholars gathered dust on the shelf for an appreciable period. Historically, it is of interest to ask why the self was for so long an unwelcome guest at the behaviorists' table. Why was it that constructs such as self, including self-esteem, ego strength, sense of omnipotence, narcissistic injury, feelings of unconscious rejection, and so on, did little to whet the behaviorists' appetite? Several related reasons appear responsible.

The very origins of the behaviorist movement rested on the identification of *observables*. Thus, hypothetical constructs were both conceptually and methodologically unpalatable. Cognitions, in general, and verbal descriptions of the self, in particular, were deemed unmeasurable since they could not be operationalized as observable behaviors. Self-report measures designed to tap self-constructs were not included on the methodological menu because people were assumed to be inaccurate judges of their own behavior. Those more accepting of introspective methodologies found the existing measures of self-concept ungratifying, in large part because their content was overly vague and general. Finally, self-constructs were not satisfying to the behaviorists' palate because their *functions* were not clearly specified. The very cornerstone of behavioral approaches rested upon a functional analysis of behavior. In contrast, approaches to the self did little more than implicate self-descriptions as *correlates* of behavior, affording them little explanatory power as causes or mediators of behavior.

Several shifts in emphasis, beginning in the second half of the 20th century, have allowed self-constructs to become more palatable. Hypothetical constructs, in general, gained favor as parsimonious predictors of behavior, often far more economical in theoretical models than a multitude of discrete observables. In addition, we witnessed a cognitive revolution, within the fields of both child and adult psychology (Bruner, 1990). For developmentalists, Piagetian and neo-Piagetian models came to the forefront. For experimental and social psychologists, numerous cognitive models found favor. With the emergence of this revolution, self theorists jumped on the bandwagon, resurrecting the self as a *cognitive* construction, as mental representations that constitute a theory of self (e.g., Brim, 1976; Case, 1985; Epstein, 1973, 1981; Fischer, 1980; Greenwald, 1980; G. A. Kelly, 1955;

Markus, 1977, 1980; Sarbin, 1962). Cognitive theories of self represented the new zeitgeist in an evolving application of modernistic scientific theory and paradigms.

Cognitive self-representations (attributes of the self described by the person) began to gain some legitimacy as clinicians, including behaviorally oriented therapists, were forced to acknowledge that the spontaneous self-evaluative statements of their clients seemed powerfully implicated in their pathology. Scholars began to conceptualize the self as a theory that the person must cognitively construct. A number of influential personality theorists contributed to the cognitive interpretations of the self-theory constructed by individuals. Many scholars placed major emphasis on the integrated, unified self (Allport 1961; Horney, 1950; C. G. Jung, 1928; Lecky, 1945; Maslow, 1954; Rogers, 1951). For Allport, the self includes all aspects of personality that make for a sense of inward unity. Lecky fashioned an entire theory around the theme of *self-consistency*, emphasizing how behavior expresses the effort to maintain the integrity and unity of the self. Epstein (1973, 1981), for example, has argued that among the criteria that one's self-theory must meet is *internal consistency*. Thus, one's self-theory will be threatened by evidence inconsistent with the portrait one has constructed of the self, or by postulates within the theory that appear to be contradictory. Epstein (1981) formalized these observations under the rubric of the "unity principle," emphasizing that one of the most basic needs of the individual is to maintain the unity and coherence of the conceptual system that defines the self.

However, the tide began to turn in the 1970s as many of the sandcastles of modernism began to crumble, and with it the belief in universal truths and rationality. James's (1890) writings were dusted off as psychologists realized that people naturally took themselves as objects of self-reflection. Thus, this distinction between the I-self as knower and the Me-self as known once again found favor. Moreover, his characterization of *multiple Me-selves* represented the reality of self development, including the challenges that such multiplicity provoked. The field began to shift toward an increasing zeal for models depicting how the self varied across situations and relational contexts (see Ashmore & Ogilvie, 1992; Gergen, 1991; Kihlstrom, 1993; Markus & Cross, 1990; S. Rosenberg, 1988; Stryker, 1987).

This realization ushered in the postmodern era that was to dominate. Postmodernism had clear and definite implications for how the self would now be conceptualized. The self shifted to an arbitrary or socially constructed identity (rather than a personally crafted self). As L. Hoffman et al. (2009) point out, the concept of a *coherent* self, in particular, came under an unprecedented attack and was in danger of annihilation at the hands of postmodern theorists such as Gergen (1991, 1998). The plurality of selves across different relational and situational contexts was viewed as an inherent threat to the modernistic concept of the unified, integrated, and coherent self, according to postmodern thought.

In contrast to the emphasis on self-unity, several social psychologists (Gergen, 1968; Mischel, 1973; Vallacher, 1980) began to argue that the most fruitful theory of self must take into account the multiple roles that people adopt. Ironically, James scooped such postmodern thinking in pointing to the conflict that the construction of multiple Me's can provoke. Gergen contended that the "popular notion of the self-concept as a unified, consistent, or a perceptually whole psychological structure is possibly ill-conceived" (p. 306). Although consistency *within* a relationship was deemed desirable, consistency *across* relationships was viewed as difficult, if not impossible, and in all likelihood damaging. That is, people are compelled to adjust their behavior in accord with the specific nature of the interpersonal relationship and its situational context. Such multiplicity is not only a response to the demand characteristics of different interpersonal contexts but also rests heavily on social comparison. As Gergen (1977) observes, "In the presence of the devout, we may discover that we are ideologically shallow; in the midst of dedicated hedonists, we may gain awareness of our ideological depths" (p. 154).

Gergen (1991, 1998) has been one of the most vocal and pessimistic proponents of this postmodern perspective, envisaging nothing but tragedy for a self that is no longer coherently organized because it cannot integrate its diverse or multiple selves, lacking a core center. Gergen argues that the concept of self during the era of modernism necessarily became eradicated, given contemporary societal forces, leading to his new conceptualization of the "saturated" or "populated" self. What is the basis for Gergen's contentions?

In developing his portrait of the "saturated" self, Gergen (1991) observes that easy access to air travel, electronic and express mail, the Internet, fax machines, cellular phones, beepers, and answering machines have all dramatically accelerated our social connectedness. As a result, contemporary life has become a dizzying swirl of social relations where the "social caravan in which we travel through life always remains full" (p. 62). For Gergen, these changes have profound implications for the self, in that they dictate the creation of multiple selves across a variety of social contexts, diverse selves that cannot be reconciled or unified.

Gergen (1991) elaborates further on this theme. The demands of these relationships produce a cacophony of multiple selves, in that their different voices do not necessarily harmonize (see Gergen, 1998, where he later refers to the "polyvocality" of the self). In the face of this multiphrenia, individuals are forced to suspend any expectation for personal coherence. Moreover, the need to craft different selves that must conform to the particular relationship at hand leads to doubt about one's true identity. That is, the sense of an obdurate core self is compromised in playing out one's role as "social chameleon." As a result, the self, in its fragile attempts at impression management, loses its *integrity*.

Lifton (1993) has developed a similar theme in his analysis of the emergence of a postmodern "protean self," named after Proteus, the Greek sea god who possessed many forms any one of which could be adopted, at will. For Lifton, the protean self in contemporary life arises out of "confusion from the widespread feeling that we our losing our psychological moorings" (p. 1). He attributes this confusion to unmanageable historical forces, rapid societal and economic changes, and social uncertainties. Lifton is a bit more sanguine, emphasizing the flexibility and resilience of the protean self. Gergen (1991) does comment on the pleasurable expansiveness that multiple selves can sometimes afford; however, his primary focus is on the difficulties that such selves pose, including how they necessarily erode the belief in a core, essential, self.

Others have pointed to potentially dangerous elements of the protean self. As May (1991) contends, the myth of Proteus as chameleon describes the ease with which many contemporary Americans play whatever role the situation demands. As a result, he finds that we typically do not speak from a sense of inner integrity nor do we have the conviction that we are expressing our true selves. The erosion of an individual's sense of an immutable, authentic core self is a topic to which we shall return, in the concluding chapter, in considering not only how the authenticity of the self can be compromised but how it can be adaptively salvaged as a major contributor to our well-being.

Cushman (1995), another postmodern theorist, offers a related perspective in identifying what he labels the "empty self." He refers to another feature of contemporary life that compromises any sense of lasting authenticity. Although he agrees with Gergen (1991) that the postmodern self has disintegrated, he views the causes as broader than the technological advances that Gergen has identified. He cites, as another major contributor, the corresponding disintegration of the traditional family, as we knew it. The collapse of what were formerly stable family structures and values has led, in Cushman's opinion, to a corresponding collapse in the structure and functioning of the self. He gives, as examples, increases in divorce, single-parent households, blended families, dysfunctional family dynamics, pathological home environments, and the mobility of today's couples and families. Mobility can disrupt contact with one's extended family that, in turn, may diminish former emotional, instrumental, and approval support that served to support the self. Moreover, if mobility requires a move from a smaller, supportive community in which one was acknowledged to a large, unfamiliar city setting in which one feels anonymous, the self can become destabilized.

In addition to concerns about the postmodern self's struggles with multiplicity, stability, coherence, and authenticity, other postmodern theorists question whether the self has lost its sense of direction, in terms of being at the helm, actively charting and navigating the unpredictable waters of life. Thus, postmodern values dealt another blow to the self, challenging its capacity for decisive action. It was Gergen's (1991) contention that "under postmodernism, processes of individual reason, intention, moral decision making, and the like—all central to the ideology of individualism—lose their status as realities" (p. 241). More radical postmodernists (e.g., M. B. Smith, 1994) have also argued that the self, as an active psychological agent has been derailed, if not destroyed (see also Vitz, 2006).

Most contemporary theorists acknowledge that the multiplicity of selves is a reality. However, many within the last decade have responded with criticism and counterarguments, challenging the postmodern claims of Gergen (1991) and others. For example, Vitz (2006) has forcefully argued for what he labels the "transmodern" person who transcends the challenges posed by postmodernism. Today's individual has the capacity to retain a vital sense of continuity across the lifespan, making meaning of a history of personal experiences that allow him/her to retain a core sense of identity that includes authenticity. Others, for example, Martin and Sugarman (2000), contend that while flux is inevitable, it need not be experienced as chaotic. Rather, the self is characterized by "emergent, changing, yet identifiable and understandable patterns" (p. 403) all of which give meaning to one's existence. The very reflective capacities of the self allow it to transcend former conceptualizations of the self, without serious threat to one's core being.

Creating and sustaining meaning is at the center of a number of counterarguments and objections to the postmodern characterization of the self. L. Hoffman et al. (2009) cite the importance of "myth making" (which is akin to the construction of a personal narrative) in providing an existential reply to postmodern theorizing. Others (see Martin & Sugarman, 2000) have countered with examples of how the contemporary self still provides a locus of action and decision making. For many of these theorists, *authenticity* can also be maintained in the face of the multiplicity of selves that most acknowledge is a contemporary reality.

Baile (2006) chides Gergen (1991) for what he considers to be Gergen's cheerfully naïve assumption that the postmodern dilemma can be "properly managed" if one only avoids looking back to the past in search of a true and enduring self. Additionally, Bechtold (2006) takes issue with Gergen's claim that the saturated self lacks coherence, even as multiple selves extend into cyberspace, where people can create alternative Internet identities that offer a virtual reality, apart from the real world. Bechtold charitably suggests that surely Gergen must know that there is an essential self that matters to people and that possesses a meaningful core sense of being. Throughout this volume, we witness how these themes have played out across each chapter. In the final chapter, we return to the claims and criticisms of postmodernism, addressing the extent to which individuals in contemporary society can adaptively adjust to, and function in, our pluralistic world, finding their true self in the process.

A Contemporary Developmental Perspective on the Construction of the Self

The above discussion frames many issues that are critical to an understanding of the self. However, it focuses primarily on adulthood, as does much of the impressive social psychological literature that has addressed the dynamics of the self, and does not speak to issues of development.

Most scholars conceptualize the self as a *theory* that must be cognitively constructed. Those theorists within the tradition of adult personality and social psychology have suggested that the self-theory should possess the characteristics of any formal theory, defined as a hypothetico-deductive system. Such a personal epistemology should, therefore, meet those criteria by which any good theory is evaluated, namely, the degree to which it is parsimonious, empirically valid, internally consistent, coherently organized, testable, and useful.

From a developmental perspective, however, the self-theories created by children cannot meet these criteria, given numerous cognitive limitations that have been identified in Piagetian (1960) and neo-Piagetian formulations (e.g., Case, 1992; Fischer, 1980). That is, the I-self, in its role as constructor of the Me-self does not, in childhood, possess the capacities to create a hierarchically organized system of postulates that are internally consistent, coherently organized, testable, or empirically valid. In fact, it is not until *late adolescence* if not early adulthood that the abilities to construct such a self-portrait potentially emerge. Therefore, in our developmental analysis of the self as a cognitive construction, it will be essential to examine how the changing characteristics of the I-self in each developmental stage directly impact the Me-self, namely, the self-theory being constructed.

The Developing Self as a Cognitive Construction

As will become evident, a cognitive-developmental analysis will focus primarily on changes in the *structure* of the self as a system, namely, how self-representations are conceptually organized. As such, primary emphasis will be given to *similarities* in self-representations among individuals at a given developmental level.

Previous ontogenetic accounts have highlighted major qualitative differences in the nature of self-descriptions associated with broad stages of development. Within the field of development, more generally defined, observers were initially struck by the most outstanding markers in the psychological landscape, namely, dramatic differences that defined the stage models of the day (e.g., Piaget, 1960). However, our traditional developmental icons such as Piaget (as well as Freud, 1952, and Erikson, 1963, 1968) have fallen from theoretical grace. The very breadth of their stages eventually held little explanatory or predictive power in furthering our understanding of specific behaviors. Moreover, these theorists did not anticipate that individual differences were damaging to their grand stage models.

More recent treatments of self-development fill in the gaps by providing a more detailed account of the progression of *substages* of self-understanding (see Harter, 2006a). As a result, the field has necessarily had to alter views about whether the development of self-representations is best viewed as a discontinuous or continuous process. In past frameworks, self-development was viewed as largely discontinuous, with an emphasis on the conceptual leaps from one broadly defined stage to another. From this perspective, investigators highlighted the dramatic differences that characterized the self-descriptions in broad developmental periods, namely, early childhood, later childhood, and adolescence (see Montemayor & Eisen, 1977). However, there has been a shift in emphasis, which is reflected in this volume. The development of self-representations is now viewed as more *continuous*. We can now specify more mini-steps or substages that occur, including how such levels build upon, and transform, one another.

Focusing on normative-developmental changes will demonstrate how cognitive development impacts two general characteristics of the self-structure, namely, the level of *differentiation* and the *integration* that the individual can bring to bear upon the postulates in his/her self-theory. With regard to differentiation, emerging cognitive abilities allow the individual to create self-evaluations that differ across various domains of experience. Moreover, they permit the older child to distinguish between real and ideal self-concepts, which can then be compared to one another, creating discrepancies that have further consequences for the self. During adolescence, newfound cognitive capabilities support the creation of multiple selves in different relational contexts.

With regard to integration, cognitive abilities that emerge across the course of development allow the individual to construct higher-order generalizations about the self in the form of trait labels (e.g., demonstrated skills in math, science, and language arts are subsumed under the self-concept of "smart"). Abilities that emerge in middle childhood also permit the individual to construct a concept of his/her worth as a person, namely, an evaluation of one's global self-esteem. Further cognitive advances in adolescence allow one to successfully intercoordinate seemingly contradictory self-attributes (e.g., "How can I be both cheerful and depressed?") into meaningful abstractions about the self (e.g., "I'm a moody person"). Each of these themes is addressed in subsequent chapters.

The Developing Self as a Social Construction

In addition to an exploration of the cognitive-developmental antecedents of the self, emphasis will be placed upon the self as a *social* construction. Thus, I devote attention to an examination of how socialization experiences in children's interactions with caregivers, peers, teachers, and in the wider sociocultural context will influence the particular *content* and *valence* of one's self-representations.

The symbolic interactionists (J. M. Baldwin, 1895; Cooley, 1902; Mead, 1934) viewed the self as socially constructed, through linguistic exchanges (i.e., symbolic interactions) with others. Several themes from Baldwin, Cooley, and Mead have found their way into contemporary treatments of the self. Paramount is the role of the opinions of others in shaping the self-concept, through social interaction. Cooley hinted at a developmental internalization process whereby the reflected appraisals of specific others become incorporated in the form of the "looking-glass self." Baldwin also described how the individual assimilates attributes, initially encouraged or identified by others, into his/her habitual sense of self. For Mead, a more generalized sense of self was internalized, although just how the opinions of various others are psychologically homogenized into a collective sense of self remained elusive. Baldwin also observed the significance of social imitative processes in fashioning a sense of self and other, founded upon the infant's realization that others have subjective experiences like the self. Baldwin anticipated later contentions concerning the infant's rudimentary "theory of mind." Moreover, Baldwin pointed to the multiplicity of the self-structure, observing that the individual can possess different self-attributes both across, as well as within, different relational contexts. He did not, however, posit that the multiple selves may produce intrapsychic conflict, as did James (1890). Finally, Cooley's observation that self-judgments are accompanied by self-*feelings* highlighted the role of affective processes in self-concept development, particularly the self-conscious emotions such as pride and shame.

This second class of antecedents—namely, *socialization* experiences—are more likely than cognitive development to impact the valence of self-attributes, resulting in both positive and negative evaluations. As the symbolic interactionists observed, the self, as a social construction, develops within the crucible of interpersonal relationships with caregivers. One outcome is that the child comes to adopt the opinions that significant others are perceived to hold toward the self. These reflected appraisals come to define one's sense of self as a person. Through an *internalization* process, the child comes to own these evaluations as his/her own judgments about the self. Internalization must itself develop according to a predictable sequence of stages; there are prerequisites to emergence of the looking-glass self. Although the symbolic interactionists pointed to critical processes in the normative construction of the self, they did not alert us to the fact that self-development could go awry. There are potential liabilities associated with the construction of a self that is so highly dependent upon social interactions with significant others.

Benevolent socializing agents will readily provide the nurturance, approval, and support that will be mirrored in self-evaluations that are positive. Approval, in the form of the reflected appraisals of others, is, therefore, internalized as acceptance of self. However, in the search for his/her image in the social mirror, the child may well gaze through a glass darkly. Caregivers lacking in responsiveness, nurturance, encouragement, and approval, as well as socializing agents who are rejecting, punitive, or neglectful, will cause their children to develop tarnished images of self. In the extreme, children subjected to severe and chronic abuse create images of the self as despicable. Attachment theorists echo this theme (see Bretherton, 1991; Bretherton & Munholland, 2008; Sroufe, 1990). They observe that the child who experiences parents as emotionally available, loving, and supportive of their mastery efforts will construct a working model of the self as lovable and competent. In contrast, a child who experiences attachment figures as rejecting or emotionally unavailable and nonsupportive will construct a working model of the self as unlovable, incompetent, and generally unworthy.

Not only do the evaluations of significant others result in representations of self, but they provoke powerful self-*affects* in the form of pride and shame. Thus, the child who receives praise and support for his/her efforts will develop a sense of pride in his/her accomplishments. However, the child who is criticized for his/her performance will develop a sense of shame that can be psychologically crippling. The ability to be proud or ashamed of the self is also defined by a developmental acquisition sequence and emerges during early to midchildhood. There are other affective consequences associated with the valence of one's self-representations. Individuals who internalize favorable views of the self are highly likely to be cheerful. Conversely, the most common affective correlate of negative self-perceptions is *depression*. In the extreme, depressive reactions associated with negative self-perceptions can result in suicidal thoughts and behaviors (see Harter & Marold, 1993).

In addition to the incorporation of the opinions of significant others, children come to internalize the *standards* and *values* of those who are important to them, including the values of the larger society, what K. Nelson (2003) has referred to as the "cultural self." For example, if it is important to meet societal standards of appearance, then perceptions of one's physical attractiveness will contribute heavily to one's overall sense of self-worth (see Harter, 1993, 2006a, and Chapter 6 in this volume). Those who feel they have the requisite physical self-attributes will experience relatively high levels of self-esteem. Conversely, those who feel that they fall short of the punishing standards of appearance that represent the cultural ideal will suffer from low self-esteem. Moreover, a related liability can be observed in the eating-disordered behavior of females, in particular, many of whom engage in symptoms (e.g., associated with anorexia) that can be life threatening.

Furthermore, if significant others provide support for who one is as a person, for attributes that the child or adolescent feels truly define the self, then one will experience the self as authentic. However, the construction of a self that is so highly dependent upon the internalization of others' opinions can, under some circumstances, lead to the creation of a false self that does not mirror one's authentic experience. False-self behavior is particularly likely to emerge if caregivers make their approval contingent upon the child's living up to his/her own unrealistic standards of behavior, as the child must adopt a socially implanted self. That is, children may suppress what they feel are true self-attributes in an attempt to garner desired but unavailable approval from caregivers.

Normative Liabilities versus Pathological Manifestations

In addition to an analysis of the primary antecedents or determinants of self-representations, this volume also examines numerous consequences. A major contribution of this volume is the distinction between normative developmental *liabilities* and more *pathological* self-manifestations during childhood, adolescence, and emerging adulthood. The very fabric of development involves advances to new substages that bring with them normative liabilities that should *not* be interpreted as pathology, since they typically dissipate as even more advanced skills and cognitive competencies are acquired.

As the reader will come to appreciate, the self serves many *positive* functions. Self-processes perform *organizational* functions in that they provide expectations, predictive structure, and guidelines that allow one to interpret and give meaning to life experiences and to maintain a coherent picture of oneself in relation to one's world. Structures that serve to define the self also cement social bonds and foster appropriate social behavior as well as self-regulation. Self-processes also perform *motivational* functions in that they energize the individual to pursue selected goals, they provide plans and incentives, and they identify standards that allow one to achieve ideals in the service of self-improvement. Finally, self-processes perform *protective* functions toward the goal of maintaining favorable impressions of one's attributes and to more generally maximize pleasure and minimize pain.

Unfortunately, the self does not always conform to this job description. Rather, there are numerous liabilities on the path to self-development. Most of these forks in the road are inevitable. Emerging cognitive-developmental structures not only pave the way for a more mature self-structure but usher in the potential for a variety of negative correlates and consequences. The path to self-development, therefore, represents a veritable minefield. As observed by others (Higgins, 1991; Leahy, 1985) there are costs to development and vulnerabilities associated with new cognitive acquisitions. These liabilities are highlighted for each level of development. For example, during toddlerhood, a positive view of oneself as an active agent, with confidence in one's abilities, will lead to a sense of *self-efficacy*, namely, the perception that one has control over certain outcomes that can be successfully performed (Bandura, 1991). Moreover, there are positive affective consequences in that such mastery produces feelings of pleasure if not elation (Case, 1991; Connell & Wellborn, 1991; Deci & Ryan, 2000; Ryan & Deci, 2009; Stipek, Recchia, & McClintic, 1992). However, there are also liabilities associated with the new cognitive-developmental acquisitions to emerge during this period. For example, the ability to differentiate the self from others, the realization that self and other are each independent agents, dramatically reduces one's sense of omnipotence and control over caregivers. If mother is her own independent agent, she may not share the same agenda, leading the toddler to experience frustration, anger, and distress as the mother engages in actions that are beyond the toddler's control.

Language represents another very potent acquisition with implications for the development of the self. It allows the toddler to craft a verbal representation of the self, including the creation of a personal narrative. However, as Stern (1985) cogently argues, language can drive a wedge between two simultaneous forms of interpersonal experience, namely, as it is lived and as it is verbally represented. The very capacity for objectifying the self through verbal representations allows one to transcend, and therefore potentially distort, one's immediate experience and to create a fantasied or false construction of the self. Language also provides descriptive labels, for example, "good" versus "bad." These allow the child to evaluate his/her behavior, evaluations that come to define the self. However, the emergence of other cognitive structures that produce all-or-none thinking may lead young children, in the face of excessive failure or censure, to conclude that they are "all bad."

During middle childhood, cognitive acquisitions allow one to differentiate one's abilities across domains (e.g., one is better in some arenas than others) and they also allow the child to compare his/her performance to that of others. These abilities lead to more realistic evaluations of one's competencies (see Chapter 2). However, social comparison also ushers in the likelihood that many who fall short of others will develop perceptions of incompetence and inadequacy. Moreover, the emerging capacity to differentiate the real from the ideal self makes possible an awareness of discrepancies that can threaten the self-system, if the ideal self far exceeds one's actual self-attributes. Newfound cognitive abilities also scaffold the construction of a more complex hierarchy of self-evaluations in which there are overarching self-schemas at the apex (e.g., global self-esteem), under which more specific attributes (e.g., cognitive competence, social skills) are conceptually nested. However, the global self-postulates at the apex are more resistant to change (Epstein, 1991), particularly if they have become highly automatized (Siegler, 1991). If such global schemas are negative, the individual will display low self-esteem that may not be responsive to specific interventions and may be associated with other liabilities such as depression.

During adolescence, the emergence of abstract thinking, introspection, and self-reflection move self-representations to a new level in that the teenager is compelled to differentiate his/her attributes into multiple, role-related selves. Simultaneously, the developing cognitive apparatus compels the individual to attempt to integrate these differing self-attributes into a coherent and consistent self-theory (Fischer, 1980; Harter & Monsour, 1992) However, those in midadolescence do not yet possess the cognitive skills to create such an integrated self-portrait. As a result, given the normative proliferation of multiple selves, he/she will experience conflict over self-attributes in different roles that are seemingly contradictory. At this particular developmental juncture, this multiplicity, in turn, provokes concern and confusion over which is the real self (Harter, Bresnick, Bouchey, & Whitesell, 1997). An appreciation for these normative liabilities, the second theme in these first chapters, can prevent us from overinterpreting what are typical developmental "anomalies" (e.g., all-or-none thinking in the young child or confusion over one's contradictory multiple selves during midadolescence) as pathological. (Moreover, such an appreciation can also result in more charitable interpretations of the obstreperous outbursts of the terrible 2-year-old or the exasperation that those in midadolescence can provoke!)

At each developmental substage, there is also the potential for serious forms of *psychopathology* that can derail the self. Typically these result from highly inappropriate child-rearing and socialization experiences. These damaging individual difference factors can be distinguished from normative developmental liabilities given their *severity*, their greater *stability*, and the extent to which they can dramatically compromise the functioning of the child, adolescent, or emerging adult. Depression, false-self behavior, conduct-disordered behavior, narcissism, and eating-disordered behavior are among the most common clinical manifestations.

Self-Processes That Undergo Developmental Change

Recurring themes in the chapters on childhood (Chapter 2), adolescence (Chapter 3), and emerging adulthood (Chapter 4) focus on developmental changes in seven different self-processes: (1) self-awareness, self-agency, self-continuity, and self-coherence (all I-self functions); (2) egocentrism; (3) accuracy of self-appraisals; (4) global self-esteem; (5) narcissism; (6) true-versus false-self behavior; and (7) self-enhancement strategies.

Self-Awareness, Self-Agency, Self-Continuity, and Self-Coherence

James (1890) distinguished between the *I-self*, as the actor, knower, or cognizer, and the *Me-self*, as the object of one's knowledge, a distinction that has remained amazingly viable. The I-self becomes aware of the Me-self, makes attributions about the agency of the Me-self, and evaluates the extent to which the Me-self displays continuity over time. From a developmental perspective, both the structure and the content of the Me-self at any given developmental level necessarily depend upon particular I-self capabilities, namely, those age-related cognitive processes that define the knower. Cognitive-developmental changes in I-self processes, therefore, will directly influence the nature of the self-theory at each substage.

The issue of establishing a sense of *self-continuity* is a particularly fascinating challenge, because, as Chandler and colleagues have pointed out, it poses the paradox of "sameness in change" (M. J. Chandler, Lalonde, Sokol, & Hallett, 2003). That is, individuals at each age level must understand the temporal persistence of the self, in the face of constant change. They must form a psychological kinship with the person one was, a bond with an enduring self that remains constant, in the face of constant developmental flux. Thus, "conservation of self" (Harter, 1983), the notion that one's self is preserved in the face of manifest transformations, becomes a challenge as children move up the ontogenetic ladder into adolescence and beyond.

M. J. Chandler et al. (2003) document the changing justifications that children and adolescents provide, in what are primarily "essentialist" verbal solutions to the problem of personal persistence. Reasons reflect increasingly mature explanations for how an essential, genotypic kernel of selfhood persists in the face of phenotypic developmental change. Young children typically supply concrete reasons such as "My name is the same," or "My fingerprints are the same." Many older children and younger adolescents provide explanations suggesting that there is an essential core self that evolves over time—for example, "I've always been athletic, I have just changed the sports that interest me"; "I am basically an artistic person, although the particular areas are different now from when I was younger."

Thus, enduring traits represent the essence of the self. More sophisticated, but less common, justifications allude to the self as a work in progress. Thus, even basic changes in the self are due to one's personal control as the self is re-created. As an example, M. J. Chandler et al. cite "I am the ship that sails through the troubled waters of my life" (p. 60) where it is implied that there is an obdurate self at the helm. Their findings reveal that their developmentally ordered justifications parallel broad differences in cognitive level, as defined by Piagetian stages.

Egocentrism

The concept of egocentrism, originally explored by Piaget (1960), refers to a singular focus on the self. The antithesis of egocentrism is observed in *perspective taking*, the ability to adopt the viewpoints of others. Perspective taking increases in complexity with development (see Selman, 1980, 2003). As such, egocentrism becomes normatively muted or transformed across the sub-substages of childhood and adolescence.

Accuracy of Self-Appraisals

The accuracy of self-evaluations will also be affected by developmental level. Advances that promote more realistic appraisals can also produce *normative liabilities* (see Harter, 2006a.) The emergence of the abilities to engage in social comparison, to construct a discrepancy between real and ideal self-images, and to recognize both positive and negative self-attributes all provoke more accurate self-evaluations. Paradoxically, they lead to more negative self-appraisals as reality-testing skills emerge.

Global Self-Esteem

The ability to verbalize a sense of one's overall worth as a person does not emerge until about the age of 8, normatively (see Harter, 2006a). Two historical scholars originally addressed the potential causes of self-esteem: James (1892) and Cooley (1902). James focused more on the cognitive prerequisites in that perceived success in domains deemed important is weighed against perceptions of actual accomplishments. If perceived successes are congruent with one's pretensions, then high self-esteem will ensue. If perceptions of success fall short of one's aspirations, then low self-esteem will be experienced. For Cooley, who proposed a "looking-glass-self" model of self-esteem, the internalization of the opinions of significant others, as social mirrors, dictated the level of global self-esteem. These processes do not emerge until middle childhood. However, in early childhood we have documented behavioral manifestations of self-esteem that reveal demonstrable individual differences. Finally, not only do children develop a concept of

their overall self-esteem in late childhood, but in early adolescence perceptions of self-esteem become differentiated as one's perceived worth as a
person differs, depending upon the particular relationship context.

Narcissism

Narcissism has historically been defined as an excessive focus on the self,
including feelings of omnipotence and grandiosity. It has developmental
origins, as Freud (1914) first illuminated, and there is a developmental
course of normative expressions of narcissism. Normative narcissism has
been contrasted to pathological manifestations, also captured by the distinction between adaptive versus maladaptive features. In adolescence and
adulthood, more pathological or maladaptive narcissism is accompanied
by defensive displays of hostility, lack of empathy, and blame, to protect
against a fragile sense of self. The precursors, residing primarily in child-
rearing experiences, will be explored.

True-Self versus False-Self Behavior and the Issue of Authenticity

A thoughtful approach to self-processes not only involves the valence
(positive vs. negative) of one's self-evaluations but the extent to which
self-representations are *authentic*. This issue also requires a developmental analysis. The emergence of language is the first precursor of the ability to display or suppress one's true self-feelings. Child-rearing practices
are instrumental in determining whether children feel safe to express their
true selves or begin to develop mechanisms that promote false-self behavior. This parallels a distinction between true or optimal self-esteem and
contingent self-esteem. A true sense of one's worth includes a balanced
perspective on one's strengths and weaknesses, is relatively stable, is not
based upon external demands, and is not a conscious pursuit. In contrast,
contingent self-esteem is highly dependent upon approval from others, is
relatively unstable, and incurs costs, one of which is the display of false-
self behavior. A verbal concept of a false self does not emerge until early
adolescence when concerns about being phony come to the fore. Individual
differences in self-reported false-self behavior can be documented, where
antecedents lie in the perceived support from parents and peers.

Self-Enhancement Strategies and Their Developmental Prerequisites

A preoccupation with the self is a contemporary cause for concern. There
are costs of self-enhancing strategies, self-serving biases, unrealistically
inflated self-perceptions, narcissistic fantasies of omnipotence, and other

illusions about the self that have been amply documented among adults (see Harter, 2012; Leary, 2004). These led Leary to refer to the "curse of the self." Adults engage in downward social comparisons: to make themselves look better, they claim to be better than average; they take more responsibility for their successes than failures (blaming external factors); they engage in the false-uniqueness effect, concluding that they are special or have unique talents; and finally, they are unaware of these biases, acknowledging them in others but not in the self. These self-serving behaviors threaten relationships with others and have negative costs to the self, one of which is *authenticity*. In addition, the true self can become seriously compromised among adults by tendencies to inflate, becloud, and distort the real inner self, in desperately seeking social approval, admiration, and associated gain.

Attention will be drawn to the developmental prerequisites necessary to engage in these processes. At each developmental level, we can ask three questions. What determines the need or *motive* to pursue various self-enhancement goals at a given substage? and Why might one be driven to enhance and protect the self? Second, at each developmental level, what cognitive *skills* or *mechanisms* are required or available to engage in these self-serving strategies? Third, what are the *consequences* of engaging in self-enhancing and self-protective behaviors?

Definitions of Self

Within such a contemporary developmental perspective, just how is the self to be defined? Self-terminology abounds: self-concept, self-image, self-esteem, self-worth, self-evaluations, self-appraisals, self-perceptions, self-representations, self-schemas, self-affects, and self-efficacy are but a few such descriptors. In fact, Leary and Tangney (2003) identify a dizzying array of 66 different terms that make reference to the self and the ego, the vast majority of which are hyphenated. As Leary and Tangney point out, the "self" prefix can take on multiple meanings and referents.

It is important to clarify how the self is defined in this volume. At the most general level, I will refer to *self-representations*. These are attributes or characteristics of the self that are consciously acknowledged by the individual through language. That is, how does one describe oneself? The terms "self-representations," "self-perceptions," and "self-descriptions" will be used interchangeably, to denote general characterizations of the self, by the self.

Narrowing the conceptualization somewhat, the primary focus in this volume will be those descriptions of the self that are specifically *evaluative* in nature; that is, they make explicit reference to the positivity or negativity of one's self-attributes. For example, how does one evaluate the self along a continuum of smart to dumb, nice to mean, popular to unpopular, attractive to unattractive, athletic to unathletic, well-behaved to bad behaved, moral to immoral? The perspective that I adopt is decidedly neo-Jamesian. That is, how does the *I-self*, as evaluator, perceive the *Me-self*, as evaluated? How do we take ourselves as an object of our own reflection? Important to this framework is a focus on how an evaluation of one's attributes, presumed self-knowledge or beliefs about one's characteristics, can be conceptualized in a verbalizable form. Thus, self-evaluations require that one can *fill in the blanks* with adjectives that convey the valence (positive to negative) of one's self-appraisals: "I think I am _____"; "I think of myself as _____"; "I see myself as a _____ person."

The focus of this volume, therefore, is somewhat narrower than the type of self-descriptions elicited by open-ended instruments that ask the participant to respond to questions such as "Who am I?" (see C. Gordon, 1968). These measures, while useful for certain theoretical and research purposes, are not as appropriate if the goal is to specify the *evaluative* component of self-representations. For example, responses such as "I am a student," "I am a wife," I am middle-aged," "I like football," or "I am a New Yorker," do not explicitly convey an evaluation of the self along a continuum of positive to negative appraisals.

The definitions put forth, therefore, may appear relatively straightforward. Why, then, do I embrace the cumbersome Jamesian language of an I-self versus a Me-self? James (1890) himself described the I-self as an incorrigible construct that he could never quite intellectually control. Why not simply provide age-related cameos of how children and adolescents of increasing age describe themselves differently, pointing to the key features that discriminate between these self-evaluations? Montemayor and Eisen (1977) provided such an interesting descriptive developmental account, a quarter of a century ago. Thus, we had rich descriptions; however, there were no compelling *explanations*.

Thus, nagging questions remained. *Why* should self-evaluations change as a function of development? At that point in the history of our discipline, as with so many intriguing fascinating developmental sequences that had been documented, we had rich descriptions but no compelling explanations. As the field has matured into the quest for specific *explanations* of the underlying developmental processes and mechanisms, it seemed appropriate to address such an inquiry. Upon reflection, it seemed that the I-self-versus-Me-self framework provided a vehicle for addressing this question with regard to the self, as the field became more appreciative of cognitive-developmental principles. First, Piagetian theory and then later neo-Piagetian models articulated the changing cognitive processes that dictated development. These processes could potentially explain changes in the I-self. Developing I-self cognitive capabilities, in turn, shape the structure and the content of the Me-self, how the self is described and evaluated differently at different ages or stages. I flesh out this perspective in Chapter 2, on childhood, and Chapter 3, on adolescence. Thus, the I-self evaluates the Me-self.

In summary, the self-terminology that is described in this volume refers to an evaluative perspective that is self-reflective and self-judgmental (see Leary & Tangney, 2003, who thoughtfully describe many different perspectives on the self and related terminology). Examples of the terms to which I refer are *self-concept* ("My concept of myself is _____"), *self-image* ("My image of who I am is that of _____"), *self-appraisals* ("I evaluate myself as someone who _____"), *self-beliefs* ("I believe that I am _____"), and *self-awareness* ("I am aware that I _____"), *self-esteem* ("Overall, I think I am a _____ person"). In each case, the responses must specify the valence of self-judgment, along a continuum of positive to negative.

The I-self, Me-self framework extends to self-affects or *self-conscious emotions* that will also be explored. What does it mean to be proud? By middle childhood, we shall come to see, the I-self can be proud of the Me-self, as witnessed by verbalizations such as "I'm so proud of myself!" To a lesser extent, in our culture, children come, through a socialization sequence, to realize that "I'm ashamed of myself" for a transgression. That said, both cognitive-developmental advances and socialization experiences, primarily in the form of parenting, are required to reach this level of self-understanding.

In laying out the definitional perspective that frames this volume, it may be instructive to ask what self-terms or constructs are ruled out? Leary and Tangney's (2003) analysis is quite helpful. For example, although self-control and self-regulation are important to developmentalists, they do not meet the definition of a conscious verbalizable evaluation of the self. Moreover, this volume does not review the burgeoning literature on *implicit* measures of the self, where unconscious evaluative dimensions are inferred from perceptual–motor responses (e.g., reaction time) to stimulus or verbal displays of potentially self-relevant content, presented in laboratory settings.

In our own work, we have tried to separate dimensions of self, so defined, from its correlates and consequences that may also bear self-hyphenated labels, a perspective that Leary and Tangney (2003) have also espoused. Many of these related constructs are emotional reactions, others are motivational correlates. For example, from our own research, participants may acknowledge that "Because I don't like myself as a person, I feel depressed"; "Because I think I am smart, I am motivated to work hard and I expect to achieve academically in the future." These issues are important to address, and indeed, we do so in our own work, but it is critical to distinguish the self-evaluative component from its correlates and consequences. Self-destruction (listed in Leary and Tangney, 2003), to take another example, is often a behavioral correlate of depression in some cases, but it does not meet our criteria as a self-evaluative judgment. However, it may be an important correlate of low self-esteem.

To recap, the "self" is defined as how one consciously reflects upon and evaluates one's characteristics in a manner that he/she can verbalize. Astute readers may well ask, "Why should we care?" As clever psychologists in the 1980s argued, people are very poor judges of their attributes; they can be totally unrealistic. This point is well taken and there is ample evidence to document such a conclusion in the adult literature, in particular (see Nisbett & Ross, 1980). So of what use are these potentially inaccurate self-evaluations that have now been identified? They may be even more unrealistic in childhood and adolescence. Why should we care about potentially inaccurate self-evaluations?

One answer lies in the findings that self-evaluations are often more predictive of outcomes than are seemingly more objective indices. Why does an all-A student, the valedictorian of her class, profess to low self-esteem, and then kill herself 2 weeks before graduation when she was to give her speech? Why does a slightly built, male middle school student from a foreign country, with poor grades, who is viciously attacked by high school students because he was different and vulnerable, come to display incredibly positive thoughts about himself and have aspirations to become a marine? These are but two dramatic and real examples. I raise them to open our eyes and minds to the predictive power of self-evaluations, independent of accuracy in the opinions of others. The point is not that self-evaluations are better or worse powerful predictors than objective indices; one must finish the sentence, predictors of what? In certain cases, self-perceptions will be very powerful predictors, in other cases, maybe not, but this is not for me to answer here. Researchers must frame their own burning question, provide a compelling rationale, and then answer it (see Harter, 2011).

Operational Definitions and Their Instrumentation

If one turns to measurement development, it is critical to operationalize one's definitions of self. For example, my own research group has developed developmentally sensitive self-report instruments (see Table 1.1), although these are not the focus of this book. Across these measures, the term "domain-specific self-concept" has been reserved for those clearly evaluative judgments of one's attributes within discrete domains such as scholastic competence, social competence, physical appearance, athletic competence, and behavioral conduct.

Beginning at age 8, older children develop the cognitive capacity to verbalize *global* evaluations of self that have typically been referred to as "self-esteem" (M. Rosenberg, 1979) or "self-worth" (Harter, 1982). In each case, the focus is on the overall evaluation of one's worth or value as a

TABLE 1.1. Domains of the Self-Concept Tapped by Our Instruments at Each Period of the Lifespan

Early childhood	Middle to late childhood	Adolescence	College years	Early through middle adulthood	Late adulthood
Cognitive competence	Scholastic competence	Scholastic competence	Scholastic competence Intellectual ability Creativity	Intelligence	Cognitive abilities
		Job competence	Job competence	Job competence	Job competence
Physical competence	Athletic competence	Athletic competence	Athletic competence	Athletic competence	
Physical appearance	Physical appearance	Physical appearance	Physical appearance	Physical appearance	Physical appearance
Peer acceptance	Peer acceptance	Peer acceptance Close friendship Romantic relationships	Peer acceptance Close friendship Romantic relationships Relationships with parents	Sociability Close friendship Intimate relationships	Relationships with friends Family relationships
Behavioral conduct	Behavioral conduct	Conduct/morality	Morality Sense of humor	Morality Sense of humor Nurturance Household management Adequacy as a provider	Morality
					Nurturance Personal, household management Adequacy as a provider Leisure activities Health status Life satisfaction Reminiscence
Global self-worth	Global self-worth	Global self-worth	Global self-worth	Global self-worth	Global self-worth

person. In this volume, I employ the terms "self-esteem" and "self-worth" interchangeably. It is important to appreciate the fact that this overall or global valuation of one's self is tapped by its own set of items that explicitly ask about one's perceived worth as a person (e.g., "I feel that I am a worthwhile person"). That is, it is *not* a summary statement of domain-specific self-evaluations across different arenas of competence or adequacy. The distinction between global self-esteem or self-worth and domain-specific self-judgments allows one to address the issue of whether evaluations in some domains are more predictive of global self-esteem than are others (see Chapter 5).

In my research group's theorizing and research, we have developed a lifespan battery of instruments that identifies age-appropriate domains across six stages of development: early childhood, middle to late childhood, adolescence, college years, middle adulthood, and late adulthood (see Table 1.1). Beginning in middle to late childhood and beyond, we have included global self-worth at each stage. (It is not included for the first period of early childhood, given that young children cannot verbalize a concept of their overall worth as a person.) Chapter 2 describes how we have developed a measure of "behaviorally manifest" self-esteem for young children that relies on teachers', or other knowledgeable adults', ratings of specific behaviors that we have determined reflect the child's overall sense of his/her global worth. For each of the stages described in Table 1.1, we have developed a self-report instrument to tap these self-evaluations. (We are currently in the process of developing an instrument for the period of emerging adulthood, given the literature reviewed in Chapter 4, revealing that the age period of 18 to 25 appears to represent a distinct stage of development.)

These instruments are *not* a primary focus of the book for a very important reason. My own review of the literature over the last decade, including dozens of studies that I have been asked to review by journal editors, as well as inquiries by individual students and researchers who have contacted me directly, has led to a disturbing conclusion. Far too many studies are now designed around *measures* rather than around thoughtful hypotheses. The advent of multidimensional measures of the self (mine and many others) has been welcome, in contrast to earlier unidimensional perspectives whose measures came up with a single score of an evaluation of the self. So what is the cause for concern?

Multidimensional measures provide (but I would argue *demand*) an opportunity to make a *pattern of predictions* across the dimensions of the self that can be assessed. The researcher must now address how an independent variable that is manipulated, how a pre–postintervention, and so on, will explicitly impact the various dimensions of the self included on a given instrument. That is, *which* domains will be affected and, equally important, which will *not* be affected? In the absence of such thoughtful a priori hypotheses, one simply uses a "let's-see-what-happens" approach, weakening any conclusions that are post hoc interpretations, at best.

In my own experience, reviewing the current studies that have emerged in the past decade, too many investigators are putting the methodological cart before the conceptual horse. That is, many studies are *not* designed around thoughtful, a priori hypotheses. They are designed around the new multidimensional instruments that are now available, but do not take advantage of what these new measures have to offer or demand. A "let's-see-what-we-might-find-out" approach *can* be the basis for pilot studies or exploratory research, although one would hope that these empirical efforts would also be guided by predictions that have some defensible rationale. Descartes became famous for his exhortation " I think, therefore I am. " I would turn his assertion on its head, and urge that "I am, therefore I think!" We need more demonstrations that a compelling thinking process has directed our research endeavors.

One Final Caveat

Armed with a battery of measures, no matter whose, it behooves us to ask to what extent is an evaluation of the Me-self on our participants' psychological radar screen? Just how interested is the I-self in scrutinizing the Me-self? To what degree is the I-self *motivated* to devote its energies to a critical appraisal of Me-self attributes? I now recall that this issue was first impressed upon me decades ago in my child clinical training where we read Anna Freud (1965) and later came to partake of her wisdom directly when she spent a year at our Yale Child Study Center. She cogently observed that a major difficulty in doing psychotherapy with children was their disinterest in reflecting on their inner psychological lives and self-attributes, given a lack of introspective proclivities. There were far more interesting activities that captured the I-self's attention.

For the contemporary child in our culture, there is a long list of choices: Hanging with friends on the mall, doing one's homework, perfecting one's skateboarding skills, worshiping pop-culture idols, engrossing oneself in video games, badgering parents to take them to McDonald's, joining a competitive sports team, occasionally doing home chores that are demanded, collecting the latest Barbie doll or GI Joe action figures, watching the latest sitcom, and maybe even, at dusk on a summer evening, catching lightning bugs in a jar (a retro nostalgic memory that intruded!). Of course, in today's world, our children are obsessively Twittering or text messaging their friends.

The concluding point is that we can cajole or coerce child participants to respond to our questionnaires and interviews, often extrinsically reinforcing them for their cooperation. However, to what extent are children truly concerned with, or engaged in, this enterprise? Just how important is the self? We would do well to address this issue directly. Children may not share our adult, cultural, preoccupation with how their I-selves are evaluating their Me-selves. There may well also be cross-cultural differences in the degree to which the self commands attention. Perhaps we should take a step back, to address the actual relevance of these self-evaluative processes directly, before we overinterpret the precious scores obtained on our psychometrically sound instruments!

Chapter 2

Developmental Differences in Self-Representations during Childhood

This chapter examines the nature of self-representations at three periods of childhood: very early childhood (ages 2 to 4), early to middle childhood (ages 5 to 7), and middle to late childhood (ages 8 to 10). Each period begins with a prototypical self-descriptive cameo that reflects the cardinal features of the content and structure of the self at that developmental level. Discussion then focuses on three topics. The first is a review of normative-developmental changes that are critical for judging whether a child's self-representations are age appropriate. Against this backdrop we examine the second topic, the normative-developmental liabilities for the construction of the self. Table 2.1 summarizes key developments at each age period for these two normative-developmental themes. Finally, the third topic addresses cognitive and social factors that can lead to distortions in self-development, in the form of disorders that can be considered more pathological in nature. Table 2.1 addresses the first two normative-developmental themes. For each period, the issue of the role of self-protective and self-enhancement strategies is also addressed, raising two questions: Do children at a given level have the need or motivation to engage in such self-serving biases, and second, do they have the requisite cognitive and social skills to enact such strategies?

27

TABLE 2.1. Normative-Developmental Changes in Self-Representations during Childhood

Age period	Salient content	Structure/organization	Valence/accuracy	Nature of comparisons	Sensitivity to others
Very early childhood	Concrete, observable characteristics; simple taxonomic attributes in the form of abilities, activities, possessions, preferences	Isolated representations; lack of coherence, coordination; all-or-none thinking	Unrealistically positive; inability to distinguish real from ideal selves	No direct comparisons	Anticipation of adult reactions (praise, criticism); rudimentary appreciation of whether one is meeting others' external standards
Early to middle childhood	Elaborated taxonomic attributes; focus on specific competencies	Rudimentary links between representations; links typically opposites; all-or-none thinking	Typically positive; inaccuracies persist	Temporal comparisons with self when younger; comparisons with age-mates to determine fairness	Recognition that others are evaluating the self; initial introjection of others' opinions; others' standards becoming self-guides in regulation of behavior
Middle to late childhood	Trait labels that focus on abilities and interpersonal characteristics; comparative assessments with peers; global evaluation of worth	Higher-order generalizations that subsume several behaviors; ability to integrate opposing attributes	Both positive and negative evaluations; greater accuracy	Social comparison for purpose of self-evaluation	Internalization of others' opinions and standards, which come to function as self-guides

28

Very Early Childhood: Ages 2 to 4

Normative Self-Representations and Self-Evaluations during Early Childhood

VERBAL CAMEO

"I'm 3 years old, I'm a boy, and my name is Jason. I live with my mommy and daddy who really love me. My mommy makes me yummy spaghetti! I am going to get my own baby sister for Christmas! I have blue eyes and a kitty that is orange and a television in my own room, it's all *mine*! I know all of my ABC's, listen: A, B, C, D, E, F, G, H, J, L, K, O, P, Q, R, X, Y, Z. I can run real fast, faster than when I was 2. And I can kick a soccer ball *real* far, all the way from one end of the field to the other. I'm a lot bigger now. When I look in the mirror at *me*, I can tell I grew. My daddy puts marks on the mirror to show how much taller I get. I have a nice teacher at preschool, she thinks I'm great at everything! I can count up to 100, want to hear me? I can climb to the top of the jungle gym, I'm not scared! I'm never scared! I'm always happy I'm really strong. I can lift this chair, watch me! My mommy and I like to make up stories about me, she helps me remember things I did or said."

Self-Awareness, Self-Agency, and Self-Continuity

As James (1892) observed, self-awareness is one of the basic functions of the I-self. The I-self, as the observer, becomes aware of the Me-self, as observed. There is no singular definition of self-awareness applicable across developmental levels; it will differ, depending upon the age or stage. Very young children (ages 2 to 4) have emerged from an earlier stage in which as toddlers, they mastered *bodily self-awareness* (see Berthenthal & Fischer, 1978; M. Lewis & Brooks-Gunn, 1979; Rochat, 2003). In the well-known self-recognition paradigm, the toddler is placed in front of a mirror, after rouge has surreptitiously been placed on his/her nose. Evidence of self-recognition comes from "mark-directed behavior" in which toddlers point to or rub the rouge. This signals a realization that the rouge violated their perceptions of what they look like, indicating physical self-awareness.

Subsequently, during very early childhood, self-awareness takes on more psychological manifestations. The I-self's awareness of the Me-self takes the form of verbalizing self-referential attributes and behaviors. That is, linguistically the young child can now *describe* the self. There are many examples in the cameo; for example, Jason calls himself by name, indicates that he has blue eyes, and describes a range of cognitive and physical competencies (e.g., knowledge of his A, B, C's, his counting ability, plus his prowess at climbing and lifting).

Such descriptions will typically be observed in 3- to 4-year-olds. The content of this particular cameo is more characteristic of young boys whose presented self is likely to be based on activities and skills. The content of the cameos of girls is more likely to be social, relational, and emotional (Fivush & Buckner, 2003) (e.g., "I'm really happy playing baby dolls with my friends," "I'm sad when grandma has to leave"). Noteworthy is the nature of the attributes selected to portray the self. Theory and evidence (see Fischer, 1980; Fischer & Canfield, 1986; S. Griffin, 1992; Harter, 2006a; Higgins, 1991; Watson, 1990) indicate that the young child can only construct very concrete cognitive representations of observable features of the self (e.g., "I'm a boy," "I have a television in my own room," "I have a kitty that is orange"). Damon and Hart (1988) label these as categorical identifications, reflecting the fact that the young child understands the self only as separate, taxonomic attributes that may be *physical* (e.g., "I have blue eyes"), *active* (e.g., "I can run real fast, climb to the top"), *social* (e.g., "My mommy and daddy love me"), or *psychological* (e.g., "I am happy"). It is noteworthy that particular skills are touted (running, climbing) rather than generalizations about abilities such as being athletic or good at sports. For girls, particular activities are specified, for example, "playing baby dolls."

Moreover, often skill descriptions will spill over into actual demonstrations of one's abilities ("I'm really strong. I can lift this chair, watch me!"), or for girls ("I could bring my baby dolls to show you, next time"), suggesting that these emerging self-representations are still very directly tied to behavior. From a cognitive-developmental perspective, they do not represent higher-order conceptual categories through which the self is defined. In addition to concrete descriptions of behaviors, the young child defines the self in terms of possessions ("I have an orange kitty and a television in my own room"). Fasig (2000) documents the young child's assertions of ownership that emerge during this age period. Possessions come to represent an extension of the self, as a defining feature. Thus, as M. Rosenberg (1979) has cogently observed, the young child acts as a demographer or radical behaviorist in that his/her self-descriptions are limited to characteristics that are potentially observable by others.

In addition to a rudimentary display of self-awareness, another manifestation of the I-self is a sense of *agency*, the conviction that one has control over one's actions and thoughts (see M. Lewis, 2008; R. A. Thompson, 2006). One's actions, as a causal agent, have a predictable impact on others or the environment. Thus, Jason describes how he "can kick a soccer ball real far" and can "count up to 100," if there is an audience to listen.

The self-representations of this period are highly differentiated or isolated from one another; that is, the young child is incapable of integrating these compartmentalized representations of self and thus self-descriptive accounts appear quite disjointed. This lack of coherence is a general cognitive characteristic that pervades the young child's thinking across a variety of domains (Fischer, 1980). As Piaget (1960) himself observed, young children's thinking is transductive, in that they reason from particular to particular, in no logical order.

Neo-Piagetians have elaborated on these processes. For example, Case (1992) refers to this level as "interrelational," in that young children can forge rudimentary links in the form of discrete event-sequence structures that are defined in terms of physical dimensions, behavioral events, or habitual activities. However, they cannot coordinate two such structures (see also S. Griffin, 1992), in part because of working memory constraints that prevent young children from holding several features in mind simultaneously. Fischer's (1980) formulation is very similar. He labels these initial structures "single representations." Such structures are highly differentiated from one another, since the cognitive limitations at this stage render the child incapable of integrating single representations into a coherent self-portrait. Thus, as the representative cameo reveals, there is little coherence to the self-descriptive narrative that constitutes piecemeal and seemingly random and unrelated features of the self.

ACCURACY OF SELF-APPRAISALS

Self-evaluations during this period are likely to be unrealistically positive (Harter, 2006a; Trzesniewski, Kinal, & Donnellan, 2010). The cameo child is naïvely unaware of inaccuracies (e.g., his inadequate knowledge of the alphabet or his unlikely kicking prowess). Moreover, experimental evidence reveals that when preschool children (4-year-olds) are asked to predict how far they could jump or how many balls they could throw in a box several feet away, they consistently overestimate their performance (Schneider, 1998). There are several reasons for this normative inaccuracy. It is important to appreciate, however, that these apparent distortions are normative in that they reflect cognitive limitations rather than conscious efforts to deceive the listener. That is, they do not represent the strategic self-presentational tactics that have been documented for adults. First, young children have difficulty distinguishing between their desired and their actual competence, a confusion initially observed by both Freud (1952) and Piaget (1932). Thus, young children cannot yet formulate an ideal self-concept that is differentiated from a real self-concept. Rather, their descriptions represent a litany of talents that may transcend reality (Harter & Pike, 1984).

For contemporary cognitive developmentalists, such overstated virtuosity or optimism (R. A. Thompson, 2006) stems from another cognitive limitation, namely, the inability of young children to bring social comparison information to bear meaningfully on their perceived competencies (Ruble & Frey, 1991). The ability to use social comparison toward the goals of self-evaluation requires that the child be able to relate one concept (his/her own performance) to another (someone else's performance), a skill that is not sufficiently developed in the young child. Thus, self-descriptions typically represent an overestimation of personal abilities.

Third, young children *do* make use of *temporal comparisons,* the awareness that today's skills greatly exceed those of their not-so-distant past. Jason, age 3, boasts that "I can run *real* fast, faster than when I was 2!" Temporal comparisons are particularly salient and gratifying given that skill levels change rapidly during this age period and thus improvement is quite noticeable. For Jason, they extend to his increasing height, which his father underscores by making marks on the mirror that chart his age-appropriate growth spurts.

Fourth, very young children lack the *perspective-taking ability* to understand and therefore incorporate the perceived opinions of significant others toward the self (Harter, 2006a; Selman, 1980, 2003). Thus, the inability to fully comprehend that significant adults may be critical of the self leads very young children to persist in overly positive evaluations of the self. The prerequisites for Cooley's (1902) looking-glass-self formulation are lacking. Furthermore, to the extent that the majority of socializing agents are relatively benevolent and supportive, the psychological scale will tip toward an imbalance of positive self-attributes. For example, in the cameo, Jason tells us that "my teacher thinks I'm great at everything," as he basks in the glow of virtuosity. Bjorklund (2007) makes a related point, observing that adults will shift or reframe the meaning of success, setting more attainable goals for very young children. As a result, and because adults offer assistance and scaffolding on difficult tasks, young children have little experience with absolute failure.

A fifth reason for inaccurate self-evaluations can be observed in young children's inability to acknowledge that they can possess attributes of *opposing valence,* for example, good and bad, or nice and mean (Fischer & Bidell, 2006; Fischer, Hand, Watson, Van Parys, & Tucker, 1984). This all-or-none thinking can be observed in the cameo, where all of the attributes appear to be positive. Young children's self-representations may also include emotion descriptors (e.g., "I'm always happy"). Findings (Fivush & Buckner, 2003) reveal that girls' descriptions are more likely to mention the emotion of sadness, as well as to provide the *causes* of an emotion (e.g., "I'm sad when Grandma has to leave").

Considerable research reveals that young children have an understanding of four such affects, namely, happy, mad, sad, and scared (see Bretherton & Beeghly, 1982; Dunn, 1988; Harris, 2008; Harter & Whitesell, 1989). However, children at this age do not acknowledge that they can experience both positive and negative emotions, particularly at the same time. Many will deny that they have certain negative emotions (e.g., "I'm never scared!"). Thus, a growing body of evidence now reveals that young children are incapable of appreciating the fact that they can experience seemingly opposing emotional reactions simultaneously (Donaldson & Westerman, 1986; Gnepp, McKee, & Domanic, 1987; Harris, 2003, 2008; Harter & Buddin, 1987; Reissland, 1985; Selman, 1980). For Fischer and colleagues (e.g., Fischer & Ayoub, 1994), this dichotomous thinking represents the natural fractionation of the mind. Such "affecting splitting" constitutes a normative form of dissociation that is the hallmark of very young children's thinking about both self and others. It is important to appreciate that the normative nature of this all-or-none thinking contributes to overly positive renditions of the young child's emotional life and does not have clinical implications.

THE IMPLICATIONS OF POSITIVITY BIASES

It is clear that very young children's self-reports are overly positive or optimistic for several reasons. To summarize, young children lack the cognitive ability to engage in *social comparison* (they rely on *temporal comparisons*), they cannot make the distinction between real and ideal self-concepts, they cannot internalize the critical opinions of others, and they cannot construct a balanced view of their strengths and weaknesses. Thus, given these biases, self-evaluations can be considered to be unrealistic.

One may question, however, whether these reflect *psychological liabilities*. That is, many of the cognitive limitations of this period may serve as *protective* factors, to the extent that the very young child maintains very positive, albeit unrealistic, perceptions of self. Positive self-views may serve as motivating factors, as emotional buffers, contributing to the young child's development. They may propel the child toward growth-building mastery attempts, they may instill a sense of confidence, and they may lead the child to rebuff perceptions of inadequacy, all of which may foster positive future development. From an evolutionary perspective, such "liabilities" may well represent critical strengths at this developmental level. Bjorklund (2007) makes a similar argument, suggesting that the positivity biases have adaptive functions at this age. Self-enhancement can serve to avert feelings of helplessness in the face of daunting challenges that accompany the mastery of many developmentally appropriate skills (e.g., learning to throw a ball, read, understand written language, understand complex social rules). Thus, children remain motivated to attempt a wide range of new tasks. The implications of *excessive* positivity are revisited as we move up the ontogenetic ladder of representations and evaluations of the self.

However, do these developmentally normative self-biases approximate the types of self-enhancing strategies that are observed in adults? Trzesniewski et al. (2010) see parallels in summarizing young children's penchant to exaggerate their capabilities, their overly optimistic expectations about the future, and their self-serving attributions, viewing the protective motives as similar. My own developmental perspective would suggest a different interpretation. That is, young children do not need to tactically or strategically enhance perceptions of competence; their self-evaluations are already normatively inflated! Thus, children do not possess the *motives* that propel adults' need to enhance the self, namely, attempts to defensively protect or conceal underlying fragile or negative images of self.

Second, the mechanisms are quite different. That is, the many cognitive limitations in early childhood (e.g., the inability to use social comparison, to construct real vs. ideal self-concepts that can be compared, the lack of perspective taking) preclude the many processes that adults draw upon to protect and enhance the self (e.g., downward social comparison, false uniqueness effects, attempts to reduce ideal–real self-images). Moreover, these strategies among adults require sophisticated perspective-taking skills in which they are aware of the potential negative perceptions of others toward the self that, in turn, require mechanisms of distortion and deception. In addition, young children do not yet have a linguistic concept of their *global self-esteem*. Adults, in contrast, may have a need, as well as the skills, to protect or enhance negative perceptions of their overall worth as a person. Finally, the *consequences* of the young child's behaviors are different, as we shall see, in the subsequent discussion of "normal narcissism." Age-appropriate narcissism is viewed as healthy, meeting needs of the young child. The exhibitionistic displays are endearing and meet with social approval from significant others. In contrast, the self-centered grandiosity among adults to protect the self blinds narcissists to their shortcomings and therefore does not elicit support from others. Rather it provokes, rebuffs, and rebukes.

THE CONCEPT OF GLOBAL SELF-ESTEEM

Cognitive limitations of this period extend to the inability of young children to create a concept of their overall worth as a person, namely, a representation of their global self-esteem or self-worth that can be verbalized (Harter, 2006a). Such a self-representation requires a higher-order integration of domain-specific attributes that have first been differentiated. Young children do begin to describe themselves in terms of concrete cognitive abilities, physical abilities, how they behave, how they look, and friendships they have formed (Harter, 1990). However, these domains are not clearly differentiated from one another, as revealed through factor-analytic procedures (Harter & Pike, 1984), nor integrated into a higher-order concept of their self-esteem.

Among securely attached young children, there are concrete acknowledgments of parental affection that represent the precursors of later perceptions of high self-esteem. As Jason describes, "my mommy and daddy really love me ... my mommy makes me yummy spaghetti!" His mother, father, and teacher all reinforce a sense of his competence. Thus, young children receive signals as to whether they are lovable and capable that will set the stage for their subsequent level of global self-esteem, when this concept can be verbalized. Before such a global concept can be cognitively constructed, very young children appear to *experience* high or low self-esteem that is exuded in *behavioral manifestations* that are observable by adults.

BEHAVIORALLY PRESENTED SELF-ESTEEM IN YOUNG CHILDREN

The fact that young children cannot cognitively or verbally formulate a general concept of their worth as a person does not dictate that they lack the experience of self-esteem. Rather, our findings (see Haltiwanger, 1989; Harter, 1990, 2006a) reveal that young children manifest self-esteem in their observable behavior. In examining the construct of "behaviorally presented self-esteem," we first invoked the aid of nursery school and kindergarten teachers who had considerable experience with young children. We found that early childhood educators frequently make reference to children's self-esteem and that this is a very meaningful concept that distinguishes children from one another.

Thus, as a first step, we conducted open-ended interviews with about 20 teachers in order to generate an item pool from which we would eventually select those items that best discriminated between high- and low-self-esteem children. Teachers were asked to describe those behaviors that characterize the high-self-esteem child, those that characterize the low-self-esteem child, and those they felt did not allow them to discriminate between the two groups. Teachers had definite opinions about behaviors that were both relevant and irrelevant to this construct.

From these interviews we culled 84 behavioral descriptors, phrases that represented behaviors ranging from those that teachers felt did discriminate between high- and low-self-esteem children as well as those they felt were not relevant. We next employed a Q-sort procedure in which we asked a separate group of teachers to sort these 84 items into those that were most descriptive of the high-self-esteem child at one end of the distribution, those that were most like the low-self-esteem child at the other end, and those that were neither like or unlike the high- or low-self-esteem child in the middle. Thus, teachers performed a single sort based on their view of the prototype of both the high- and low-self-esteem child. Reliability analyses indicated very substantial agreement among teachers.

There were two primary categories of items that defined the high-self-esteem child:

1. *Active displays of confidence, curiosity, initiative, and independence.* Examples include trusts his/her own ideas, approaches challenge with confidence, initiates activities confidently, takes initiative,

sets goals independently, is curious, explores and questions, is eager to try doing new things. Two other behaviors seemed to convey the more general manifestation of these attributes: describes self in positive terms and shows pride in his/her work.

2. *Adaptive reaction to change or stress.* Examples include able to adjust to changes, comfortable with transitions, tolerates frustration and perseveres, able to handle criticism and teasing.

Similar categories describing the low-self-esteem child, representing the converse of these two sets of items, emerged:

1. *Failure to display confidence, curiosity, initiative, and independence.* Examples include: doesn't trust his/her own ideas, lacks confidence to initiate, lacks confidence to approach challenge, is not curious, does not explore, hangs back, watches only, withdraws and sits apart, describes self in negative terms, does not show pride in his/her work.

2. *Difficulty in reacting to change or stress.* Examples include gives up easily when frustrated, reacts to stress with immature behavior, reacts inappropriately to accidents.

This content analysis is particularly illuminating given what it reveals about the nature of self-esteem as seen through the collective eyes of experienced teachers. It suggests two primary dimensions: one active and one more reactive. The active dimension represents a style of approach rather than the display of skills per se. That is, the high-self-esteem child manifests confidence and interest in the world, whereas the low-self-esteem child avoids challenge, novelty, and exploration. The reactive dimension involves the response of the child to change, frustration, or stress. The high-self-esteem child reacts more adaptively, whereas the low-self-esteem child reacts with immature, inappropriate, or avoidant behaviors. (Empirically, these two dimensions are highly correlated.)

Of particular interest are the categories of behaviors that do *not* seem to discriminate between high- and low-self-esteem children, according to teachers. Most noteworthy, if not striking, was the fact that *competence* per se is not a correlate of overall self-esteem in young children, although confidence was a marker. It would thus appear that *confidence*, as a behavioral style, is not synonymous with competence, at least at this age level. This is illuminating because it suggests that the origins of a sense of confidence during early childhood do not necessarily reside in the display of skills, more objectively defined. During later childhood, the link between confidence in the self and one's level of competence apparently becomes stronger. In early childhood, the developmental path to high self-esteem will be facilitated by parental support, sensitivity, and contingent responsiveness. In addition, specific support for exploration, mastery, and curiosity that all promote a sense of confidence will also contribute. In middle childhood, competence will become a much more critical factor, contributing to self-esteem. We would argue, in bridging these two developmental periods, that socialization practices that reward displays of confidence will lead the young child to engage in behaviors that would allow him/her to begin to develop skills and competencies that will subsequently become a defining predictor of self-esteem.

ADDITIONAL FUNCTIONS OF THE SOCIALIZING ENVIRONMENT

In addition to the effect of parenting on behavioral manifestations of self-esteem, Higgins (1991), building upon the efforts of Case (1985), Fischer (1980), and Selman (1980, 2003), also focuses on how self-development during this period involves the interaction between the young child's cognitive capacities and the role of socializing agents (see also R. A. Thompson, 2006). He provides evidence for the contention that during Case's stage of interrelational development and Fischer's stage of single representations, the very young child can place himself/herself in the same category as the parent who shares his/her gender, which forms an initial basis for identification with that parent. Thus, the young boy can evaluate his overt behavior with regard to the question: "Am I doing what daddy is doing?" The young girl focuses on what mommy is doing. Attempts to match that behavior, in turn, will have implications for which attributes become incorporated into the young child's self-definition (see Ruble, Martin, & Berenbaum, 2006). Thus, these processes represent one process through which socializing agents impact the self.

Higgins (1991) observes that at the interrelational stage, young children can also form structures allowing them to detect the fact that their behavior evokes a reaction in others, notably parents, which in turn causes psychological reactions in the self. These experiences shape the self to the extent that the young child chooses to engage in behaviors designed to please the parents. Stipek et al. (1992), in a laboratory study, have provided empirical evidence for this observation, demonstrating that slightly before the age of 2, children begin to anticipate adult reactions, seeking positive responses to their successes and attempting to avoid negative responses to failure. Thus, in early childhood, young children show a rudimentary appreciation for adult standards; for example, by turning away from adults and hunching their shoulder in the face of failures (see also Kagan, 1984, who reports similar distress reactions). Although young children are beginning to recognize that their behavior elicits a reaction from significant others, their perspective-taking skills are extremely limited (see Harter, 2006a;

Selman, 1980, 2003; R. A. Thompson, 2006). Thus, they are unable to incorporate or internalize others' opinions of the self, which precludes a realistic self-evaluation that can be verbalized.

THE ROLE OF NARRATIVE IN THE CO-CONSTRUCTION OF THE SELF

Another arena in which socialization agents in general, and parental figures, in particular, impact children's self-development involves the role of narratives in promoting the young child's autobiographical memory, namely, a rudimentary story of the self. These narratives greatly contribute to the young child's emerging self-understanding in the form of a sense of *continuity* or physical *permanence* over time (K. Nelson, 2003; Rochat, 2003). There is the realization that the self is invariant over time, even given changes in outward appearance (e.g., wearing different clothes). There is considerable agreement (Fivush & Haden, 2003) that autobiographical memory is critical to a sense of continuity and requires the retention of memories that are personally meaningful to the self (K. Nelson, 2003). Nelson elaborates with regard to the unique function of autobiographical memory, which is to establish one's personal history that can be contrasted to the narratives of others. In so doing, the child comes to appreciate the continuity of the self over time, what Nelson and others (see Harter, 1983) refer to as the "conservation of self."

For most developmental memory researchers, language is a critical acquisition allowing one to establish a personal narrative (Fivush & Hamond, 1990; Hudson, 1990; K. Nelson, 1990, 2003; K. Nelson & Fivush, 2004). Between the ages of 18 and 27 months, the child begins to refer to the self in linguistic terms such as "I," "me," "my," and "mine." The mastery of language, in general, and of personal pronouns, in particular, enables young children to think and talk about the I-self and to expand their categorical knowledge of the Me-self (Bates, 1990; P. J. Miller, Potts, Fung, Hoogstra, & Mintz, 1990). That young children wrestle with the I-self–Me-self distinction, at a more rudimentary level than James's (1890) loftier deliberations, was evidenced by a question that a 30-month-old once asked the author, "Am I me?"

For K. Nelson (2003), these processes lead to the construction of the *representational self*. She observes that such a representation is not merely the experiencing self, or the self in action, but also the conceptual self. Thus, in the parlance of this chapter, the representational self consists of both an appreciation for the active I-self as well as the Me-self that is constructed. Moreover, representations of the autobiographical self in language are further facilitated by acquisition of the past tense, which occurs toward the latter half of the third year and functions to solidify the continuity of the self in time.

Howe (2003) and Howe and Courage (1993) bolster these arguments, but contend that the emergence of language is not sufficient to explain the emergence of an ability to create autobiographical memories. They note that self-knowledge—that is, an appreciation for the self as an independent entity with actions, attributes, affects, and thoughts that are distinct from those of others—is required for the development of autobiographical memory. Without the clear recognition of an independent I-self and Me-self, there can be no referents around which personally experienced events can be organized. Thus, for Howe and Courage, the emergence of the infant's sense of self is the cornerstone in the development of autobiographical memory that further shapes and solidifies one's self-definition. Moreover, the fact that the infant's self-development, in the form of the experience of both an I-self and Me-self, does not emerge until the end of the second year of life is taken as one explanation for the phenomenon of childhood amnesia; namely, that adults can rarely recall memories from their first 2 years of life.

Parents play a critical role in young children's development of their autobiographical self through the construction of personal narratives. Initially, parents recount to the child stories about his/her past and present experiences. For the young child, such narratives are highly scaffolded by the parents, who reinforce aspects of experience that they feel are important to codify and remember (Fivush & Hudson, 1990; Haden, 2003; K. Nelson, 1989, 2003). With increasing age and language facility, children come to take on a more active role in that parent and child co-construct the memory of a shared experience (A. Eisenberg, 1985; Hudson, 1990; K. Nelson, 1993, 2003; K. Nelson & Fivush, 2004; Reese, 2002; Rogoff, 1990; Snow, 1990). Through these interactions, an autobiographic account of the self is created.

K. Nelson (2003) cites evidence that parents initially provide the linguistic and conceptual framework that dictates the conventional components of a narrative. In this formula, the narrative consists of a *setting* (time and place), a central *goal*, a *motivation*, an element of *surprise*, *success* or *failure*, *emotions*, and a *conclusion* with evaluative connotations (e.g., good or bad, right or wrong). These components influence the child's structure of the remembered episode, and carry over into the child's later more independent and active construction of his/her narratives (see also Reese, 2002).

Of further interest are findings demonstrating individual differences in parental styles of narrative construction (see Bretherton, 1993; Haden, 2003; Hayne & MacDonald, 2003; K. Nelson, 1990, 1993, 2003; Tessler, 1991). A major distinction contrasts a highly elaborative style and a low elaborative approach to narrative construction. A highly elaborative style places emphasis on long, embellished accounts of previously experienced events that are rich in descriptive material and are highly reminiscent. In contrast, a low elaborative style leads to much shorter narratives that provide more impoverished descriptions of the event. These tend to provide a more pragmatic account that is repetitive in nature, focusing more on the "correctness" of memories as well as useful information.

Parents who are highly elaborative early in the child's development facilitate their children's ability to report on their past experiences in a richer, more descriptive, account (Haden, 2003). Haden concludes that as these linguistic and narrative skills are modeled by parents, children come to understand and represent their personal experiences in more elaborative forms. Thus, elaborative parents are more effective in establishing and eliciting autobiographical memories in their young children. Reese (2002) provides further evidence that the young children of mothers who provide more terms to orient the narrative (who, where, when themes) and employ more evaluative terminology (how, why) and emotion labels, similarly use more such linguistic constructions in their own narratives (see also Farrant & Reese, 2000).

Moreover, both mothers and fathers have been found to exhibit a more elaborated style when discussing shared events with their daughters, compared to their sons (Hayne & MacDonald, 2003). Mothers also talk more to girls about emotions, particularly sadness, and focus on the causes of emotions (Fivush & Buckner, 2003). Social relationships are also more evident in mothers' conversations with their daughters.

These differences are likely to be one factor contributing to gender differences in the content and structure of young children's narratives (see Fivush & Buckner, 2003). Compared to boys' narratives, the autobiographical stories of girls are longer and more detailed, reflect more internal state language, make more references to emotions, and place greater emphasis on relationships and the importance of interpersonal connection. In contrast, the presented self in boys' narratives emphasizes activities that involve skill development. Although parental narrative styles may contribute to the demonstrated gender differences, Fivush and Buckner as well as Hayne and MacDonald (2003) also observe that the prevalent gender stereotypes in our society (witnessed in the media, advertising, television, movies, children's books, children's toys, children's clothing) are not lost on our young children. These latter influences intensify in the subsequent periods of childhood that are discussed, reflecting what K. Nelson (2003) describes as the emergence of the *cultural* self.

Attachment theory and research add another dimension to our understanding of children's narratives. Attachment security has been found to be associated with mothers' reminiscing style (see Reese, 2002). Securely attached young children of those mothers who utilized more elaborative descriptions later produced more independent autobiographical memories whose themes were also more connected and coherent. Bretherton and

Munholland (2008) describe a more recent longitudinal study of mother–child memory talk of children at 19, 25, 32, 40, and 51 months (Newcombe & Reese, 2004). Mothers of securely attached infants (at 19 months) employed more evaluative language (e.g., internal state labels, intensifiers, affect modifiers, and emotional emphasis), whereas the opposite was documented for mothers of insecurely attached infants. At all five age levels, children in the secure group used more such evaluative language than their insecure peers. Moreover, beginning at 25 months, maternal and child evaluative language scores in secure (but not insecure) mother–child dyads became correlated.

Bretherton and Munholland (2008) indirectly place many of the findings discussed in this section on narratives into a historical attachment theory perspective. They remind us that Bowlby (1973, 1988) put considerable emphasis on the quality of the parent–child relationship as well as on frank and open parent–child communication about themselves and significant others. Emotions and other mental states were paramount in these discussions. Bowlby was particularly concerned with deliberate parental *miscommunication* because he observed the detrimental consequences, namely, confusing and disorganizing children's attempts to construct working models of self and others.

It was central to Bowlby's (1973, 1988) theorizing that evolution prepared the infant to *expect* appropriate and caring parental responses to attachment signals (see Bretherton & Munholland, 2008). If parents ignored or deliberately misinterpreted their infant's emotional communications, then this would not convey that these signals were meaningless. Rather, it would constitute overt *rejection*. If such rejection is consistent and pervasive, then it will lead to the development of a working model of self signifying that "My needs (or I myself) don't count" (Bretherton, 1990; Bretherton & Munholland, 2008). As a result, the child concludes that he/she is worthless, which has tremendous emotional significance for the child's developing self. These observations anticipate our subsequent discussion where findings reveal that inappropriate parental communications, coupled with conditionality ("Behave as I demand or you will lose even the contingent support we offer"), cause children to engage in false-self behavior.

Normative Liabilities for Self-Development during Early Childhood

Many of the normative liabilities of this period can be inferred from the previous description and thus will only be briefly reviewed here. Once very young children are able to verbally describe the self, linguistic self-representations emerge but are limited in that they reflect only concrete descriptions of behaviors, abilities, emotions, possessions, and preferences that are potentially observable by others. These attributes are also highly differentiated or isolated from one another, leading to rather disjointed accounts, because at this age, young children lack the ability to integrate such personal characteristics. For some adult observers, this lack of a logical self-theory may be cause for concern if not consternation. However, these features are normative in that the I-self processes, namely the cognitive structures available at this developmental period, preclude a more coherent organization of Me-self characteristics. Moreover, self-evaluations are unrealistically positive, although discussion earlier focused on whether this should be considered a liability because at this age it may have adaptive functions.

Egocentrism

For very young children, egocentrism is defined as a cognitive-developmental limitation in that they cannot separate their own perspectives from others' points of view (Piaget, 1960). Piaget concentrated on young children's inability to adopt the *spatial* perspective of another, imposing their own. Later investigators extended this analysis to *cognitive* perspective taking, demonstrating the inability of very young children to appreciate the thoughts or minds of others (see reviews by Harris, 2008; R. A. Thompson, 2006). Moreover, young children lack the capacity to take the *emotional* perspective of others (see Saarni, Campos, Camras, & Witherington, 2006). In all cases, the focus is singularly on one's own egocentric perspective, as a normal developmental process, and *not* a personality characteristic.

I recently had an opportunity to observe a rather endearing example of childhood egocentrism in a young child friend of mine who was born in Hawaii and given the unique name of *Kanani*. Kanani is a rather petite child with short blond hair. In the January 2011 catalogue of the currently popular American Girl doll, the girl of the year portrayed on the cover proudly displayed the name *Kanani*, quite a coincidence. She was an older and therefore taller child, with long dark hair. Knowing how passionate my child friend was about these dolls, I was excited to share this catalogue and gave it to her mother to show to her. Her response was one of perplexity and utter indignation! She looked up at her mother and bitterly complained, "But she doesn't look *anything like me*!"

Narcissism

For Freud (1914), primary normative narcissism represented an investment of energy in the self, in the service of self-preservation. Infants experience a sense of *omnipotence,* if benevolent parents respond relatively promptly to the infant's demands (Winnicott, 1965). Kohut (1977, 1986) and Erikson (1963) considered these omnipotent narcissistic illusions to be critical precursors of positive feelings about the self. Integrating Kohut's formulation with an attachment theory perspective, Shaver and Mikulincer (2011) have argued that security-enhancing interactions with caregivers facilitate for young children what Kohut identified as "healthy narcissism." Secure attachment facilitates a sense of the stability, permanence, and coherence of self that will provide resilience in the face of future stress, disappointments, and frustrations.

Others (Bleiberg, 1984; Kernberg, 1975) have also viewed narcissistic illusions of grandeur as primitive defense mechanisms that protected the infant/toddler from separation anxiety, frustration, and disappointment. However, if the infant's needs are severely denied, he/she is at risk for extreme frustration and rage. These more negative experiences sow the seeds for the development of a pathological narcissistic disorder to emerge more clearly during the next period of childhood.

Kernberg (1975) has provided the most systematic analysis of the criteria that distinguish normal from pathological narcissism (see also Bardenstein, 2009; Lapsley & Stey, in press). Several are particularly relevant to early childhood. The very young child's desire to be the center of attention is age appropriate, compared to pathological forms of narcissim where these concerns are excessive. The exhibitionism among healthy children is typically warm and engaging, whereas in pathological narcissism, the demands for constant admiration are defensive. Jason makes endearing bids for attention, demonstrating his professed skills at the alphabet, counting, and lifting, in an account replete with personal pronouns (e.g., "I," "me," and "mine"). Finally, the needs of well-adjusted young children are *real* and can be fulfilled, whereas with pathological narcissism, the demands are excessive, unrealistic, and impossible to meet.

Pathological Self-Processes and Outcomes during Early Childhood

A critical goal of this chapter is to distinguish between normative liabilities in the formation of the self and more pathological processes, at each developmental level. Thus, what, in very early childhood, could serve to seriously derail normative self-development, leading to outcomes that would seriously compromise the very young child's psychological development? Typically, the causes of pathology involve an interaction between the child's level of cognitive development and chronic, negative treatment at the hands of caregivers.

The Contribution of Attachment Theory

A central tenet for those studying psychopathology is that there are multiple pathways to a given disorder (Cicchetti & Rogosh, 1996; DeKlyen & Greenberg, 2008). Insecure styles of attachment (e.g., avoidant or anxious ambivalent), in and of themselves, do not necessarily lead directly to pathological outcomes. Rather, attachment styles interact with other risk factors and, in conjunction, produce pathological disorders. Examples of high-risk environmental factors include harsh and ineffective child-rearing practices, family stress and trauma, lack of instrumental resources, and diminished social support.

In high-risk social environments, those who exhibit insecure attachment styles are likely to display poor peer relations. For example, young children with an avoidant attachment style, in reaction to unresponsive caregivers, may redirect their anger toward peers, exhibiting a hostile, antisocial pattern. DeKlyen and Greenberg (2008) cite research revealing that avoidant children, particularly boys, are more likely to be disruptive preschoolers, and in the extreme, may exhibit oppositional defiant disorder.

Disruptive behaviors at home may represent strategic attempts to regulate unresponsive caregivers' neglect. Insecurely avoidant young children may engage in misbehavior designed to attract parental attention. However, such a strategy is likely to have only short-term effectiveness and will not be adaptive in the larger social environment, for example, preschool. Ambivalently attached children who also display a wary temperament as infants are likely to exhibit chronic anxiety in the face of continued, inconsistent parenting, expressing concern that their needs will not be met.

Those displaying the disorganized–disoriented attachment style may react negatively to parental pathology, for example, a traumatizing mother. Such a parent is frightening to the child, rendering the child conflicted and confused because caregivers are supposedly a source of safety rather than fear. Moreover, poor emotion regulation may be an associated outcome (see also Lyons-Roth & Jacobvitz, 2008). These various illustrations demonstrate how insecure attachment styles, in conjunction with social stressors, confer risks for pathological outcomes. In contrast, a secure attachment style, in the face of stressors, serves as a buffer, thereby reducing the risk for disordered behavior (DeKlyen & Greenberg, 2008).

Contemporary treatments of attachment theory (see Bretherton & Munholland, 2008; R. A. Thompson, 2006) review findings revealing that attachment styles and their related working models are not necessarily stable over time, in contrast to the original contentions of Bowlby, 1973). Thus, the attachment styles laid down in early childhood will not necessarily persist into subsequent periods of development. Several factors would appear to be responsible. These include unanticipated stressors (e.g., parental divorce, illness, child maltreatment), initially nonstressful changes (e.g., mother returning to work, a shift to nonmaternal care), or the birth of a sibling where the mother diverts her attention to the new infant. Thus, related changes in the quality or sensitivity of caregiving are predictive of changes in attachment security status and resulting working models of self.

The Effects of Abuse

It should first be noted that it is common for children who experience severe and chronic sexual abuse to have also been subjected to other types of maltreatment, including verbal, physical, and emotional abuse (see Cicchetti, 2004; Cicchetti & Toth, 2006; Harter, 1998; Rossman & Rosenberg, 1998). The normative penchant for very young children to engage in all-or-none thinking (e.g., all good vs. all bad) will lead such children, who have a rudimentary sense of negative parental attitudes toward the self, to view the Me-self as *all bad*. As noted earlier, the more typical pattern for children who are socialized by benevolent, supportive parents, is to view the self as all good. Abuse, as well as severe neglect can, in turn, produce early forms of depression in which the very young child eventually becomes listless, unconnected to caregivers, and eventually numb, emotionally (Bowlby, 1979).

Abuse or maltreatment can also affect I-self functions, for example, self-awareness, one of the basic functions of the I-self as originally described by James (1892). (See Harter, 1998, in which an entire chapter is devoted to the deleterious effects of abuse on both I-self and Me-self functions.) Briere (1992) points to a feature of abusive relationships that interferes with the victim's lack of awareness of self and related I-self process. The fact that the child must direct sustained attention to external threats draws energy and focus away from the developmental task of self-awareness. Thus, the hypervigilance to others' reactions, what Briere (1989) terms "other directedness," interferes with the ability to attend to one's own needs, thoughts, and desires.

Research findings with children support these contentions. Cicchetti and colleagues (Cicchetti, 1989, 2004; Cicchetti & Toth, 2006) found that maltreated children (ages 30–36 months) report less internal-state language, particularly negative internal feelings and physiological reactions, than do their nonmaltreated, securely attached counterparts. Similar findings have been reported by Beeghly, Carlson, and Cicchetti (1986). Coster, Gersten, Beeghly, and Cicchetti (1989) have also reported that maltreated toddlers use less descriptive speech, particularly about their own feelings and actions. Gralinsky, Fesbach, Powell, and Derrington (1993) have also observed that older, maltreated children report fewer descriptions of inner states and feelings than children with no known history of abuse. Thus, there is a growing body of evidence that the defensive processes that are mobilized by maltreated children interfere with one of the primary tasks of the I-self, namely, a verbal awareness of inner thoughts and feelings. Moreover, lack of self-awareness should also interfere with the ability to develop autobiographical memory, as those who have documented the role of narratives have indicated.

Many attachment theorists also contribute to our understanding of how maltreatment in early childhood can adversely influence self-development. There is considerable consensus that the vast majority of maltreated children form insecure attachments with their primary caregivers (Cicchetti & Toth, 2006; Crittenden & Ainsworth, 1989; Westen, 1993). More recent findings have revealed that maltreated infants are more likely to develop disorganized–disoriented attachment relationships (Barnett, Ganiban, & Cicchetti, 1999; V. Carlson, Cicchetti, Barnett, & Braunwald, 1989; Cicchetti & Toth, 2006). Thus, the effects of early sexual and/or physical abuse, coupled with other forms of parental insensitivity, disrupt the attachment bond, which in turn interferes with the development of positive working models of self and others.

The foundation of attachment theory rests on the premise that if the caregiver has fairly consistently responded to the infant's needs and signals, and has respected the infant's need for independent exploration of the environment, the child will develop an internal working model of self as valued, competent, and self-reliant. Conversely, if the parent is insensitive to the infant's needs and signals, inconsistent, and rejecting of the infant's bid for comfort and exploration, the child will develop an internal working model of the self as unworthy, ineffective, and incompetent (Ainsworth, 1979; Bowlby, 1973; Bretherton, 1993; Bretherton & Munholland, 2008; Crittenden & Ainsworth, 1989; Sroufe & Fleeson, 1986). Clearly, the parental practices that have been associated with child abuse represent precisely the kind of treatment that would lead children to develop insecure attachments, as well as a concept of self as unlovable and lacking in competence.

As described earlier, one critical function of parenting is to assist the young child in creating a narrative of the self, the beginnings of one's life story, as it were, an autobiographical account that includes the perceptions of self and other (see Hudson, 1990; K. Nelson, 1986, 2003; Snow, 1990). Initially, these narratives are highly scaffolded by parents, who reinforce aspects of experience that they, the parents, feel are important to codify and to remember or else to forget (Fivush & Hudson, 1990; Hudson, 1990; K. Nelson, 1986, 1990, 1993; Rogoff, 1990; Snow, 1990). More recent findings have revealed that the narratives of maltreated children contain more negative self-representations as well as more negative maternal representations compared to nonmaltreated children (Toth, Cicchetti, Macfie, & Maughan, Vanmeenen, 2000). Moreover, such narratives show less coherence; that is, the self that is represented is more fragmented (Cicchetti & Toth, 2006; Crittenden, 1994). These findings reveal greater signs of dissociative symptoms that reflect disruptions in the integration of memories and perceptions about the self. Thus, maltreatment at the hands of caregivers severely disrupts normative self-development. In turn, this disruption produces associated pathological symptoms, where it has been found that conflictual themes in young children's narratives predicts externalizing problems, in particular. Moreover, severe and chronic abuse has been associated with disorders such as borderline personality where symptoms emerge during adulthood (Putnum, 1993; Westen, 1993).

False-Self Behavior

Language clearly promotes heightened levels of relatedness and allows for the creation of a personal narrative. Stern (1985), however, also alerts us to the liabilities of language. He argues that language can drive a wedge between two simultaneous forms of interpersonal experience, as it is lived and as it is verbally represented. The very capacity for objectifying the self through verbal representations allows one to transcend, and therefore potentially distort, one's immediate experience and to create a fantasized construction of the self. As noted in the previous section, there is the potential for incorporating the biases of caregivers' perspectives on the self, since initially adults dictate the content of narratives incorporated in autobiographical memory (Bowlby, 1979; Bretherton, 1991; Crittenden, 1994; Pipp, 1990). Children may receive subtle signals that certain episodes should not be retold or are best "forgotten" (Dunn, Brown, & Beardsall, 1991). Bretherton describes another manifestation, namely, "defensive exclusion," in which highly negative information about the self or other is not incorporated because it is too psychologically threatening (see also Cassidy & Kobak, 1988). Wolf (1990) further describes several mechanisms such as deceit and fantasy, whereby the young child, as author of the self, can select, edit, or change the "facts" in the service of personal goals, hopes, or wishes (see also Dunn, 1988).

Such distortions may well contribute to the formation of a self that is perceived as unauthentic if one accepts the falsified version of experience. Winnicott's (1958) observations alert us to the fact that intrusive or overinvolved mothers, in their desire to comply with maternal demands and expectations, lead infants to present a false outer self that does not represent their own inner experiences. Moreover, such parents may reject the infant's "felt self," approving only of the falsely presented self (Crittenden, 1994). Bretherton and Munholland (2008) point to certain parents who deliberately misinterpret their infant's emotional communications. Such practices may well lead to the display of false-self behaviors, and, as Stern notes such displays incur the risk of alienating oneself from those inner experiences that represent one's true self (see also Main & Solomon, 1990). Thus, linguistic abilities not only allow one to share one's experiences with others but also to withhold or distort them, as well.

The Impoverished Self

As noted in the preceding discussion of normative development during early childhood, an important function of parenting is to scaffold the young child's construction of autobiographical memory in the form of a narrative of one's nascent life story. However, clinicians observe that maltreatment and neglect sow the seeds for children to lack such constructions. In once speaking to a group of astute child clinicians about the causes of high and low self-esteem, they raised a question I had never before encountered: "But what if the child doesn't *have* a self?" This led to the identification of what we have labeled an "impoverished self" (Harter, 2006a). Such a self has its roots in the early socialization practices of caregivers who fail to assist the child in the co-construction of a positive, rich, and coherent self-narrative. Research described earlier in this chapter has revealed individual differences among mothers in that some help their children to construct an embellished narrative, whereas others focus on more restricted conversations that target useful information leading to fewer autobiographical memories. Our clinical observations reveal that there is another group of parents who, because of their own dysfunction (e.g., depression) and parental inadequacies, do little to nothing in the way of co-constructing a self-narrative with their child. The seeds of an impoverished self, therefore, begin in early childhood and continue into middle childhood and beyond, if such children do not receive therapeutic intervention.

When these children later come to the attention of family therapists, they lack a descriptive, evaluative vocabulary to define the self and there is little in the way of autobiographical memory or a personally meaningful narrative. An impoverished self represents a liability in that the individual has few personal referents or self-concepts around which to organize present experiences. As a result, the behavior of such children will often appear to be disorganized, without purpose. Moreover, to the extent that a richly defined self promotes motivational functions in terms of guides to regulate behavior and to set future goals, such children may appear aimless, with no clear pursuits.

A clinical colleague, Donna Marold, has astutely observed that these children do not have dreams for the future, whereas most children do have future aspirations (Marold, personal communication, August 1998). For example, the prototypical child in early to midchildhood will share occupational aspirations; for instance, he/she wants to be on a sports team someday, or wants to be a firefighter, or a teacher. Marold notes that the families of children with an impoverished self typically do not create or construct the type of narratives that provide the basis for autobiographical memory and a sense of self. Nor do such parents provide the type of personal labels or feedback that would lead to the development of semantic memory that codifies self-attributes. Often, these are parents who do not take photographs of their children or the family, nor do they engage in such activities as posting the child's artwork or school papers on the refrigerator door. Marold has also observed that such parents do not have special rituals, such as cooking the child's favorite food or reading (and rereading) cherished bedtime stories.

What type of therapeutic interventions might be applicable, and how can they be guided by developmental theory and research? Child therapists (myself included) have learned through trial and error that one cannot, with older children, simply try to instill, teach, or scaffold the self-structures appropriate for their age level, namely, trait labels that represent generalizations that integrate behavioral or taxonomic self-attributes. With such children, there are few attributes to build upon. Thus, one must go back to the beginning, utilizing techniques that help the child create the missing narratives, the autobiographical memory, and rudimentary self-descriptive labels.

Marold (personal communication, August 1998) has employed a number of very basic techniques to address these challenges, interventions that necessarily enlist the aid of parents. She has suggested that the parent and child create a scrapbook in which there may be any available mementos (the scant photograph, perhaps from the school picture; a child's drawing; anything that may make a memory more salient) are collected and discussed. Where such materials are not available, Marold suggests cutting pictures out of magazines that represent the child's favorite possessions, activities, preferences—the very features that define the young child's sense of self. If there have been no routines that help to solidify the child's sense of self, Marold recommends that parents be counseled to establish routines, establishing some family rituals around a child's favorite food, for example, Friday night pizza. Obviously, these techniques require collaboration with the parents and depend upon their ability to re-create their child's past experiences, something that inadequate parents may not be equipped to do. In this regard, the therapist can serve as an important role model. From the standpoint of our developmental analysis, an impoverished self ideally requires this type of support in early childhood, continuing into subsequent stages.

Early to Middle Childhood: Ages 5 to 7

Normative Self-Representations and Self-Evaluations during Early to Middle Childhood

VERBAL CAMEO

"I have made a lot of friends, in my neighborhood and at school. One is my very best friend. I'm good at schoolwork, I know my words, and letters, and my numbers, and now I can *read*! When I was littler, I could climb to the top of the jungle gym, but *now* I can climb to the top of the diving board, that's a lot higher! And I can jump into the water, if my parents are watching. I'm happy and excited when they watch me. I can run even farther than when I was 3. I can also throw a football farther, and catch it too! I'm going to be on a team some day when I am older and later when I grow up, I want to play for the Denver Broncos! My best friend wants to be a Bronco, too, it would be cool to be teammates. I can do lots of stuff, real good, lots! If you are good at things you can't be bad at things, at least not at the same time. I know some other kids who are bad at things but not me! (Well, maybe sometime a little later I could be sort of bad, but not a whole lot or not very often). If my parents know I did something bad, they might be ashamed of me. But mostly, my parents are real proud of me, like when they watch me dive. I want to make them proud of me. They also make sure I know how to be nice and behave myself. I'm learning more about how girls and boys are supposed to act differently and why that is important. I like to make up stories about me. Some parts are kind of make-believe but mostly they are true! They're really good stories! I tell them to my parents (who sometimes make a few changes) and at 'show-and-tell' time in school. My teacher makes sure we all get a turn, to be fair. I'm a good story teller! I might also want to be a famous actor when I grow up."

Self-Awareness, Self-Agency, and Self-Continuity

These I-self processes undergo several advances at this next developmental level that Rochat (2003) describes as one of *metacognitive self-awareness.* Some of the features of the previous stage persist in that self-representations are still typically very positive and the child continues to overestimate his/her virtuosity. References to various competencies (e.g., social skills, cognitive abilities) and athletic talents, are common self-descriptors. Consistent with the gender analysis provided for the previous developmental stage, girls will be more likely to elaborate on interpersonal themes such as their best friend (e.g., "my best friend Rebecca and I usually play together after school"). Ruble et al. (2006) provide a detailed analysis of the dynamics and processes underlying various related gender differences.

Gender differences in self-descriptions are consistent with K. Nelson's (2003) concept of a "cultural self," an advance that emerges between the ages of 5 and 7. The child's autobiographical self-history, as codified in narratives, begins to be crafted in accordance with a cultural framework that dictates cultural roles, institutions, and values. Occupational choices are likely to reflect gender stereotypes such as firefighter, doctor, and professional athlete (as in the case of the male cameo child) and teacher, nurse, and mother, for female children. Behavioral norms are also salient (e.g., "I'm learning more about how girls and boys are supposed to act differently and why that is important"). As Bem (1985) has argued, gender schemas not only dictate the *content* of stereotypes but highlight the importance of adhering to these directives.

In the construction of *narratives*, children take an increasingly active role in telling their autobiographical story, displaying a greater sense of *self-agency*. They incorporate their own personal experiences, although parents are still given some editorial license. As the cameo child indicates about his self-stories, "sometimes my parents make a few changes." Children, as architects of their narratives, are more likely to underscore intentions and *future plans*. Finally, there is a greater sense of *self-continuity* as children project their narratives into the future. They also provide concrete justifications for why there are the same person, in the face of obvious physical and psychological changes (Chandler et al., 2003). For example, a child may highlight the fact that "I still have the same name."

Cognitive-Developmental Advances and Limitations

With regard to the cognitive-developmental advances of this age period, children begin to display a rudimentary ability to intercoordinate concepts that were previously compartmentalized (Case, 1985; Fischer, 1980). For example, they can form a category or representational set that combines a number of their competencies (e.g., good at running, jumping, climbing, and throwing, or knowing letters, words, and numbers). However, all-or-none thinking persists. In Case's model and its application to the self (S. Griffin, 1992), this stage is labeled "unidimensional" thinking. At this age, such black-and-white thinking is supported by another new cognitive process that emerges at this stage. The novel acquisition is the child's ability to link or relate representational sets to one another, to "map" representations onto one another, to use Fischer's terminology. Of particular interest to self-development is one type of representational mapping that is extremely common in the thinking of young children, namely, a link in the form of *opposites*. For example, in the domain of physical concepts, young children can oppose up versus down, tall versus short, and thin versus wide or fat, although they cannot yet meaningfully coordinate these representations.

Opposites can also be observed within the descriptions of self and others, where the child's ability to oppose "good" and "bad" is especially relevant. As observed earlier, the child develops a rudimentary concept of the self as good at a number of skills. Given that good is defined as the opposite of bad, this cognitive construction typically precludes the young child from being "bad," at least at the same time. Thus, an oppositional "mapping" (Fischer's [1980] term), takes the necessary form of "I'm good and therefore I can't be bad." However, other people may be perceived as bad at these skills, as the cameo description reveals ("I know some other kids who are bad at things but not me!"). Children at this age may acknowledge that they might be bad at some earlier or later time ("Well, maybe sometime a little later I could be sort of bad, but not very often"). However, the oppositional structure typically leads the child to overdifferentiate favorable and unfavorable attributes, as demonstrated by findings revealing young children's inability to integrate attributes such as nice and mean (Fischer & Bidell, 2006; Fischer et al., 1984) or smart and dumb (Harter, 1986). This mapping structure leads to the persistence of self-descriptions laden with virtuosity.

These principles also apply to children's understanding of their emotions, in that they cannot integrate emotions of opposing valence such as happy and sad (Harter & Buddin, 1987). There is an advance over the previous period in that children come to appreciate the fact that they can have two emotions of the same valence (e.g., "I'm happy and excited when my parents watch me"). They can also develop representational sets for feelings of the same valence, but these are separate emotion categories; namely, one for positive emotions (happy, excited) and one for negative emotions (sad, mad, scared). However, children at this stage cannot yet integrate the sets of positive and negative emotions; sets that are viewed as conceptual opposites are therefore incompatible.

The inability to acknowledge that one can possess both favorable and unfavorable attributes, or that one can experience both positive and negative emotions, represents a cognitive liability that is a hallmark of this period of development. Due to greater cognitive and linguistic abilities, the child is now able to verbally express his/her staunch conviction that one cannot possess both positive and negative characteristics at the same time. As one 5-year-old interviewee vehemently asserted: "Nope, there's no way you could be smart and dumb at the same time. You only have one mind!"

Although children may describe themselves in such terminology as good or bad, nice or mean, smart or dumb, these characteristics do not represent "traits," given their typical psychological meanings. From a cognitive-developmental perspective, traits represent *higher-order generalizations,* as we see at the next stage where abilities in specific school subjects combine to represent the inference that one is smart. From the perspective of *personality* theorists, traits represent characteristics that are stable across time and situation and typically converge with external ratings or manifestations. At this age, the use of such terms are more likely to reflect the use of self-labels that have been modeled by others (e.g., parents or teachers).

THE ROLE OF THE SOCIALIZING ENVIRONMENT

Socializing agents also have an impact on self-development, in interaction with cognitive acquisitions. Children become more cognizant of their self-presentation, how they are viewed in the "public eye," as they attempt a simulation of how the minds of others construct an image of the self (Rochat, 2003). Thus, children's increasing cognitive appreciation for the perspective of others influences their self-development (e.g., "My parents are real proud of me when I'm good at things"). The relational processes of this level allow the child to realize that socializing agents have a particular viewpoint (not merely a reaction) toward them and their behavior (Higgins, 1991). As Selman (1980, 2003) has also observed, the improved perspective-taking skills typical of this age permit children to realize that others are actively evaluating the self, although children have not yet internalized these evaluations sufficiently to make independent judgments about their attributes (see Deci & Ryan, 2000; Ryan & Deci, 2009). Nevertheless, as Higgins argues, the viewpoints of others begin to function as "self-guides" as the child comes to further identify with what he/she perceives socializing agents expect of the self. These self-guides function to aid the child in the regulation of his/her behavior.

One can recognize in these observations mechanisms similar to those identified by Bandura (Bandura, 1991; Bandura, Caprara, Barbaranelli, Gerbino, & Pastorelli, 2003) in his theory of the development of self-regulation. Early in development, children's behavior is more externally controlled by reinforcement, punishment, direct instruction, and modeling. Gradually, children come to anticipate the reactions of others and to incorporate the rules of behavior set forth by significant others. As these become more internalized personal standards, the child's behavior comes more under the control of evaluative self-reactions (self-approval, self-sanctions). This aids in self-regulation and the selection of those behaviors that promote positive self-evaluation.

Cognitive-developmental theory identifies those cognitive structures making such developmental acquisitions, such as the initial incorporation and later internalization of the values of caregivers, possible (Deci & Ryan, 2000). Structures underlying such a shift require processes allowing for the incorporation of the evaluative opinions of significant others leading to self-evaluations. However, during early to middle childhood, cognitive-developmental limitations preclude a solidified internalization of others' standards and opinions toward the self. Internalization, in which the child comes personally to "own" these standards and opinions, awaits further developmental advances (see Deci & Ryan, 2000; Ryan & Deci, 2009).

As Higgins (1991) and Selman (1980, 2003) have pointed out, although children at this age do become aware that others are critically evaluating their attributes, they lack the type of perspective taking, the hallmark of *egocentrism*, that is required to develop self-awareness, allowing them to be critical of their own behavior. In I-self, Me-self terminology, the child's I-self is aware that significant others are making judgments about the Me-self, yet the I-self cannot directly turn the evaluative beacon on the Me-self. These processes will only emerge when the child becomes capable of truly internalizing the evaluative judgments of others for the purpose of self-evaluation (Deci & Ryan, 1991, 2000). Thus, children at this age period will show little interest in scrutinizing the self. As Anna Freud (1965) cogently observed, young children do not naturally take themselves as the object of their own observation, particularly if negative self-evaluations may be involved. They are much more likely to direct their inquisitiveness toward the outside world of events rather than the inner world of intrapsychic experiences.

With regard to other forms of interaction between cognitive-developmental level and the socializing environment, there are certain advances in the ability to utilize social comparison information, although there are also limitations. Evidence (reviewed in Ruble & Frey, 1991) now reveals that younger children do engage in certain forms of social comparison; however, it is directed toward different goals than for older children. For example, young children use such information to determine whether they have received their fair share of rewards, rather than for purposes of self-evaluation. Moreover, findings reveal that young children show an interest in others' performance to obtain information about the task demands that can facilitate their understanding of mastery goals and improve their learning (Ruble & Dweck, 1995). However, they do not yet utilize such information to assess their competence, in large part due to the cognitive limitations of this period; thus, their self-evaluations continue to be unrealistic.

Frey and Ruble (1990) as well as Suls and Sanders (1982) provide evidence that at this stage children are still more likely to focus on *temporal* comparisons (how I am performing now, compared to when I was younger) and age norms, rather than individual difference comparisons with agemates. As our prototypical subject tells us, "I can climb a lot higher than when I was little and I can run faster, too." Suls and Sanders observe that such temporal comparisons continue to be gratifying to young children given that skills are still rapidly developing at this age level. As a result, such comparisons contribute to the highly positive self-evaluations that typically persist at this age level.

Normative Liabilities for Self-Development during Early to Middle Childhood

The Inaccuracy of Self-Appraisals

Many of the features of very early childhood persist, in that self-representations are typically very positive, and the child continues to overestimate his/her abilities. Thus, inaccurate self-appraisals persist, due to five limitations. First, children still lack the ability to engage in *social comparison* that would allow them to conclude that they may be less competent than peers. Second, the use of *temporal comparisons* contributes to their perceptions of virtuosity. Third, they do not yet have the ability to construct separate concepts of a *real* and an *ideal* self-concept in which discrepancies contribute to more realistic self-evaluations. Fourth, immature perspective-taking skills do not allow children to internalize the negative perceptions of significant others that would lead to more accurate self-appraisals. Fifth, the persistence of all-or-none thinking favors the conclusion that one is "all good" at age-appropriate skills. These beliefs are even more intractable than in the previous period given cognitive and linguistic advances that bring such beliefs into consciousness, allowing them to be verbalized, and given benevolent adults who support such positivity. However, as children move toward middle childhood, inaccuracy becomes less adaptive, as one has to face the consequences of self-appraisals that do not conform to reality.

The Lack of a Concept of Global Self-Esteem

Children at this period still lack the ability to develop an overall concept of their worth as a person; they are still unable to verbalize a concept of their *global self-esteem*. Although they are becoming more aware of the evaluations of significant others, they still lack the perspective-taking skills necessary to internalize others' attitudes in the form of a global judgment about their overall self-worth. Moreover, they cannot yet combine perceptions of their adequacy across domains where the importance of success is also taken into account (James, 1892). This ability requires the construction of separate constructs of real and ideal self-concepts, which are not yet in the repertoire of children at this age level. In this transitional period, children still lack the sociocognitive skills that would allow for the construction of a concept of their global self-esteem.

Implications for Self-Enhancement

The arguments advanced for very early childhood are still applicable to this period of development. The overestimation of one's abilities, in conjunction with the lack of a concept of one's self-esteem, renders it unnecessary to engage in self-enhancement or self-protective strategies of the type that adults display. Self-perceptions of competence are already normatively inflated given the five limitations described above. Thus, there is little need for most to engage in defensive psychological maneuvers to protect fragile or negative self-images. That is, the *motives* of adults are quite different. Second, children at this age do not have the *mechanisms* to distort or conceal the self (e.g., self-comparison, the construction of both real and ideal self-images that can reflect disparities). Finally, the display of normal narcissism as exemplified by exhibitionism does not have the negative impact on others that the grandiosity of adult narcissists produces.

Children at this age may continue to lie or blame a sibling in an attempt to conceal a transgression. However, these attempted self-serving strategies are typically quite transparent to parents, and thus not that effective. Abused children do not fit the normative mold, in that their all-or-none thinking is likely to lead to the conclusion that they are "all bad," not "all good." However, they do not yet have the cognitive capabilities to develop strategies to protect themselves against the negative implications for the self.

Normative Narcissism

The normative, narcissistic demand for attention becomes tempered as children become more aware of the social reactions of others. The need to be admired is balanced by genuine expressions of gratitude toward the caring adults in their lives, as children display a sense of *reciprocity* in giving back affection (Kernberg, 1975). The cameo child feels "really happy and excited when my parents watch me dive" and wants to make his parents proud. In contrast, narcissistic children display little gratitude or affection toward their caregivers; rather, they express disdain.

Normal manifestations of narcissism at this age also include fantasies of success, wealth, power, and fame that may be less than realistic. The cameo child wants to play football for the Denver Broncos when he grows up or become a famous actor. What differentiates these fantasies from those of dysfunctional narcissistic children is the willingness to share these visionary goals with others (see Bardenstein, 2009; Kernberg, 1986; Lapsley & Stey, in press). The cameo child's best friend also wants to be a Bronco, "it would be cool to be teammates." At show-and-tell time, "we all get a turn, to be fair." In contrast, the child with pathological narcissistic tendencies is likely to be envious, possessive of grandiose fantasies, and resentful of others.

At this age level, normative narcissism is associated with more conscious *exhibitionism*. That is, there is more awareness of the impact on one's audience, how one is presenting oneself, and the child often displays some budding showmanship. The cameo child acknowledges that he tells "good stories" and has aspirations to be an actor when he grows up. Nevertheless, these behaviors are still within the normative bounds of age-appropriate narcissism.

Pathological Self-Processes and Outcomes during Early to Middle Childhood

The potentials for pathological self-development that were identified for very early childhood exist for this subsequent period of development, particularly if the caregiving of socializing agents remains chronically negative or inconsistent (see Cicchetti & Toth, 2006). Thus, the attachment processes identified during the previous developmental period, the dynamics of an *impoverished self*, as well as the effects of abuse, continue to be applicable at this age period. These effects may be amplified because cognitive and linguistic acquisitions make such effects more evident. The child is now more able to verbalize negative self-evaluations. Concerns over the development of *false-self* behavior plus the emergence of pathological *narcissistic* patterns also represent serious threats to the self.

From an attachment theory perspective, the processes outlined in the preceding section will continue to negatively impact the self-development of children, to the extent that caregiving practices of lack of sensitivity, neglect, noncontingent responsiveness, and other forms of maltreatment leading to insecure attachment styles continue. As noted earlier, should circumstances lead to changes in parental sensitivity and responsiveness, attachment styles and corresponding working models of self may be altered (see R. A. Thompson, 2006). The impact of parenting practices may be amplified because children can now *verbalize* their sense of inadequacy and lack of lovability. These now become etched in the child's conscious realization and expression of their negative sense of self. These should readily translate into experiences of profound sadness and lack of energy, symptoms of depression at this age level. Although no research has yet to examine our "behaviorally presented self-esteem" construct in depressed children, we predict that there would be strong relationships between observable depression and behaviorally manifested low self-esteem at this age level.

The preceding section on very early childhood described the rudimentary antecedents of the *impoverished self* that reside in the fact that caregivers do not adequately support the child's construction of an autobiographical narrative or self-story. The effects of such lack of scaffolding should become more evident as children moving into middle childhood where normatively a child should be able to verbally express an autobiographical sense of self, a narrative of his/her past life story, with implications for the future. However, the failure to express one's dreams for the future, positively describe one's capabilities, or express pride in one's accomplishments all reflect pathological distortions of self-development. These symptoms should represent serious red flags that require clinical intervention.

The Potential for False-Self Behavior

Processes identified in very early childhood will continue to set the stage for the development of false-self behavior. The emergence of language provides the linguistic vehicle through which the child can falsify his/her experiences. The increasingly active role that the child at this age level plays in constructing his/her narrative becomes relevant. As the cameo child reveals in describing his stories, "Some parts are kind of make-believe but mostly they are true!" Thus, he has the basic notion that the content can be distorted. Wolf (1990) describes several mechanisms, such as deceit and fantasy, whereby the young child, as author of the self-narrative, can select, edit, or change the "facts" in the service of personal goals, hopes, or wishes (see also Dunn, 1988). Against this linguistic-cognitive backdrop that paves the way for a lack of authenticity, child-rearing practices that foster the display of individual differences in false-self behavior continue to apply, particularly if the negative parental behavior persists.

The Effects of Abuse

Abuse will detrimentally affect both I-self processes (e.g., self-awareness, self-agency, and self-coherence) as well as Me-self processes (e.g., positive self-perceptions, high self-esteem, true-self behavior), effects that have been detailed in Harter (1998). In the case of chronic and severe abuse, the major coping strategy is "dissociation" in which the child attempts to cognitively split off traumatic events from consciousness, to detach the self from excessively stressful experiences (Herman, 1992; Putman, 1993; Terr, 1991). When such abuse occurs at this period of childhood, it conspires with the natural or normative penchant for cognitive dissociation, splitting, or fragmentation (Fischer & Ayoub, 1994). Moreover, the very construction of cognitive structures that consciously lead the child of this age to think in terms of opposites (e.g., one must be all good or all bad), lead to the painful conclusion that one must be *all bad,* that the self is totally flawed. This, in turn, can lead to compromising symptoms of low self-esteem, hopelessness, and depression.

Briere (1992), based upon clinical cases, provided a complementary analysis of the sequential "logic" that governs the abused child's attempt to make meaning of his/her experiences. Given maltreatment at the hands of a parent or family member, the child first surmises that either "I am bad or my parents are bad." However, the assumption of young children that parents or adult authority figures are always right leads to the conclusion that parental maltreatment must be due to the fact that they, as children, are bad, that the act was their fault. Therefore they believe that they deserve to be punished. When children are repeatedly assaulted, they come to conclude that they must be "very bad" or "all bad," which contributes to the sense of fundamental badness at their core (see Cicchetti & Toth, 2006).

From a cognitive-developmental perspective, the young child who is abused will readily blame the self (Herman, 1992; Piaget, 1932; Watson & Fischer, 1993; Westen, 1993). That is, given young children's natural egocentrism, they will take responsibility for events they did not cause or cannot control. Moreover, as Piaget (1960) demonstrated, young children focus on the deed (e.g., the abusive act) rather than on the intention (e.g., the motives of the perpetrator). As Herman points out, the child must construct some version of reality that justifies continued abuse and therefore inevitably concludes that his/her innate badness is the cause. Moreover, the child will suppress true-self attributes, to the extent that they are viewed as causes of maltreatment.

Middle to Late Childhood: Ages 8 to 10

Normative Self-Representations and Self-Evaluations during Middle to Late Childhood

VERBAL CAMEO

"I'm in fourth grade this year. It's a little tougher than when I was younger, in the 'baby' grades. I'm pretty popular, at least with the girls who I spend time with, but not with the super-popular girls who think they are cooler than everybody else. With my friends, I know what it takes to be liked, so I'm nice to people and helpful and can keep secrets. I'm usually happy when I'm with my close friends but I can get sad if they are not there to do things with. Sometimes, if I get in a bad mood I'll say something that can be a little mean and then I'm ashamed of myself. At school, I'm feeling pretty smart in certain subjects like language arts and social studies, someday I will probably get a job that depends on having good English skills. I know I can do well, I mostly get A's in these subjects on my last report card, which makes me feel really proud of myself. But I'm feeling pretty dumb in math and science, especially when I see how well a lot of the other kids are doing. I now understand that I can be both smart and dumb, you aren't just one or the other. Even though I'm not doing well in certain subjects, I still like myself as a person, because math and science just aren't that important to me. Language arts and social studies are what I really want to be good at. So if I do well at what I want to be good at, I'll still like myself as a person. I also like myself because I know my parents like me and so do the other kids in my classes, I take their opinions of me seriously. That helps you like who you are, you have higher self-esteem. But you also have to look and dress a certain way, if you want other kids to like you. My parents don't really understand how important this is. At school, I try not to act like I'm better than other people. But some kids are show-offs and they make fun of others in class who aren't doing as well as they are. They put them down in front of everyone, just so they can feel superior. If you ask me, they are just *acting* like they're totally awesome but I think they really aren't that sure of themselves."

Self-Awareness, Self-Agency, Self-Coherence, and Self-Continuity

In contrast to the more concrete behavioral self-representations of younger children, older children are much more likely to describe the self in such terms as "popular," "helpful," "nice," "mean," "smart," and "dumb." Children moving into late childhood continue to describe themselves in terms of their competencies (e.g., "smart," "dumb"). However, self-attributes become increasingly interpersonal as relations with others, particularly peers of the same gender, become a more salient dimension of the self (see also Brown, 1990; Damon & Hart, 1988; Harter, 2006a; M. Rosenberg, 1979).

Personal relationships are typically more important to girls who are more likely to describe socially relevant emotional reactions, including the causes of such affective experiences, as the cameo reveals. Boys are more likely to include physical activities with male peers, such as sports-team play, skateboarding, dirt-bike riding, and so forth. This developmental period represents the pinnacle of gender segregation (Maccoby, 1990, 1994, 1998; Ruble et al., 2006) during which children not only prefer same-sex friends, but may actively show disdain for interactions with the opposite gender. K. Nelson's (2003) concept of the "cultural self," reflected here in adherence to appropriate gender roles, becomes even more pronounced.

Narratives reflect a more mature sense of *agency* as well as *self-coherence*. Autobiographical memory now is primarily dictated by the child's own experiences, as the child becomes the author and owner of his/her life story, not merely the narrator. If there is a conflict between the child's version of an experience and the parents', the child's account is likely to predominate (K. Nelson, 2003). Parents are less likely to be the ultimate authority (Kitchner, 1986; Piaget, 1932). The cameo child recounts how her parents don't understand the importance of certain peer values. A sense of *self-agency* can also be observed in perceptions of *self-efficacy*, future expectations about what one can achieve in challenging circumstances (Bandura, 1977; Maddux & Gosselin, 2003). Academic, as well as social, self-efficacy beliefs become particularly salient. The cameo child knows she "can do well" in certain school subjects and understands "what it takes to be liked."

The personal ownership of narratives, in contrast with greater memory capacities, increased linguistic abilities, and sense of self-efficacy, all provide an increasing sense of *self-continuity*. The cameo child projects her prowess at language arts into future job possibilities. Moreover, self-continuity at this age will be justified by the fact that in the face of obvious self-changes, one's fingerprints or DNA remains the same (Chandler et al., 2003). The child's *cultural self* (K. Nelson, 2003) also expands during these years, as the child adopts the standards and values of the larger society.

For example, perceptions of one's attractiveness are highly determined by cultural standards of appearance, given its importance in contemporary American society (see Chapter 5). These observations are not lost on older children, as the cameo child indicates in addressing how critical it is to look and dress a certain way. (Our daughter once babysat for an 8-year-old who professed that she needed a tummy tuck!)

COGNITIVE-DEVELOPMENTAL ADVANCES

From the standpoint of emerging cognitive developmental processes, self-attributes represent traits in the form of higher-order generalizations or concepts, based upon the integration of more specific behavioral features of the self (see Fischer, 1980; Siegler, 1991). Thus, in the representative cameo, the higher-order generalization that she is "smart" is based upon the integration of scholastic success in both language arts and social studies. That she also feels "dumb" represents a higher-order construction based on her math and science performance. "Popular" also combines several behaviors, namely, being nice, helpful, and keeping secrets. Moreover, these trait labels are more likely to reflect great stability across time and situation, as personality characteristics.

A major cognitive-developmental advance at this age is the realization that one's self-attributes can be both positive *and* negative, in contrast to the all-or-none thinking that dominated the two earlier periods of childhood. As the cameo child thoughtfully observes, "I now understand that I can be both smart *and* dumb, you aren't just one or the other." Thus, what were former contradictory opposing attributes that could not coexist in one's self-portrait can now be acknowledged as realistic self-descriptors that can simultaneously define the self. Thus, self-attributes also become more integrated.

The preceding developmental analysis has focused primarily upon advances in the ability to conceptualize self-attributes. However, the processes that emerge during this age period can also be applied to emotion concepts. Thus, the child develops a representational system in which positive emotions (e.g., "I'm usually happy with my friends") are integrated with negative emotional representations (e.g., "I get sad if my friends aren't there to do things with"), as a growing number of empirical studies reveal (Carroll & Steward, 1984; Donaldson & Westerman, 1986; Fischer, Shaver, & Carnochan, 1990; Gnepp et al., 1987; Harris, 2003, 2008; Harter, 1986; Harter & Buddin, 1987; Saarni et al., 2006; Selman, 1980, 2003).

This represents a major conceptual advance over the previous two age periods during which young children deny that they can have emotions of opposing valences. Our own developmental findings (see Harter & Buddin, 1987) reveal that at the beginning of this age level, the simultaneous experience of positive and negative emotions can initially only be brought to bear on different targets. As one child participant observed, "I was sitting in school, worried about all of the responsibilities of a new pet but I was happy that I had gotten straight A's on my report card." In Fischer's (1980) terms, the child demonstrates a "shift of focus," directing the positive feeling to a positive target or event and then shifting to the experience of a negative feeling, which in the example is worry about being able to care for a new pet.

The concept that the very same target can simultaneously provoke both a positive and a negative emotion is not yet cognitively accessible. However, by later childhood (at the end of this age period), positive and negative emotions can be brought to bear on one target given the emergence of representational systems that better allow the child to integrate emotion concepts that were previously differentiated. Sample responses from our empirical documentation of this progression (Harter & Buddin, 1987) were as follows: "I was happy that I got a present but mad that it wasn't what I wanted; "If a stranger offered you some candy, you would be eager for the candy but worried about whether it was OK." The ability to combine attributes and emotions of opposing valence facilitated in those children who have a secure attachment style (see R. A. Thompson, 2006).

Another new affective acquisition is reflected in the newfound ability to appreciate self-conscious emotions (e.g., pride and shame). As the cameo child observes, "I mostly get A's in these subjects [language arts and social studies] on my last report card, which makes me feel really proud of myself." She also indicates that "I'll say something that can be a little mean and then I'm ashamed of myself." Major contributors are cognitive-developmental advances that include the ability to take the perspective of parental figures who display feelings of pride and shame about their children's behavior. A four-stage developmental sequence, documented by research from our own laboratory, is presented in Chapter 6, which is devoted to self-conscious emotions.

SOCIAL PROCESSES

A more balanced view of self, in which positive as well as negative attributes of the self are acknowledged, is also fostered by social comparison. As our prototypical participant reports, "I'm feeling pretty dumb in math and science, especially when I see how well a lot of the other kids are doing." A number of studies (see Frey & Ruble, 1990; Ruble & Frey, 1991) have presented evidence revealing that it is not until middle childhood that the child can apply comparative assessments with peers in the service of *self-evaluation*. From a cognitive-developmental perspective, the ability to use social comparison information for self-evaluation requires that the child have the ability to relate evaluations of both self and other simultaneously. This ability is not sufficiently developed at younger ages. In addition to the contribution of advances in cognitive development (see also Moretti & Higgins, 1990), age stratification in school stimulates greater attention to individual differences between agemates (Higgins & Bargh, 1987). These more recent findings reveal that children in this age period primarily utilize social comparison for personal competence assessment.

Social comparison is also underscored by the socializing environment. For example, evidence reveals that as children move up the academic ladder, teachers make increasing use of social comparison information (Eccles & Midgley, 1989; Eccles, Midgley, & Adler, 1984; Eccles & Roeser, 2009) and that students are well aware of these educational practices (Harter, 1996). Moreover, parents may contribute to the increasing salience of social comparison, to the extent that they make comparative assessments of how their child is performing relative to siblings, friends, or classmates. (The negative effects of the increasing emphasis on social comparison as children move through the educational system are explored in Chapter 7).

Another major developmental acquisition during this age period is the ability to formulate an evaluation of one's global *self-esteem*. One's overall worth as a person can now be expressed verbally (Harter, 2006a). Prior to this age level, children could only formulate self perceptions within specific domains (e.g., scholastic competence, athletic competence, social acceptance, physical attractiveness) but could not yet integrate these self-appraisals into an overall evaluation of their self-esteem. In mid- to late childhood, children come to appreciate that success in domains of personal importance promotes high self-esteem, whereas failure in critical domains not only undermines their sense of competence but takes its toll on their global self-esteem (as James, 1892, contended, and our own research, Harter, 2006a, has documented). Thus, the child at this age has a basic understanding of the reasons why a positive evaluation of the self might result. For example, the cameo participant cites the fact that the school subjects in which she is excelling contribute to her self-esteem. She is then able to *discount* the importance of the subjects in which she is not doing well. Moreover, she realizes that the approval of both parents and peers also contributes to her liking herself as a person, consistent with Cooley's (1902) looking-glass self-theorizing, as described in Chapter 1.

Normative Liabilities for Self-Development during Middle to Late Childhood

The Greater Accuracy as Well as Negativity of Self-Appraisals

A cardinal thesis of this chapter is that cognitive advances paradoxically bring about normative liabilities for the self-system. The ability to be able to construct a global perception of one's worth as a person represents a major developmental acquisition, a milestone, as it were in terms of a shift from mere domain-specific self-perceptions to an integrated sense of one's overall self-esteem. However, other cognitive-developmental acquisitions can serve to lower the valence of this global perception of self, leading to lowered self-esteem. Findings clearly reveal (see Harter, 2006a; Jacobs, Lanza, Osgood, Eccles, & Wigfield, 2002) that beginning in middle childhood, self-perceptions become more negative, normatively, compared to the very positive self-perceptions of the majority of young children. As a result, self-appraisals also become more *accurate* as older children develop better reality-testing skills.

The emergence of four cognitive skills are noteworthy in leading to more accurate but more negative self-appraisals for many at this age level: (1) an appreciation for one's negative as well as positive attributes, (2) the ability to use social comparison for the purpose of self-evaluation, (3) the ability to differentiate real from ideal self-perceptions, and (4) increases in social perspective-taking skills.

First, cognitive-developmental acquisitions that cause older children to realize that they simultaneously possess negative in addition to positive self-attributes, seriously dampens the perceived virtuosity of the previous two periods of earlier development. Thus, perceptions become more realistic and potentially more negative.

Second, the ability to employ social comparison for the purpose of self-evaluation (see Maccoby, 1980; Moretti & Higgins, 1990; Ruble & Frey, 1991) leads many, with the exception of the most competent or adequate in any given domain, to fall short in their self-evaluations. If one therefore judges oneself deficient compared to others, in domains that are deemed important to the self, then self-perceptions in specific domains as well as global self-esteem will be eroded. Thus, the very ability and penchant, supported by the culture (e.g., family, peers, schools, the media) to compare oneself to others makes one vulnerable in valued domains (e.g., appearance, popularity, scholastic competence, athletic performance, and behavioral conduct) and negatively impacts global self-esteem.

A third newfound cognitive ability to emerge in middle to late childhood involves the capacity to make the distinction between one's real and one's ideal self. From a Jamesian perspective, this skill involves the ability to distinguish between one's actual competencies or adequacies and those to which they aspire, namely, those that they deem important. The cognitive realization that one is not meeting his/her expectations (an ability that young children do not possess) will necessarily lower one's overall level of self-esteem, as James' (1890) formulation accurately predicts. Moreover, findings (see Glick & Zigler, 1985; Leahy & Shirk, 1985; Oosterwegel & Oppenheimer, 1993) reveal that the real–ideal discrepancy tends to increase with development. Two causes of such an increase can be identified. As noted above, social comparison processes lead older children to lower the valence of their self-perceptions, viewing themselves less positively. Second, given increasing perspective-taking skills, children are becoming increasingly cognizant of the standards and ideals that socializing agents hold for their behavior. Moreover, parents, teachers, and peers may normatively raise the bar in terms of their expectations, leading to higher self-ideals, which children adopt in an attempt to please significant others.

Finally, increased perspective-taking skills can *directly* impact self-perceptions, leading them to be more realistic. Protected by limitations in the ability to divine what others truly think of the self, younger children can maintain very positive self-perceptions. The developing ability to more accurately assess the opinions that others hold about one's characteristics, coupled with increasing concern about the importance of the views of others toward the self, normatively leads many older children to realistically lower their self-evaluations.

We can ask whether these processes that lead to more realistic and potentially negative self-evaluations, in fact, represent liabilities. Many have argued that realistic self-evaluations are more adaptive beginning in middle to late childhood. Thus, the initial liabilities, in terms of psychological blows to one's self-image, may be temporary as the child seeks to realistically readjust his/her self-perceptions and pursue more adaptive paths of development that are consistent with his/her actual attributes (see Chapter 7 for a review of the controversy over attempts to enhance self-perceptions and self-esteem in the classroom.)

Self-Enhancement Strategies and Self-Serving Biases

Advances heralded as hallmarks of development usher in the potential for various self-protective strategies to emerge. First and foremost, the newfound capacity to forge a concept of one's global self-esteem raises the psychological specter that feelings or work may need to be protected, defended, or enhanced. Greater perspective-taking skills allow the older child to realize that there is a wider, observing audience. This, in turn, can provoke self-consciousness and the need to develop strategies to ensure positive self-evaluations. The increased ability to engage in social comparison also makes self-appraisals more vulnerable. Thus, advances during the period paradoxically may produce new *needs*, demanding that new *skills* be devoted to the protection and enhancement of the self.

For example, sensitivity to social comparison allows one to capitalize on this awareness and to submit others to the *downward social comparison* strategy. Thus, one can implicitly or explicitly compare oneself to peers considered inferior, thereby enhancing the self. Older children can now also adopt the *better than average* strategy as well as make attributions that one is more successful than others in areas of greater social importance (e.g., attractiveness, if realistic), thereby elevating their self-esteem.

The greater social awareness that emerges at this period does not necessarily ensure that it will be utilized toward the greater good of peers. It might be employed in the service of *impression management*, playing to the prevailing peer standards of what is "cool." Newfound perspective-taking skills can also be used to one's advantage, by manipulating peers in order to meet the needs of the self (Selman, 1980, 2003). The older child can now engage in psychological attempts at persuasion, convincing others to view things from his/her perspective. One is reminded of Tom Sawyer who conned his peers into believing that his job of painting the fence was a desirable enterprise, a tour de force in impression management.

Thus, the period of middle to late childhood ushers in two critical acquisitions that forecast the emergence of self-enhancement strategies. First, the concept of one's global self-esteem and the potential for negative self-appraisals presents new *motives*. Second, new cognitive-developmental skills (e.g., social comparison abilities, enhanced perspective-taking skills) equip the older child with the *capacity* to engage in self-protection, self-enhancement, and self-presentation. Our cameo child tries to resist these temptations: "I try not to act like I'm better than other people." However, she shows an awareness of others who may deviate from this path. "Some kids are show-offs and they make fun of others in class who aren't doing as well as they are." She provides some insight into their motivations. "They put them down in front of everyone, just so they can feel superior. If you ask me, they are just *acting* like they're totally awesome but I think they really aren't that sure of themselves."

Pathological Self-Processes and Outcomes during Middle to Late Childhood

A central tenet of neo-Piagetian models is that movement to a new stage of development can be fostered by socializing agents, or alternatively, can be delayed if caregiving support is not forthcoming (see Fischer & Bidell, 2006). One can imagine scenarios in which there would be little environmental support for the integration of positive and negative attributes or positive and negative emotions. Parents who are inattentive, neglectful, or depressed may simply not attend to experiences of the child that can realistically be interpreted as the simultaneous displays of skills as well as lack of competence where improvement is in order (e.g., a thoughtful discussion of their report cards). In the extreme, in child-rearing situations where children are chronically and severely abused, family members typically reinforce negative evaluations of the child that are then incorporated into the self-portrait (Briere, 1992; Fischer & Ayoub, 1994; Harter, 1998; Herman, 1992; Terr, 1991; Westen, 1993). As a result, there may be little scaffolding for the kind of self-structure that would allow the child to develop, as well as integrate, both positive and negative self-evaluations. Abused children, therefore, display a less coherent self-structure (Cicchetti & Toth, 2006).

Moreover, the negative self-evaluations that are instilled become automatized (Siegler, 1991), leading them to become even more resistant to change. Thus, to the extent that there is little or no support for the normative integration of positive and negative attributes, children will not advance cognitively. If the majority of feedback from socializing agents is negative, then children in this age range may remain at the previous level of all-or-none thinking, viewing their behavior as overwhelmingly negative. In addition, neglectful parents who do not support the development of their children's autobiographical memory, through the construction of narratives, will produce children who manifest an *impoverished self* that not only lacks substance and self-coherence but reflects little future orientation.

Caregivers lacking in responsiveness, nurturance, encouragement, and approval, as well as socializing agents who are rejecting, punitive, or neglectful, will cause their children to develop tarnished images of self. Abusive parents, in particular, set unrealistic performance expectations that, because they are unattainable, lead children to feelings of personal failure. Overly controlling or intrusive parents rob their children of the experience of competence and autonomy, basic needs that Deci and Ryan (1991, 2000) have deemed essential to healthy, psychological functioning. In undermining these needs, such parents also derail children's opportunities to construct a self-image that reflects competence, a developmental goal that is also underscored in attachment theory (Bowlby, 1973; Bretherton, 1991; Bretherton & Munholland, 2008; Sroufe, 1990). Attachment theorists observe that the child who experiences parents as emotionally available, loving, and supportive of their mastery efforts will construct a working model of the self as lovable and competent. In contrast, a child who experiences attachment figures as rejecting, emotionally unavailable, and nonsupportive will construct a working model of the self as unlovable, incompetent, and generally unworthy.

In the extreme, children subjected to severe and chronic abuse create images of the self that are despicable (Briere, 1992; Fischer & Ayoub, 1994; Herman, 1992; McCann & Pearlman, 1992; Terr, 1991; van der Kolk, 1987; Westen, 1993; Wolfe, 1989). More than merely constructing negative self-perceptions, they view the self as fundamentally flawed. The excessively high and unrealistic parental standards that are unattainable contribute to these negative views of self. Thus the Me-self, both at the level of domain-specific self-perceptions and one's sense of global self-esteem, may be irrevocably damaged. Moreover, Cicchetti and Toth (2006) report that sexually abused children have more negative self-representations than those who are physically abused, presumably because the latter group of children receive occasional positive feedback. In addition, sexually abused children are also more likely to generalize their negative representational models of attachment figures to future relationship partners.

A considerable body of research (see Harter & Marold, 1993) has revealed that there is a very robust relationship between negative self-perceptions, including low self-esteem and depression. Depressive symptoms include lack of energy, profound sadness in the form of depressed affect, and hopelessness. Depression, in turn, is highly predictive of suicidal ideation and suicidal behavior. Thus, caregiving practices resulting in very negative perceptions of the self put children at risk for serious forms of depressive pathology (see also Harter, 2006b).

Moreover, not only do the evaluations of significant others influence representations of self, but also they provoke powerful self-affects in the form of pride and shame (see Harter, 2006a). Thus, the child who receives praise and support for his/her efforts will develop a sense of pride in his/her accomplishments. However, the child who is chronically criticized for his/her performance will develop a sense of shame that can be psychologically crippling. At this level of development the child has internalized shame as a self-affect, carrying the burden of being ashamed of the self.

These processes are exacerbated for children who have experienced severe and chronic abuse, and extend to guilt, in addition to shame. Closely linked to abuse victims' perceptions of low self-esteem, self-blame, and a sense of inner badness are emotional reactions of guilt as well as humiliation (see Briere, 1992; Herman, 1992; Kendall-Tackett, Williams, & Finkelhor, 1993; McCann & Pearlman, 1992; Terr, 1991; Westen, 1993; Wolfe, 1989). Normatively, such self-affects are intimately related to evaluative self-perceptions, both of which result from the internalization of the opinions of significant others (Cooley, 1902; Harter, 1998, 2006a). Thus, the blame, stigmatization, condemnation, and ostracism that parents, family, and society express toward the abuse victim are incorporated not only into attributions of self-blame but also result in other powerful negative self-conscious emotions directed toward the self. The sexual abuse victim is made to feel humiliated for his/her role in shameful acts. Moreover, guilt and shame are also fueled by the perception that one's personal badness led to the abuse, rather than that the unjustified abuse at the hands of cruel perpetrators was the cause of one's negative self-views.

In addition to the incorporation of the opinions of significant others, children come to internalize the standards and values of the larger society, as K. Nelson (2003) describes in her concept of the cultural self. For example, perceptions of one's physical attractiveness can contribute heavily to one's overall sense of worth as a person (see Harter, 1993, 2006a, and Chapter 5 in this volume, which is entirely devoted to a discussion of these issues.) Those who feel they have attained the requisite physical attributes will experience relatively high levels of self-esteem. Conversely, those who feel that they fall short of the punishing standards of appearance that represent the cultural ideal will suffer from low self-esteem and depression.

Unfortunately, we see these processes occurring at earlier and earlier ages during childhood.

Moreover, a related liability can be observed in the eating-disordered behavior of females in particular, many of whom display symptoms (e.g., associated with anorexia) that are life threatening. Our own recent findings (Kiang & Harter, 2006) provide support for a model in which endorsement of the societal standards of appearance leads to low self-esteem that in turn predicts both depression and eating-disordered behavior (see Chapter 5). Finally, genetic factors that may lead to physical characteristics that do not meet cultural standards of attractiveness will also contribute to this pattern that may be particularly resistant to change.

False-Self Behavior

True-self behavior may become eroded at this stage, as older children are better able to evaluate both domain-specific competencies as well as their self-esteem negatively. This vulnerability may provoke the manipulation of the self that is presented to the social world, leading to displays of false-self behavior. Here it is instructive to distinguish between *optimal* or *true self-esteem* and *contingent self-esteem* that is more reflective of a false sense of self. Optimal self-esteem is grounded in reality, based on a balanced perspective of one's personal strengths and weaknesses (J. Crocker, 2006a, 2006b; J. Crocker & Park, 2004). It reflects an inherent sense of the self as worthy (Ryan & Brown, 2006) and is relatively stable. It does not become inflated when one succeeds nor does it crumble in the face of failure. Furthermore, it is characterized by greater personal integrity and authenticity.

Optimal self-esteem can be contrasted with contingent and often false self-esteem in which feelings of self-worth are highly dependent upon external approval. One must meet the goals that others dictate and seek constant validation (J. Crocker & Park, 2004; Deci & Ryan, 2000). Contingent self-esteem is unstable and invariably quite fragile. In the face of a setback, it can plummet dramatically, leading to frantic efforts to regain favor in the eyes of others.

Ryan & Deci (2000, 2009) find the roots of contingent self-esteem in child-rearing practices. Thus, parents, heavily invested in specific child outcomes, purposely or unwittingly convey love, regard, or support that is contingent upon the child attaining often unrealistic, socially implanted goals. As a result, the child only garners favor if he/she meets the typically unrealistic expectations such as being smart, athletic, attractive, or other outcomes demanded by parents. Our own findings (Harter, Marold, Whitesell, & Cobbs, 1996) reveal that unhealthy levels of false-self behavior are particularly liken to emerge if parents make their approval *conditional* on the child's ability to live up to unattainable standards of behavior. Our term "conditional support" is somewhat of a misnomer in that older children do not perceive it as supportive. Rather, it dictates the psychological hoops through which they must jump in order to conform to the parental agenda. As a result, they suppress their true-self attributes, in an attempt to garner the desired approval from parents. Not only do such children engage in high levels of false-self behavior, but report low self-esteem and hopelessness about ever pleasing parents.

Chronic and severe abuse puts children at even more extreme risk for suppressing their true self and for displaying false-self behavior. Parenting practices that allow abusive acts to occur and that reflect conditional support, lack of validation, threats of harm, coercion, and enforced compliance all cause the true self to go underground (Bleiberg, 1984; Stern, 1985; Sullivan, 1953; Winnicott, 1958, 1965). For the maltreated child, secrecy pacts around sexually abusive interactions provoke the child to defensively exclude such episodic memories from awareness, setting the stage for the loss of one's true self (Bretherton & Munholland, 2008).

Narcissism

Earlier *normative* narcissistic features begin to fade, as children become better able to accept their flaws and adopt a more balanced perspective on their strengths and weaknesses (Bardenstein, 2009). However, new *pathological* manifestations of narcissism emerge. The older narcissistic child lacks empathy for others' feelings and intentions (see also Kohut, 1977). Grandiosity, an inflated sense of self, and impulsivity all preclude a tolerance for outcomes that are not immediately successful. Others are blamed for one's personal deficits, compromising peer relationships (see Bardenstein, 2009; Kernberg, 1986). The narcissist's sense of superiority and entitlement leads to the exploitation and manipulation of peers. Preoccupied with protecting a fragile sense of self, these narcissistic children devalue others and if criticized, display rage. Narcissists may self-select relationships with weaker peers who will reinforce their grandiose self-views (K. S. Carlson & Gjerde, 2009). They seek to dominate social interactions, impress others, and gain admiration rather than establish genuine friendships or close relationships (Thomaes, Bushman, Stegge, & Olthof, 2008).

Additional *causes* of narcissism surface, complementing the two patterns previously described (see Thomaes, Bushman, De Castro, & Stegge, 2009): (1) parental overevaluation, overindulgence, and excessive praise; as well as (2) parental coldness and lack of support, in conjunction with unrealistically high expectations. Bardenstein (2009) identifies several other family determinants. First, certain *adoptive* parents may compensate for the child's sense of rejection by their biological parents and be overly indulgent, emphasizing the specialness of the adopted child. Second, children of the *wealthy* may be overindulged when a sense of entitlement is reinforced.

Third, children of highly *successful* parents who have achieved fame may suffer from the expectation that they should be blessed with genetically determined talent. Deficits precluding the same success lead to narcissistic compensation for a sense of inadequacy. Finally, children of *divorce* are at risk for narcissistic pathology, to the extent that each parent attempts to curry their favor. In the process, parents may overindulge the child with praise as well as excessive privileges and possessions.

Findings reveal the high stability of narcissistic symptoms beginning in late childhood, continuing into adolescence and adulthood (see Crawford, Cohen, & Brook, 2001). Barry, Frick, Adler, and Grafeman (2007), in a longitudinal study of children ages 8 to 11, have reported that symptoms of maladaptive narcissism (i.e., exploitativeness, entitlement, and exhibitionism) predicted delinquent behavior 3 years later. These researchers identified negative parenting patterns such as harsh or inconsistent discipline and the lack of supervision.

Chapter 3

Developmental Differences
in Self-Representations
during Adolescence

Adolescence represents a dramatic developmental transition, with pubertal and related physical changes, cognitive-developmental advances, and changing social expectations. With regard to cognitive-developmental acquisitions, adolescents develop the ability to think abstractly (Case, 1985; Fischer, 1980; Fischer & Bidell, 2006; Flavell, 1985; Harter, 2006a; Higgins, 1991). From a Piagetian (1960) perspective, the capacity to form abstractions emerges with the stage of formal operations in early adolescence. These newfound acquisitions, according to Piaget, should equip the adolescent with the hypothetico-deductive skills to create a formal theory. This observation is critical to the topic of self-development, given the claims of many (e.g., Epstein, 1973, 1981, 1991; Greenwald, 1980; G. A. Kelly, 1955; Markus, 1980; Sarbin, 1962) that the self is a personal epistemology, a cognitive construction, a theory that should possess the characteristics of any formal theory. Therefore, a self-theory should meet those criteria by which any good theory is evaluated. These criteria include the degree to which it is parsimonious, empirically valid, internally consistent, coherently organized, testable, and useful. Given Piaget's frame of reference, entry into the period of formal operations should make the construction of such a theory possible, be it a theory about elements in the world or a theory about the self.

As will become apparent, however, the self-representations during early and middle adolescence fall far short of these criteria. The self-structure of these periods is not coherently organized, nor are the postulates of the self-portrait internally consistent. Moreover, many self-attributes fail to be subjected to tests of empirical validity; as a result, they can be extremely unrealistic. Nor are self-representations particularly parsimonious. Thus, the Piagetian framework fails to provide an adequate explanation for the dramatic developmental changes in the self-structure that can be observed across the substages of adolescence. A neo-Piagetian approach is needed to understand how changes in cognitive-developmental I-self processes result in very different Me-self organization and content at each three age levels: early adolescence, middle adolescence, and late adolescence. As in Chapter 2, three topics are examined for each age level. The first describes the normative-developmental changes in self-representations and self-evaluations that are summarized in Table 3.1. Second, the normative liabilities of each age period are explored. Third, the implications for pathological self-development at each age are discussed.

Early Adolescence. Ages 11 to 13

Normative Self-Representations and Self-Evaluations during Early Adolescence

Verbal Cameo

"I'm an extrovert with my friends. I'm talkative, cheerful, and funny. My friends really like me. So I like myself a lot when I'm around my friends but not so much when I'm with my mom and dad. I'm more likely to be depressed and feel pretty hopeless. They think I spend too much time at the mall, with my friends. So when they get on my case, I get down on myself and don't like who I am as a person. I spend a lot of time worrying about what other people think of me, mostly the kids at school, particularly the ones who are popular, but I still care about how grown-ups look at me, like my parents, teachers, and the supervisor at my part-time job. Sometimes it can be hard to know what others think because everyone seems to have a different opinion of me. Who should you believe? My best friend Sharon and I try to figure things out together, that helps, and it brings us closer together. But if we spend too much time thinking about how the other kids might not like us, we both get confused and depressed. I'm not so sure of myself right now, in fact, sometimes I feel like I'm in a fog. In school, it seems like I'm pretty intelligent, because I feel smart, am curious, and sometimes creative. I think I am intelligent, my teachers say so. But then how do you ever know for sure? I get better grades than most kids; I don't brag about it because that's not cool. The other kids know that I am at the top of the class. It's really hard *not* to compare yourself to other kids because the teachers really emphasize how we are doing, compared to others. They post everybody's grades, they split us into groups, based

TABLE 3.1. Normative-Developmental Changes in Self-Representations during Adolescence

Age period	Salient content	Structure/organization	Valence/accuracy	Nature of comparisons	Sensitivity to others
Early adolescence	Social skills, attributes that influence interactions with others or one's social appeal; differentiation of attributes according to roles	Intercoordination of trait labels into single abstractions; abstractions compartmentalized; all-or-none thinking; opposites; don't detect, integrate, opposing abstractions	Positive attributes at one point in time; negative attributes at another; leads to inaccurate overgeneralizations	Social comparison continues although less overt	Compartmentalized attention to internalization of different standards and opinions of those in different relational contexts
Middle adolescence	Further differentiation of attributes associated with different roles and relational contexts	Initial links between single abstractions, often opposing attributes; cognitive conflict caused by seemingly contradictory characteristics; concern over which reflect one's true self	Simultaneous recognition of positive and negative attributes; instability, leading to confusion and inaccuracies	Comparisons with significant others in different relational contexts; personal fable	Awareness that the differing standards and opinions of others represent conflicting self-guides, leading to confusion over self-evaluation and vacillation with regard to behavior; imaginary audience
Late adolescence	Normalization of different role-related attributes; attributes reflecting personal beliefs, values, and moral standards; interest in future selves	Higher-order abstractions that meaningfully integrate single abstractions and resolve inconsistencies, conflict	More balanced, stable view of both positive and negative attributes; greater accuracy; acceptance of limitations	Social comparison diminishes as comparisons with one's own ideals increase	Selection among alternative self-guides; construction of one's own self-standards that govern personal choices; creation of one's own labels toward which the self aspires

on how well we are doing, and it can be really embarrassing. All they talk about is how we need to show that we are intelligent and that we have to do better than other schools on the stupid achievement tests they keep making us take. So if I do well on them, I tell myself it's because I am smart. If I don't do well, it's because the test was too hard or the teacher didn't teach us what we needed to know. Socially, I can be a real introvert around people I don't know well. I'm shy, uncomfortable, and nervous. Sometimes I'm simply an airhead. I act really dumb and say things that are just plain stupid. Then I worry about what they must think of me, probably that I am a total dork! I just hate myself when that happens. How much I like myself really depends on what other kids think about me, I have to admit it. One day, like if I get invited to a party, I'll feel great about myself. But then the next day, if somebody I know ignores me in the hall or doesn't say something nice to me, then I feel terrible about myself. Sometimes I think too much about this during my classes and I don't concentrate on what the teacher is saying. If I don't care about the subject, it doesn't matter to me, what's important is doing well in those classes I care about, where I get A's. How much I like myself as a person also depends on how I look. I'd like to be good-looking, like the movie and TV stars, but that's impossible. I'm too short and weigh too much and don't wear a size 2. I try to tell myself that what *I* think is the most important, that I should just be my true self. I shouldn't be phony and act like I'm somebody else. But sometimes you have to because it's very important to *seem* as if you really like yourself, it's a big deal to show that you have high self-esteem."

Self-Awareness, Self-Agency, Self-Coherence, and Self-Continuity

For young adolescents, interpersonal attributes and social skills that influence one's social appeal are typically quite salient (Damon & Hart, 1988). Thus, our prototypical young adolescent admits to being talkative, cheerful, and funny. These characteristics enhance one's acceptance by peers. Self-representations also focus on competencies such as one's scholastic abilities (e.g., "I'm intelligent"), as well as affects (she is both cheerful and depressed).

From a developmental perspective, there is considerable evidence that the self becomes increasingly differentiated (see Harter, 2006a), an awareness that challenges a sense of *self-coherence*. A sense of *self-agency* is also compromised, as shifting views of self cause the young adolescent to question just who is at the helm. There is also a threat to *self-continuity* in the face of one's shifting persona (see M. J. Chandler et al., 2003). One strategy for preserving a sense of continuity over time is to claim obdurate traitlike characteristics that underlie more superficial behavioral changes

("I'm basically an artistic person, it just takes different directions as I grow older").

Early adolescence brings with it clear proliferation of selves that vary as a function of social context. These include self with father, mother, close friends, romantic partners, and peers, as well as the self in the role of student, on the job, and as an athlete (N. Griffin, Chassin, & Young, 1981; Hart, 1988; Harter, Bresnick, et al., 1997; Harter & Monsour, 1992; Smollar & Youniss, 1985). As the cameo reveals, the adolescent may be cheerful with friends, depressed and hopeless with parents, intelligent, as a student, and shy, uncomfortable, and nervous around people whom she does not know. A critical developmental task, therefore, is the construction of multiple selves that will undoubtedly vary across different roles and relationships, as James (1892) observed over a century ago. From the point of view of attachment theory, adolescent development brings major growth in the ability to create and sustain a diverse array of relationships that meet correspondingly different attachment needs (J. P. Allen, 2008).

Both cognitive and social processes contribute to this proliferation of selves. Cognitive-developmental advances promote greater differentiation (see Fischer, 1980; Fischer & Bidell, 2006; Fischer & Canfield, 1986; Harter, 2006a; Harter & Monsour, 1992; Keating, 1990). Moreover, these advances conspire with socialization pressures to develop different selves in different relational contexts (see Erikson, 1968; Grotevant & Cooper, 1983; Hill & Holmbeck, 1986; M. Rosenberg, 1986). For example, bids for autonomy from parents make it important to define oneself differently with peers in contrast to parents (see also Steinberg & Silverberg, 1986; White, Speisman, & Costos, 1983). Another component of the differentiation process is the realization that one is more likely to be treated differently by those in different relational contexts (see Harter, Bresnick, et al., 1997; Harter & Monsour, 1992).

This realization is accompanied by intense self-consciousness, a heightened concern with the reflected appraisals of others (Harter, 1990, 2006a). *Social awareness* increases dramatically, leading to a greater self-awareness of how one's attributes are viewed through the eyes of others. Because these others hold differing opinions of the self, there is necessarily variability in the self-concept across relational contexts (e.g., the admiration of peers in contrast to the criticalness of parents, for our cameo adolescent). She laments that "I spend a lot of time worrying about what other people think of me ... but sometimes it can be hard to know what others think because everyone seems to have a different opinion of me. Who should you believe?"

As Selman (1980, 2003) points out, the young adolescent is desperately trying to figure out what others think of the self in order to make decisions about which perspectives to internalize as defining features of the self. This preoccupation and uncertainty contributes to intense introspection or self-reflection, and, for many adolescents, excessive rumination, particularly about one's negative characteristics. Introspection can represent *shared reflection* within a close relationship that can border on corumination. The cameo adolescent discloses that "My best friend Sharon and I try to figure things out together, that helps, and it brings us closer together. But if we spend too much time thinking about how the other kids might not like us, we both get confused and depressed. I'm not so sure of myself right now, in fact, sometimes I feel like I'm in a fog." Thus, corumination is a mixed blessing because although it may strengthen personal bonds, it can also lead to confusion and depression.

For Kitchner and colleagues (Kitchner, 1986; Kitchner, King, & DeLuca, 2006), this period of "existential doubt" is characterized by the conclusion that knowledge is *uncertain*. Because different, supposedly knowledgeable adult "authorities" (e.g., parents, teachers, supervisors, scientists, politicians, pop cultural icons) make contradictory claims about the same issues, there is no clear pathway for the young adolescent to discern the real truth. In trying to fathom the different opinions of significant others, the young cameo adolescent ponders about just who you should believe. In trying to assess how bright she is, she surmises that she is pretty intelligent because "my teachers say so. But then how do you ever know for sure?" Thus, doubt and uncertainty are pervasive during early adolescence and becloud a sense of awareness.

COGNITIVE-DEVELOPMENTAL ADVANCES AND CONSEQUENCES

Many (although not all) of the self-descriptions to emerge in early adolescence represent abstractions about the self, based upon the newfound cognitive ability to integrate trait labels into higher-order self-concepts (see Case, 1985; Fischer, 1980; Flavell, 1985; Harter, 1983; Higgins, 1991). For example, as the prototypical cameo reveals, one can construct an abstraction of the self as "intelligent" by combining such traits as smart, curious, and creative. Alternatively, one may create an abstraction that the self is an "airhead" given situations where one feels dumb and "just plain stupid." Similarly, an adolescent could construct abstractions that he/she is an "extrovert" (integrating the traits of talkative, cheerful, and funny) as well as that he/she is also an "introvert" in certain situations (when one is shy, uncomfortable, and nervous). Thus, abstractions represent more cognitively complex concepts about the self in which various trait labels can now be appropriately integrated into even higher-order generalizations.

Although the ability to construct such abstractions reflects a cognitive advance, these representations are highly compartmentalized; that is, they are quite distinct from one another (Case, 1985; Fischer, 1980; Fischer & Bidell, 2006; Higgins, 1991). For Fischer, these "single abstractions" are therefore overdifferentiated, and therefore the young adolescent can only think about each of them as isolated self-attributes. According to Fischer, structures that were observed in childhood reappear at the abstract level. Thus, just as single representations were compartmentalized during early childhood, Fischer argues that when the adolescent first moves to the level of abstract thought, he/she lacks the ability to integrate the many single abstractions that are constructed to define the self in different relational contexts. As a result, adolescents will engage in all-or-none thinking at an abstract level. For Fischer, movement to a qualitatively new level of thought brings with it lack of "cognitive control" and, as a result, adolescents at the level of single abstractions can only think about compartmentalized self-attributes, one at a time, but not simultaneously. Thus, contrary to earlier models of mind (Piaget, 1960), in which formal operations usher in new-found cognitive-developmental abilities that should allow one to create an integrated theory of self, fragmentation of self-representations during early adolescence is more the rule than the exception (Fischer & Ayoub, 1994; Harter & Monsour, 1992).

Compartmentalization of these abstract attributes can also be observed in the tendency for the young adolescent to be unconcerned about how certain postulates appear inconsistent across different roles, as the prototypical self-description implies (in contrast, at middle adolescence there will be considerable concern). Thus, the self-portrait lacks consistency and coherence but at this age, it is not distressing. During early adolescence, the inability to integrate seemingly contradictory characteristics of the self (intelligent vs. airhead, extrovert vs. introvert, depressed vs. cheerful) has the psychological advantage of sparing the adolescent conflict over opposing attributes in his/her self-theory (Harter & Monsour, 1992). Moreover, as Higgins (1991) observes, the increased differentiation functions as a cognitive buffer, reducing the possibility that negative attributes in one sphere may spread or generalize to other spheres (see also Linville, 1987; Simmons & Blyth, 1987). Thus although the construction of multiple selves sets the stage for attributes to be contradictory, most young adolescents do not identify potential contradictions or experience conflict, given the compartmentalized structure of their abstract self-representations.

Evidence for these claims comes from our own research (see Harter, Bresneck, et al., 1997; Harter & Monsour, 1992), in which we asked adolescents at three developmental levels, early adolescence (seventh grade), middle adolescence (ninth grade), and late adolescence (eleventh grade) to generate self-attributes across several roles and then indicate whether any of these attributes represented opposites (e.g., cheerful vs. depressed, rowdy vs. calm, studious vs. lazy, at ease vs. self-conscious). After identifying any such opposites, they were asked whether any of these pairs caused them conflict; namely, were they perceived as clashing within their personality? The specific roles we ask about have varied across studies. They have included self with a group of friends, with a close friend, with parents (mother vs. father), in romantic relationships, in the classroom, and on the job. Across a number of converging indices (e.g., number of opposites, number of conflicts, percentage of opposites in conflict), attributes identified as *contradictory* and experienced as *conflicting* were infrequent among young adolescents.

An examination of the responses of young adolescents has revealed that there are potential contradictions that go undetected. Examples not identified by young adolescents (but that appeared contradictory to our research team) included being talkative as well as shy in romantic relationships, being uptight with family but carefree with friends, being caring and insensitive with friends, being a good student as well as a troublemaker in school, being self-conscious in romantic relationships but easygoing with friends, being lazy as a student but hardworking on the job. These observations bolster the interpretation, derived from Fischer's (1980) theory, that young adolescents do not yet have the cognitive ability to simultaneously compare these attributes to one another, and therefore they tend not to detect, or be concerned about, self-representations that are potential contradictions. One young adolescent when confronted with his description of himself as both caring and rude retorted, "Well, you are caring with your friends and rude to people who don't treat you nicely. There's no problem. I guess I just think about one thing about myself at a time and don't think about the other until the next day." Another young adolescent was asked why opposite attributes did not bother her; she succinctly exclaimed, "That's a stupid question. I don't fight with myself!" As will become apparent, this pattern changes dramatically during middle adolescence.

SELF-ESTEEM

The very term "self-esteem" becomes more salient in the young adolescent's vocabulary. As the cameo adolescent concludes, "It's a big deal to show that you have high self-esteem." Moreover, young teenagers begin to form metatheories about the causal nature of constructs that involve the self and others. For example, they speculate about the directionality of perceived attractiveness and self-esteem or about the causal links between peer approval and self-esteem.

From a Jamesian (1892) perspective, perceived adequacy in domains of importance is highly predictive of self-esteem, as young adolescents come to appreciate (Harter, 2006a). A preoccupation with the congruence or discrepancy between ideal and real self-representations intensifies during early adolescence. Moreover, perceptions of physical appearance head the list in terms of the correlation with feelings of overall worth (see Chapter 5). The majority of young adolescents admit that they base their self-esteem on their perceived appearance. Those whose self-esteem is dependent on meeting the punishing societal standards report lower perceptions of their appearance, lower global self-worth, and greater feelings of depression (Harter, 2000). The cameo youth admits that "How much I like myself as a person also depends on how I look. I'd like to be good-looking, like the movie and TV stars, but that's impossible. I'm too short and weigh too much and don't wear a size 2."

Young adolescents who are preoccupied with the importance of the opinion of peers are also at risk (Harter, Stocker, & Robinson, 1996). They admit to greater *fluctuations* in both approval and self-esteem, lower *levels* of both approval and self-esteem, and are more distracted in the classroom. The cameo adolescent admits that how much she likes herself is dependent on what other kids think of her, documenting the basic for fluctuations: "One day, like if I get invited to a party, I'll feel great about myself. But then the next day, if somebody I know ignores me in the hall or doesn't say something nice to me, then I feel terrible about myself." She also documents the pattern of distraction that teachers' ratings have demonstrated. "Sometimes I think too much about this during my classes and I don't concentrate on what the teacher is saying." These adolescents, drawn like magnets to the social mirror, are also more likely to report being depressed.

The differentiation of role-related selves, beginning in early adolescence, can also be observed in the tendency to report differing levels of self-esteem across relational contexts. In the prototypical description, the young adolescent reports that she likes herself a lot with peers but "not so much when I'm with my mom and dad." Although the concept of self-esteem has traditionally been reserved for perceptions of global self-esteem, we have introduced the construct of "relational self-esteem" (Harter, Waters, & Whitesell, 1998). Beginning in the middle school years, adolescents discriminate their level of perceived self-esteem, namely, how much they like themselves as a person, across relational contexts. We have examined these perceptions across a number of such contexts including self-esteem with parents, teachers, male classmates, and female classmates. Factor-analysis revealed a clear factor pattern with high loadings on the designated factors (i.e., each relational context) and negligible cross-loadings. We have also examined the discrepancy between individuals' highest and lowest relational self-esteem scores. Although a minority of adolescents (approximately one-fourth) reported little variation in self-esteem across contexts, the vast majority (the remaining three-fourths) report that their self-esteem did vary significantly as a function of the relational context. In the extreme, one female participant reported the lowest possible self-esteem score with parents and the highest possible self-esteem score with female classmates.

In addition to documenting such variability, our goal has been to identify potential causes of these individual differences. In addressing one determinant, we adopted Cooley's (1902) looking-glass self-perspective, in which the opinions of significant others are incorporated into one's sense of personal worth. Building upon our previous empirical efforts (see Harter,

1990), we hypothesized that context-specific validation for who one is as a person, should be highly related to self-esteem within the corresponding context. The findings corroborated the more specific prediction that support within a given relationship was more highly associated with relational self-esteem in that relationship, compared to self-esteem in the other three contexts (Harter, Waters, & Whitesell, 1998). The pattern of results suggests a refinement of the looking-glass-self formulation; support as validation from particular significant others will have its strongest impact on how one evaluates one's sense of worth in the context of those particular others.

Normative Liabilities for Self-Development during Early Adolescence

Inaccuracies in Self-Appraisals

As with the entry into any new developmental level, there are liabilities associated with these emerging self-processes. For example, although abstractions are developmentally advanced cognitive structures, they are removed from concrete, observable behaviors and therefore more susceptible to distortion. The adolescent's self-concept, therefore, becomes more difficult to verify and is often less realistic. As to change, frustration, M. Rosenberg (1986) observes, when the self comes to be viewed as a collection of abstractions, uncertainties are introduced, as there are "few objective and unambiguous facts about one's sensitivity, creativity, morality, dependability, and so on" (p. 129). Moreover, the necessary skills to apply hypothetico-deductive thinking to the postulates of one's self-system are not yet in place. Although the young adolescent may have multiple hypotheses about the self, he/she does not yet possess the ability to correctly deduce which are true, leading to distortions in self-perceptions. The all-or-none thinking of this period, in the form of overgeneralizations that the young adolescent cannot cognitively control, also contributes to unrealistic self-representations, in that at one point in time, one may feel totally intelligent, whereas at another point in time, one may feel like a complete dork.

Fluctuations in Self-Appraisals

The adolescent sense of self will vacillate, given the inability to cognitively control one's self-representations. In describing this "barometric self" during adolescence, M. Rosenberg (1986) points to a different set of causes. He cites considerable literature indicating that adolescents experience an increased concern with what their peers think of them, findings that are relevant to Cooley's (1902) looking-glass-self model. This heavy dependence on the perceptions of other's opinions sets the stage for volatility in one's assessment of the self. Moreover, there is inevitable ambiguity about others' attitudes toward the self, since one can never have direct access to the mind of another. Thus, attributions about others' thought processes may change from one time period to another. The second reason for fluctuating self-evaluations stems from the fact that different significant others have different opinions of the self, depending on the situation or moment in time. Third, adolescents' concern with what others think of them leads to efforts at impression management, provoking variations in the self across relational contexts. Finally, at times, adolescents are treated as more adultlike (e.g., on a job), whereas at other times, they are treated as more childlike (e.g., with parents at home). Thus, the self fluctuates in tandem.

Our own findings on how self-esteem varies as a function of one's relationships (what we have termed "relational self-esteem") is consistent with M. Rosenberg's (1986) analysis (Harter, 2006a). The young adolescent is not yet troubled by what could be viewed as inconsistent self-representations because he/she cannot simultaneously evaluate them as contradictory. However, there are liabilities associated with this inability. The compartmentalization of abstractions about the self precludes the construction of an integrated portrait of self. The fact that different significant others may hold differing opinions about the self makes it difficult to develop the sense that one's self is coherent. With movement into midadolescence, abstract self-descriptors become far less isolated or compartmentalized. However, new liabilities then follow.

Finally, there are domain-specific normative liabilities that are associated with educational transitions. Young adolescents all shift from an elementary school to either a middle school or junior high school that typically draws upon several elementary feeder schools. Thus, they must now move into a group of peers, many of whom they have previously not known (typically two-thirds to three-fourths of the peer group will be new). Given the young adolescent's heightened concern with how others view the self, an important source of global self-esteem, there may be understandable shifts in global self-esteem across the transition. Individuals may perceive that their academic competence and social acceptance is higher or lower than when they were in elementary school (Harter, 1990, 2006a).

Social Comparison

In addition to new social reference groups, the nature of social comparison takes on new dimensions. While the *use* of social comparison is heightened, young adolescents shift from more conspicuous to more subtle acknowledgments, as they become aware of the negative social consequences of overt comparisons. They may be accused of boasting about their superior performance (Pomerantz, Ruble, Frey, & Greulich, 1995). As the prototypical young adolescent observes, "I get better grades than most kids; I don't brag about it because that's not cool."

Eccles and colleagues (Eccles & Midgley, 1989; Eccles & Roeser, 2009) have pointed to different educational emphases during the transition to middle school and junior high school. They observe that teachers place considerably more emphasis on comparisons with others (e.g., public posting of grades, ability grouping, announcing to their students the personal results of performance at competitive activities). These educational practices represent a mismatch given the adolescent's needs. At a time when young adolescents are painfully self-conscious, the school system heightens the salience of social comparison in conjunction with publicizing each student's performance.

In addition to the greater emphasis on social comparison, the standards of evaluation shift from *effort* to *ability*, according to Eccles and colleagues (Eccles & MIdgley, 1989; Eccles & Roeser, 2009). They note that in elementary school, there is more emphasis on effort; that is, "try harder and you can do better." In middle and junior high schools, however, poorer performance is attributed to lack of scholastic ability, leading the young adolescent to feel that he/she does not have the aptitude to succeed, that he/she lacks intelligence. These educational changes are not lost on young adolescents, as revealed in the cameo: "The other kids know that I am at the top of the class. It's really hard *not* to compare yourself to other kids because the teachers really emphasize how well or poorly we are doing, compared to others. They post everybody's grades, they split us into groups, based on how well we are doing, and it can be really embarrassing. All they talk about is how we need to show that we are intelligent and that we have to do better than other schools on the stupid achievement tests they keep making us take." The emphasis on social comparison is a pernicious new influence that leads to the conclusion that everyone but those at the top of the academic ladder is intellectually incapable. This, in turn, ushers in a need to protect the self.

Self-Enhancing Strategies and Self-Serving Biases

Normative strategies to protect and enhance the self are evident in early adolescence. The heightened preoccupation with others' perceptions of the self, coupled with a focus on the discrepancy between the real and ideal self, conspire to produce an escalation in the *need* to protect and enhance the self. As the cameo adolescent observes, "it's very important to *seem* as if you really like yourself." Thus, there is the recognition of the powerful motives for self-protection and self-enhancement. Moreover, young adolescents have certain requisite skills.

The increasing emphasis on the comparison with others at this juncture provides a psychological stimulus for the strategy of downward social comparison. Although overt comparisons are frowned upon, successful students have the information to conclude that they are more scholastically competent than others, thereby protecting or enhancing the self. The criteria for social acceptance are quite clearly communicated by peers, leading the more popular young teenagers to conclude, through downward social comparison, that they are higher on the totem pole of popularity. Since only a few can rise to the top of the scholastic and social ladders, the average young adolescent self is vulnerable, fueling the motivation to enhance, or at least protect, one's image. One mechanism can be found in the formation of cliques that provide personal support, even though one's in-group, itself, may not achieve status in the overall hierarchy.

Cognitive skills to engage in certain adult attributional biases become available to the young adolescent. For example, successes can be attributed to internal, stable characteristics such as intelligence, whereas failures are due to external factors such as excessively difficult tests. The cameo adolescent recounts that "If I do well on them, I tell myself it's because I am smart. If I don't do well, it's because the test was too hard or the teacher didn't teach us what we needed to know." Another attribution for lack of success is the claim that one simply didn't study hard enough, implying that one could have done better, with increased personal effort.

The cameo young adolescent also makes use of Greenwald's (1980) concept of "beneffectance," a self-protective strategy in which one's central or important attributes are viewed as positive, whereas negative characteristics are relegated to the periphery of the self. In admitting that she gets distracted in certain classes, the cameo adolescent asserts that "If I don't care about the subject, it doesn't matter to me, what's important is doing well in those classes I care about, where I get A's."

Pathological Self-Processes and Outcomes during Early Adolescence

False-Self Behavior

Early adolescence brings (1) a greater appreciation of the meaning of false-self behavior, (2) its greater salience in one's vocabulary, and (3) a preoccupation with its detection. It is not until about the age of 12 or 13 that young adolescents can clearly define false-self behavior (Harter, 2006a). Definitions focus on concealing what you really think or feel and saying things you don't really believe. The cameo adolescent struggles with this issue: "I try to tell myself that what *I* think is the most important, that I should just be my true self. I shouldn't be phony and act like I'm somebody else." Young adolescents also appear to be highly sensitive to the detection of hypocrisy. While they acknowledge some false-self behavior in themselves, they are far more likely to observe it in others (e.g., parents and peers). Anthony describes a new vocabulary that emerges at this stage of development; young adolescents subject others' beliefs to scrutiny and criticism, attempting to expose the inconsistencies and contradictions in parental arguments, values, and behaviors. Thus, parents are accused of hypocrisy, deflecting blame from the self. These processes are normative manifestations to emerge in early adolescence but can set the stage for more pathological processes. If significant others provide support for whom one is as a person, for those attributes that the young adolescent feels truly define the self, then one will experience the self as authentic.

However, the construction of a self that is too highly dependent upon the internalization of the opinions imposed by others can lead to the creation of a false self that does not mirror one's authentic experience. Our own findings (Harter, Marold, et al., 1996) reveal that unhealthy levels of false-self behavior are particularly likely to emerge if caregivers make their approval conditional upon the young adolescent living up to unrealistic standards of behavior. We have labeled this phenomenon "conditional support." We have learned, however, that this term is a misnomer. In the face of such demands, adolescents do not perceive parental responses as "supportive." Rather, conditionality specifies the psychological hoops through which adolescents must jump in order to please parents. Those adolescents who experience such a conditional atmosphere are forced into adopting a socially implanted self. That is, they must learn to suppress what they feel are true-self attributes, in an attempt to garner the needed approval from parental caretakers, a process that can first be observed in mid- to late childhood.

Here, the terminology purposely switches from "caregiver" to "caretaker" in a metaphorical effort to convey the fact that such socialization practices "take away" from the care for whom one is as a person, from true-self development. Our findings reveal that those experiencing high levels of conditionality from parents will express hopelessness about their ability to please the parents. Hopelessness then translates into high levels of false-self behavior in an attempt to garner some level of needed parental support. Of particular relevance is that high levels of false-self behavior are directly related to low levels of self-esteem. Low levels of self-esteem are highly correlated with self-reported depressive symptomatology that can, for some adolescents, lead to suicidal thoughts and actions.

Chronic and severe abuse puts one at even more extreme risk for suppressing one's true self and displaying various forms of inauthentic, or false-self, behavior. Such a process has its origins in childhood, given the very forms of parenting that constitute psychological abuse. As described in Chapter 2, parenting practices that represent lack of attunement to the child's needs, empathic failure, lack of validation, threats of harm, coercion, and enforced compliance all cause the true self to go underground (Bleiberg, 1984; Stern, 1985; Winnicott, 1958, 1965) and lead to what Sullivan (1953) labeled "not-me" experiences.

Furthermore, as described in Chapter 2, the ability to express oneself verbally allows one to falsify what is shared with others. For the maltreated child, secrecy pacts around sexually abusive interactions further provoke the child defensively to exclude such episodic memories from awareness (see also Bretherton, 1993; Bretherton & Munholland, 2008). Thus, sexual and physical abuse cause the child to split off experiences, either consciously or unconsciously, relegating them to either a private or inaccessible part of the self. The very disavowal, repression, or dissociation of one's experiences, coupled with psychogenic amnesia and numbing as defensive reactions to abuse, therefore, set the stage for loss of one's true self.

Herman (1992) introduces other dynamics that represent barriers to authenticity among victims of abuse. She notes that the malignant sense of inner badness is often camouflaged by the abused child's persistent attempts to be good. In adopting different roles designed to please the parent, to be the perfect child, one comes to experience one's behavior as false or inauthentic (see also A. Miller, 1990). Thus, one develops a socially acceptable false self that conforms to the demands and desires of others in an attempt to obtain their approval (see Harter, Marold, et al., 1996). If a child believes that his/her true self is corroded with inner badness, it would be met with scorn and contempt if it were revealed. Therefore, the true self must be concealed at all costs, also eroding positive feelings of self-esteem. Although these dynamics have their origins in childhood, beginning in adolescence there is much more conscious awareness of these dynamics and the realization that one is being false or phony.

A Broader Model of Self-Esteem

Our overall model of the determinants, correlates, and consequences of self-esteem (see Figure 3.1) becomes increasingly relevant at early adolescence and beyond where there is strong empirical support across numerous studies (see Harter, 2006b, Harter & Marold, 1993). Findings reveal that lack of both parental support as well as peer support can lead to pathological levels of low self-worth, depressed affect, and hopelessness, that in turn may provoke suicidal ideation if not suicidal behaviors. Moreover, in the first edition of this book we reported on six different profiles, reflecting different combinations of competence/adequacy perceptions as well as peer versus parent support, as they impact the adjustment/depression composite (self-esteem, hopelessness, and depressed affect).

Our own findings (see Harter, 2006a) indicate that although peer support increases in its predictability of global self-esteem between late childhood and early adolescence, the impact of parental support does *not*

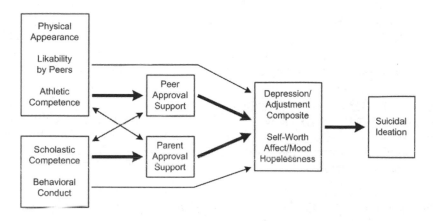

FIGURE 3.1. Predictors and consequences of the depression/adjustment composite.

decline. Historically, textbook portrayals of adolescence imply that parental influences wane as one moves into adolescence. However, nothing is further from the truth when one examines the impact of parental support, including conditionality, upon self-processes that extend from false-self behavior and global self-esteem, to the related correlates of depressed affect, hopelessness, and suicidal ideation.

That said, the peer culture does come to loom large in adolescence. From an attachment perspective, early adolescence marks the process of transferring dependencies on parents to peer relationships (J. P. Allen, 2008). Needs for companionship, intimacy, and enhancement of personal worth are now more likely to be met by classmates and friends (H. K. Rubin, Bukowsly, & Parker, 2006). Peer support and approval, or its absence, is a powerful predictor of what we have labeled the depression/adjustment composite that includes self-esteem or self-worth, affect/mood, along a continuum of depressed to cheerful, hope (hopeless to hopeful), that has empirically been demonstrated to predict suicidal thinking. Lack of peer approval appears to be more directly predicted by perceived inadequacies in what we have labeled as more *peer-salient* domains, namely, physical appearance, likability by peers, and athletic competence. In contrast, lack of parent support is more highly associated with perceived inadequacies in the more *parent-salient* domains of scholastic competence and behavioral conduct.

Dubois and colleagues (2002) have also reported evidence for the distinction between *peer-salient* domains and what they refer to as *adult-oriented* domains (i.e., school and family). Of particular interest is their emphasis on the *balance* between these categories and their corresponding support levels from peers and parents in predicting adjustment. For example, they report that a pattern of perceived success in the peer-oriented domains, in contrast to less positive evaluations in the adult-oriented arenas, was consistently linked to higher levels of externalizing problems in early adolescence. They suggest that when adult-oriented domains provide relatively weak sources of support and esteem, youth may be deprived of the capacities to cope successfully with stressors such as parent–child conflict or the increased academic demands that accompany the transition to adolescence. Thus, a balance between these two sources is the healthier pathway to adjustment.

Peer Rejection, Humiliation, and Implications for the High-Profile School Shootings

More recently, we have become more focused on the role of peer *rejection*, not merely the lack of peer approval (Harter, Low, & Whitesell, 2003). Our initial interest in this construct came from an analysis of the emerging profiles of the now 11 high-profile cases in which White, middle-class older children and adolescents, from small cities or suburbs, have gone on shooting sprees killing peers, and in a few cases, school officials who were random targets, rather than specifically identified individuals. What became evident, in the analysis of media reports, is that all of these male youth killers had a history of peer rejection and *humiliation*. As a psychologist who for many years has contributed to (and kept up with) the literature on emotional development in children and adolescents, I was astounded to realize, upon further exploration, that we have virtually no research literature on humiliation, until very recently. There is ample literature on shame, guilt, and embarrassment, but little about humiliation (see Chapter 6). Yet we can all appreciate the fact that humiliation is a daily event in the lives of many children. As the media accounts document, for the school shooters, extreme feelings of chronic humiliation by peers due to excessive teasing, taunting, and physical insults eventually led them to psychologically "snap," resulting in random killings and in the case of the Columbine teens, to suicide.

An examination of the media accounts of the school shooters made it obvious that many of the determinants in our model could be found in the lives of these adolescents (see Harter, Low, et al., 2003). As a result, we revised the model by the addition of angry aggression, as well as violent ideation. We examined the revised model in a normative sample of middle school students. Through path-analytic techniques we demonstrated that the data fit the model exceedingly well. That is, the antecedents in the model, perceived lack of competence and social inadequacies, predicted lack of approval from peers and parents alike. Bellmore and Cillessen (2006) have also reported that adolescents perceived as victims of bullying and harassment came to view themselves as disliked by peers, lacking peer support, and generally unlikable and socially inadequate, a negative social self-concept. In our own model, these determinants, in turn, predicted low self-esteem, depressed affect, angry affect, and hopelessness, all of which predicted suicidal ideation *and* violent ideation. Consistent with the clinical literature on the comorbidity of internalizing and externalizing symptoms, we found a correlation of $r = .55$ between suicidal and violent ideation toward others. Thus, the determinants in our model, if negative, put adolescents at pathological risk for endangering their own, as well as others' lives.

We have further examined the role of humiliation and its role in contributing to violent ideation. In the Harter, Low, et al. (2003) study we wrote vignettes that simulated some of the types of humiliating events that were experienced by the school shooters. We then asked middle school students what other emotions they might experience (e.g., anger, depression) as well as what actions they might take, along a continuum from doing nothing to acting violently toward the perpetrators and/or toward anyone. The majority of students reported that they would be humiliated, as predicted, given that the vignettes were designed to provoke humiliation. We identified two groups: violent ideators (in the minority) who indicated that they would engage in violent revenge, and those who did *not* report that they would think about such revenge. We then sought to determine what distinguished the two groups, finding that those entertaining violent thoughts expressed higher levels of anger and depression. In addition, the violent ideators reported higher levels of the negative determinants in the model, for example, more peer rejection, less parental support, lower self-concept scores (appearance, peer likability), lower self-worth, and greater hopelessness. Thus, certain factors in the histories of violent ideators propel them to thoughts of seriously harming others as well as themselves. These pathological outcomes may require clinical interventions given that they put themselves and others at serious risk.

In a subsequent study, we sought more specifically to investigate what are some of the factors that lead humiliation to result in violent ideation as well as suicidal ideation. Our findings revealed that the role of an *audience that mocks the victim* is a particularly critical determinant. Prototypical reactions include revenge, wanting to hide, or attempts to minimize the humiliation (Harter, Kiang, Whitesell, & Anderson, 2003). We have continued to pursue this prototypical approach to humiliation currently (see Chapter 6 on self-conscious emotions for further recent work on humiliation).

Is There a Dark Side to High Self-Esteem?

Our own modeling efforts, reported above, reveal that it is *low* self-esteem that is consistently related to suicidal and violent thinking. These findings are consistent with the broader literature revealing that high self-esteem is a psychological commodity associated with positive adjustment and mental health outcomes. Low self-esteem, in contrast, has been viewed as a liability and has been associated with poor adjustment in the literature (e.g., depression, anxiety, conduct problems, teen pregnancy). However, there is current controversy over whether there may also be a dark side to high self-esteem.

Just what is the controversy? One vocal group of theorists (Baumeister, Smart, & Boden, 1996) has argued that there is a subset of individuals with high but fragile self-esteem who are often aggressive in response to perceived ego threats. Baumeister et al. contend that individuals who report high self-esteem in combination with high narcissism, low empathy, and sensitivity to rejection will exhibit violent tendencies in the face of threats to the ego.

We (Harter & McCarley, 2004) believe that Baumeister et al.'s (1996) composite of predictors has some merit, with the exception of the role of self-esteem. Specifically, we predicted that high narcissism, low empathy, and sensitivity to rejection coupled with *low* self-esteem (not high self-esteem) would lead young adolescents, in the face of threats to the ego, to violent ideation. To assess violent ideation, we asked participants to read humiliating scenarios that represented threats to the ego and then to rate how they would typically respond in such a situation, ranging from doing nothing to seriously harming the perpetrator. Self-esteem was measured by our Global Self-Esteem subscale (Harter, 1985). Narcissism, empathy, and sensitivity to rejection were assessed by adaptations of previously developed measures, all of which were found to be reliable (alphas ranging from .76 to .87). Regression analyses revealed that high narcissism and low empathy significantly predicted violent ideation. However, in contrast to Baumeister et al.'s claims, higher self-esteem was associated with lower levels of violent ideation. Furthermore, when self-reported conduct (positive to negative) and the frequency of experiencing humiliating events were included in the model, they both explained a substantial proportion of the variance in violent ideation.

In addition, we identified two extreme groups, those high and low on violent ideation. Findings revealed that violent ideators reported significantly higher narcissism, lower empathy, and greater sensitivity to rejection, as Baumeister would predict. However, violent ideators reported *lower* self-esteem, which is inconsistent with his formulation. In a subsequent study, we added fluctuating self-esteem, conduct, and the frequency of humiliating, rejection events (McCarley & Harter, 2006). These increased the predictability of violence ideation, both in regression analyses and in comparisons of violent and nonviolent ideators. Violent ideators reported fluctuating self-esteem, greater conduct problems, and a greater frequency of humiliating experiences that were ego threatening. Thus, our findings of the precursors of violent thoughts qualifies as well as broadens our understanding, given that lack of empathy and narcissism are clear predictors of humiliation, although high self-esteem is not. In fact, self-esteem and narcissism correlated −.01, revealing that these are different constructs both conceptually, as scales define the two constructs, as well as empirically. Narcissism entails a sense of entitlement, superiority, and exhibitionism, whereas high self-esteem is defined as liking and respecting who one is as a person. Clearly there is a need to distinguish between these two concepts, conceptually, methodologically, and empirically.

Finally, in this study we uncovered an interesting finding that is cause for concern. In the actual high-profile cases of the school shooters most had not been in any major trouble with the law and had *not* come to the attention of teachers or school personnel as potential troublemakers. In fact, many teachers and school officials, as well as students were astounded that these boys committed such violent acts. Debriefing efforts of the surviving students and families at Columbine, conducted by University of Denver clinicians and some in private practice, revealed that students and their families became realistically fearful that they would not be able to detect who, in the future, might commit such acts because there were few public warning signs that the shooters were capable of such behavior.

These concerns are real, given findings from our own research (Harter & McCarley, 2004). In this study we asked teachers to rate student conduct (getting in trouble, potential for violence) and among the subgroup of violent ideators who had rated their own conduct as quite negative, teachers misrated one-third of the group, giving them positive scores on conduct. This is concerning and highlights the difficulty in assessing which students are at risk. Not all violent ideators may be at risk for violent *action* (given the low percentage of such acts in most schools). However, violent ideation represents another kind of pathological risk factor to the extent that it interferes with attention to, and concentration on, scholastic endeavors and with socially appropriate behaviors that would promote positive peer interactions.

The very presence of this subgroup of violent ideators suggests that they represent a type of adolescent who is different from those students with demonstrable histories of conduct problems, delinquency, and acting-out patterns, all of whom readily come to the attention of teachers, school officials, and students. Those not showing these obvious and observable patterns escape identification. One of our goals is to devise a short form of our instruments that will allow schools to identify those who may have escaped the attention of school personnel but are nevertheless at pathological risk. Many of these processes begin in early adolescence (and for some, in late childhood) but continue into middle and later adolescence, as the range of ages of the actual school shooters (9 to 18) reveals.

Pathological Narcissism

The specific features of narcissistic personality disorders begin to crystallize during early adolescence (Bleiberg, 1994; Bukowski, Schwartzman, Santo, Bagwell, & Adams, 2009). These include an omnipotent sense of self, refusal to acknowledge one's shortcomings, and unrealistic demands for public affirmation. Narcissists' inflated sense of self is revealed in their perception of themselves as far more intellectually and socially competent than is warranted by objective criteria. Thus, it is the *discrepancy* between highly positive evaluations of self that are not shared by others. Bukowski et al. have demonstrated these processes among young adolescents in the domain of social acceptance. Their findings reveal that the discrepancy between peer sociometric ratings of popularity and self-evaluations of social acceptance was markedly higher for narcissistic adolescents, compared to those low in narcissism.

Furthermore, narcissistic individuals are heavily invested in maintaining these unrealistic positive views of self, and are thus motivated to defend against threats to these beliefs. The defense against these threats to an inflated sense of self often take the form of peer aggression. Bukowski et al. (2009) have demonstrated a clear relationship between aggression and narcissistic behavior among young adolescents. Of particular interest are their findings that narcissistic individuals are more likely to demonstrate *reactive* and *relational* or indirect forms of aggression than *proactive*, direct attacks on others. Presumably, retaliation in the form of more covert or indirect forms of aggression is not as evident, and therefore may give the illusion that one is viewed less negatively than if one blatantly displays more proactive aggression.

Narcissistic disturbances also invariably stem from concerns that one is ignored or not given sufficient attention, typically covered by doubts about one's ability to evoke positive responses from others. Those adolescents who present an inflated sense of self to peers will incur negative social feedback, provoking a vicious cycle in which they blame others and display retaliatory aggression that exacerbates peer relationship problems (Barry & Malkin, 2010). Moreover, narcissistic distortions in the self, related to defensive forms of peer aggression, become quite stable during early adolescence (Bukowski et al., 2009).

Another source of narcissism vulnerability is some realization that one's actual self does not conform to one's lofty aspirations (Joffe & Sandler, 1967). These clinicians observe that narcissistic vulnerability evokes *shame* given the deflation that accompanies the inability to measure up to one's ideal. Their self-narrative contains illusions of power, omnipotence, control, perfection, and invulnerability resulting in a highly distorted sense of self. They cannot see past their own reflection. These self-aggrandizing fantasies conceal very fragile and unstable self-esteem, requiring "high-maintenance" personal efforts to obtain compensatory attention and admiration (Rhodewalt, 2006). Bleiberg (1994) cites another mechanism. To rid themselves of the specter of any negative self-evaluations, narcissists *project* their limitations onto others, holding them in contempt, accusing *them* of being worthless, weak, or incompetent.

Pathological Eating-Disordered Behavior

Our model identifies one self-concept domain that robustly affects global self-esteem across ages and cultures, namely, perceived physical appearance or attractiveness. This link is profoundly impacted by cultural standards of appearance for each gender, given that the culture touts physical attractiveness as the measure of one's worth as a person (see Chapter 5). The empirical findings have revealed that the correlation between perceived attractiveness and global self-esteem range from the .40s to the .80s, in our own research. Moreover, investigators have demonstrated that these relationships are not merely statistical but are very much embedded in the consciousness of individuals who are aware of this link. In our own work (Kiang & Harter, 2006), we have found strong support for a model in which contemporary cultural values are highly endorsed. These values include the perceptions that being attractive will lead to higher self-esteem, meeting standards of appearance will make people more popular, and that people who are overweight are discriminated against. However, there is enough variability in these scores to determine that such awareness predicts perceptions of one's own appearance, which in turn predict level of self-esteem and eating-disordered behaviors. Specifically, those endorsing these cultural values reported more negative views of their appearance, lower self-esteem, more psychological correlates of eating disorders, and more eating-disordered behaviors.

This particular study was conducted with college students. However, the seeds of such a model are sown in early adolescence, if not earlier. Children and teenagers of both genders are well aware of the prevailing norms for desirable appearance. For adult females in the 2000s, one must be tall, very thin, weigh very little (around 110–115 pounds), have ample breasts, and of course a pretty face and stunning hair, an unattainable combination for more than 90% of the female population. However, the average American woman is 5'4" and weighs 140 pounds. Standards have been exceedingly punishing for females across the decades. What is new within the last two decades is the fact that the bar has been raised for males in our society. No longer is appeal to be judged primarily by status, wealth, position, and power but by physical standards of attractiveness, as well. Muscular build, abs, biceps, physique, hair, on head as well as face, have all come to define the new ideals for men (see Chapter 5).

These standards are not lost on our young adolescents. Children succumb to the same discouragement of not being able to emulate the looks of models, singers, and movie stars in the limelight. Meeting these standards becomes particular critical during early adolescence as teenagers face inevitable pubertal changes that signal their impending adulthood. Thus, they look to adult standards as the physical markers for what defines attractiveness, appeal, and social acceptability, all of which determine one's self-esteem.

The genetic throw of the dice lead some young adolescent males and females to fare better than others on the competitive battleground, a minefield on the road to winning the attractiveness wars. For example, early-maturing girls are at a distinct disadvantage given the current emphasis on thinness and height because on average they are typically heavier and shorter, compared to later-maturing girls who tend to be thinner and taller. The pattern is just the opposite for adolescent males. Earlier-maturing boys tend to be taller and more muscular, which gives them a physical edge. Thus, beginning in earnest at this age, evaluations of one's appearance take on critical implications for one's global self-esteem. Those not meeting the gold standard are at serious risk for pathological forms of depression and possibly suicide, as well as for eating disorders that can be life threatening. While this preoccupation initially becomes quite salient in early adolescence, it continues throughout the lifespan.

Middle Adolescence: Ages 14 to 16

Normative Self-Representations and Self-Evaluations during Middle Adolescence

VERBAL CAMEO

"What am I like as a person? You're probably not going to understand. I'm complicated! With my really close friends, I am very tolerant. I mean, I'm understanding and caring. With a group of friends, I'm rowdier. I'm also usually friendly and cheerful but I can get pretty obnoxious and intolerant if I don't like how they're acting. I'd like to be friendly and tolerant all of the time, that's the kind of person I want to be, and I'm disappointed in myself when I'm not. Part of me would like to have a boyfriend but then, on the other hand, it would interfere with the time I spend with my close friends. At school, I'm serious, even studious every now and then, but I'm also a goof-off too, because if you're too studious, you won't be popular. So I go back and forth, which means I don't do all that well in terms of my grades. But that causes problems at home, where I'm pretty anxious when I'm around my parents. They expect me to get all A's, and get pretty annoyed with me when report cards come out. I care what they think about me, and so then I get down on myself, and get confused about how well I should do at school. I mean I worry about how I probably should get better grades, but I'd be mortified in the eyes of my friends if I did too well. So, I'm usually pretty stressed out at home, and can even get very nasty, especially when my parents get on my case. It's not like they are so perfect! They can be real hypocrites, sometimes. But I really don't understand how I can switch so fast from being cheerful with my friends, then coming home and feeling anxious, and then getting frustrated and nasty to my parents. Which one is the real me? I have the same question when I'm around boys. Sometimes, I feel phony. Say I think some guy might be interested in asking me out. I try to act different, like Beyoncé, she's a really hot singer. I'll be a real extrovert, fun-loving and even flirtatious, and think I am the best-looking girl in the room, the guys will really notice me! It's important to be good-looking like the music and movie stars. That's what makes you popular. I know in my heart of hearts that I can never look like Beyoncé, so why do I even try? It makes me hate myself and feel depressed. Plus, when I try to look and act like her, then everybody, I mean *everybody* else is looking at me like they think I am totally weird! They don't act like they think I'm attractive so I end up thinking I look terrible. I just hate myself when that happens! Because it gets worse! Then I get self-conscious and embarrassed and become radically introverted, and I don't know who I really am! Am I just acting like an extrovert, am I just trying to impress the other kids, when really I'm an introvert? But I don't really care what they think, anyway. I mean I don't want to care, that is. But you have to, because what all of the other kids think of you is important to how much you like yourself as a person, although I go back and forth on that, too. My self-esteem is higher with kids who know me than with my parents. I can be my true self with my close friends. I can't be my real self with my parents. They don't understand me. What do *they* know about what it's like to be a teenager? They treat me like I'm still a kid and don't realize that I am growing up and don't need them as much now. At least at school, people treat you more like you're an adult. That gets confusing, though. I mean, which am I? When you're 15, are you still a kid or an adult? I have a part-time job and the people there treat me like an adult. I want adults to approve of me, so I'm very responsible at work, which makes me feel good about myself there. But then I go out with my friends and I get pretty crazy and irresponsible. So, which am I, responsible or irresponsible? How can the same person be both? If my parents knew how immature I act sometimes, they would ground me forever, particularly my father. I do things that they would say are risky, but I know I would never be the one who was hurt or got in trouble. I'm real distant with my father. I'm pretty close to my mother though. But it's hard being distant with one parent and close to the other, especially if we are all together, like talking at dinner. Even though I am close to my mother, I'm still pretty secretive about some things, particularly behavior that my parents wouldn't approve of. Let's face it, at my age you have to be different with your parents, even though you still want to have a good relationship with them. But you have to try things with other *kids* to see what fits who you are. It can be confusing. So I think a lot about who is the real me, and sometimes I try to figure it out when I write in my diary, but I can't resolve it. In fact, I spend a lot of time and energy thinking as hard as I can about who I am and who I will become. How hopeless it all seems! There are days when I wish I could just become immune to myself!"

Self-Awareness, Self-Agency, Self-Coherence, and Self-Continuity

Development is not necessarily a linear progression toward some teleological endpoint. There is clearly a blip on the psychological radar screen at midadolescence. This point is missed in classic treatments of development. For example, Piaget (1960) asserted that the stage of formal operations, beginning at about age 13, was the final period of cognitive development, and did not posit further advances or refinements. However, there are not only additional acquisitions but significant setbacks, particularly during midadolescence.

Dawson, Fischer, and Stein (2006) articulate a number of these processes. They observe that knowledge is increasingly elaborated, given the transition to new complexity levels. Individuals can now detect the limitations of previous strategies and are likely to reject them. As a result, their perceptions of self can be derailed. During this period of disequilibrium, they have not yet developed new strategies to overcome the limitations of the earlier, inadequate, solutions.

The unreflective self-acceptance of earlier periods of development clearly vanishes. What were previously unexamined self-truths, the basis for a durable self-image, now become unproven and troublesome self-hypotheses. The tortuous search for the self is made more difficult given the painful recognition of the proliferation of multiple Me-selves that now crowd the self-landscape and do not speak with a single voice (Harter, Bresnick, et al., 1997). The cameo adolescent describes a self with really close friends (e.g., tolerant), with a group of friends (e.g., intolerant), as well as a self with mother (e.g., close) versus father (e.g., distant). Additional roles, for example, self at a job, also require the construction of novel context-specific attributes (e.g., responsible). Self-awareness, therefore, is quite intense; however, the images are not stable or enduring. It is much like a lighthouse beacon that flits from buoy to buoy, providing only fleeting glimpses of potentially troubled waters. By analogy, awareness quickly shifts from role to role where one's image of self is defined quite differently. Thus, a new *kaleidoscopic* self emerges.

Additional cognitive I-self processes emerge that give the self-portrait a very new look (Case, 1985; Fischer, 1980; Fischer & Bidell, 2006). Whereas, in the previous stage, single abstractions were isolated from one another, during middle adolescence one acquires the ability to make comparisons between single abstractions, namely, between attributes within the same role-related self as well as across role-related selves. Fischer labels these new structures "abstract mappings," in that the adolescent can now "map" constructs about the self onto one another; that is, directly compare them. Therefore, mappings force the individual to compare and contrast different attributes. It should be noted that abstract mappings have features in common with the "representational" mappings of childhood, in that the cognitive links that are initially forged often take the form of opposites. During adolescence, these opposites can take the form of seemingly contradictory abstractions about the self (e.g., tolerant vs. intolerant, extrovert vs. introvert, responsible vs. irresponsible, good looking versus unattractive, as in the cameo).

However, the abstract mapping structure has limitations as a means of relating two concepts to one another, in that the individual cannot yet truly integrate such self-representations in a manner that would resolve apparent contradictions. Therefore, at the level of abstract mappings, the awareness of these opposites causes considerable intrapsychic conflict, confusion, and distress (Fischer et al., 1984; Harter & Monsour, 1992; Higgins, 1991), given the inability to coordinate these seemingly contradictory self-attributes. For example, our prototypical adolescent agonizes over whether she is an extrovert or an introvert ("Am I just acting like an extrovert, am I just trying to impress the other kids, when really I'm an introvert? So which am I, responsible or irresponsible? How can the same person be both?") Such cognitive-developmental limitations contribute to the emergence of what James (1892), over a century ago, identified as the *conflict of the different Me's*.

In addition to such confusion, these apparent contradictions lead to very *unstable* self-representations that are also cause for concern (e.g., "I really don't understand how I can switch so fast from being cheerful with my friends, then coming home and feeling anxious, and then getting frustrated and nasty to my parents. Which one is the real me?") The creation of multiple selves, coupled with the emerging ability to detect potential contradictions between self-attributes displayed in different roles, naturally ushers in concern over which attributes define the true self. However, from a normative perspective, the adolescent at this level is not equipped with the cognitive skills to fully solve the dilemma (e.g., "So I think a lot about who is the real me, and sometimes I try to figure it out when I write in my diary, but I can't resolve it").

Other I-self functions are also compromised, given the contradictory multiple selves that cannot be integrated. Thus, there is little sense of *self-coherence*, precluded by the many conflicting persona. *Self-continuity* becomes more of a challenge, subjecting some to thoughts of suicide, as will soon be described. *Self-agency* is hampered given that there is no efficacious self at the helm, no causal agent in control. Kitchner's (1986) developmental theory of reflective judgment is also relevant to the issue of agency. Her stage, corresponding to Fischer's (1980) level of abstract mappings, is characterized by reasoning in which knowledge is viewed as contextual or *relative*; that is, it depends upon the situation. Thus, the expression, "It's all relative." There is the awareness that different people, in different situations, will propose different arguments and that these can conflict. Thus, there is no basis on which to determine just who is correct, no ability to compare actual evidence that bears on contradictory claims of the truth. If one needs to make a decision, the adolescent at this stage will be perplexed, confused, and potentially paralyzed. If an action is required, there is no basis on which to make a clear judgment that would guide one's behavior. Thus, the belief that knowledge is relative can negatively impact a sense of agency.

Developmental Evidence

As introduced in the section on early adolescence, our own research has examined the extent to which adolescents at three developmental levels both identify opposing self-attributes and report that they are experienced as conflictual (Harter, Bresnick, et al., 1997; Harter & Monsour, 1992). We have determined, across several studies, that young adolescents infrequently detect opposites within their self-portrait. However, we predicted that during midadolescence there would be a dramatic rise in the detection of opposing self-attributes as well as an acknowledgment that such apparent contradictions lead to conflict within the self-system.

Our procedure for examining these issues is illustrated in the protocol presented in Figure 3.2. Adolescents are first asked to generate several attributes for each role or interpersonal context. These contexts have varied from study to study; however, in the sample protocol, we asked them to generate attributes for four roles: self with parents, with friends, with a romantic interest, and in their role as student, in the classroom. They wrote each attribute in one of three concentric circles, based on their *importance* to the self. In this procedure (see Harter & Monsour, 1992), respondents were then asked to identify any pairs of attributes they perceived to reflect *opposites* in their personality, by connecting them with lines. Next, they indicated whether any of these opposites were experienced as clashing or in *conflict* with each other, by putting arrowheads on the lines connecting those pairs of opposites.

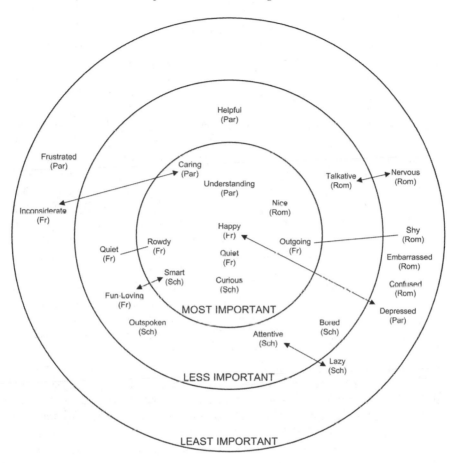

FIGURE 3.2. Prototypical self-portrait of a 15-year-old girl.

Across three different studies (see Harter, Bresnick, et al., 1997) we have found that the number of opposing self-attribute pairs, as well as the number of opposites in conflict, increases between early and middle adolescence. This pattern of findings supports the hypothesis that the abstract mapping structures that emerge in middle adolescence allow one to detect, but not to meaningfully integrate, these apparent contradictions. Thus, they lead to the phenomenological experience of intrapsychic conflict. We have asked teenagers to verbally elaborate on the opposites and conflicts that they reported on our task. As one 14-year-old put it, "I really think I am a happy person and I want to be that way with everyone, not just my friends; but I get depressed with my parents, and it really bugs me because that's not what I want to be like." A 15-year-old, in describing a conflict between self-attributes within the realm of romantic relationships, exclaimed, "I hate the fact that I get so nervous! I wish I wasn't so inhibited. The real me is talkative. I just want to be natural, but I can't." Another 15-year-old girl explained, "I really think of myself as friendly and open to people, but the way the other girls act, they force me to become an introvert, even though I know I'm not." In exasperation, one ninth grader observed of the self-portrait she had constructed, "It's not right, it should all fit together into one piece!" These comments suggest that at this age level, there is a need for coherence; there is a desire to bring self-attributes into harmony with one another, yet in midadolescence, the cognitive abilities to create such a self-portrait have yet to be developed.

An examination of the protocol in Figure 3.2 illustrates the fact that adolescents can identify two types of opposing attributes: those occurring *within* a given role (e.g., quiet and rowdy with friends or talkative and nervous with a romantic interest), and those occurring across relational contexts (e.g., happy with friends and depressed with parents or fun loving with friends but serious in school). We became curious about whether there were more opposing attributes and associated conflict *within* particular role contexts or *across* contexts. Among those social psychologists who have focused on the adult self, it has been argued that consistency within a particular relationship is critical; therefore, perceived violations of this consistency ethic, where one displays opposing attributes within a role, should be particularly discomforting to the individual (Gergen, 1968; Vallacher, 1980). According to these theorists, the adoption of different behaviors in different roles should be less problematic or conflictual for adults, because differences represent appropriate adaptation to different relational contexts rather than inconsistencies.

From a developmental perspective, we did not expect these processes to be in place during adolescence. Adolescents are actively concerned with creating, defining, and differentiating their role-related selves, and thus there is relatively little overlap in the self-attributes associated with different roles. Moreover, opposing attributes across relational contexts become more marked or salient in midadolescence, when teenagers develop the cognitive ability to detect seeming contradictions. Thus, heightened awareness of these opposites leads to a greater focus on contradictions across roles rather than within roles. Perceived conflict caused by opposing attributes should also be greater across roles, particularly with the onset of midadolescence, when teenagers can begin to compare characteristics across such roles but cannot integrate these salient and seemingly contradictory self-attributes. We confirmed these hypotheses. The number of opposites identified at mid- and late adolescence is far greater for attributes identified *across* roles than within each role. The same pattern was obtained for opposites in conflict.

For both across-role opposites, at every age level, females detected significantly more contradictory attributes than did males. These findings were replicated in two other studies in which similar gender differences were obtained (see Harter, Bresnick, et al., 1997). Moreover, in one study in which we asked participants to indicate how upset they were over conflicting attributes, we found that females become more upset over conflicting attributes across early, middle, and late adolescence, whereas males become less upset. Elsewhere (Harter & Monsour, 1992) we have offered a general interpretation of this pattern, drawing upon those frameworks that emphasize the greater importance of relationships for females than males (Chodorow, 1989; Eichenbaum & Orbach, 1983; Gilligan, 1982; Jordan, 1991; J. B. Miller, 1986; L. Rubin, 1985; Ruble, Martin, & Berenbaum, 2006). These theorists posit that the socialization of girls involves far more embeddedness within the family, as well as more concern with connectedness to others. Boys, in contrast, forge a path of independence and autonomy in which the logic of moral and social decisions takes precedence over affective responses to significant others.

In extrapolating from these observations, we have suggested that in an effort to maintain the multiple relationships that girls are developing during adolescence, and to create harmony among these necessarily differentiated roles, opposing attributes within the self become particularly striking as well as problematic. Boys, in contrast, can move more facilely among their different roles and multiple selves to the extent that such roles are logically viewed as more independent of one another. However, these general observations require further refinement, including an empirical examination of precisely which facets of the relational worlds of adolescent females and males are specifically relevant to gender differences in perceiving opposing attributes displayed across different contexts.

Closer examination of the gender effects reveals that it is a subset of female adolescents who report more opposites and greater conflict compared to males. We have determined that adolescent females who endorse a traditionally feminine gender orientation (eschewing masculine traits) may be particularly vulnerable to the experience of opposing attributes and associated conflict. Feminine adolescent females, compared to females who endorse an androgynous orientation, report more conflict, particularly in roles that involve teachers, classmates, and male friends (in contrast to roles involving parents and female friends).

Several hypotheses would be worth pursuing in this regard. Is it that feminine girls report more contradictions in those public contexts where they feel they may be acting inappropriately by violating feminine stereotypes of behavior? Given that femininity as assessed by sex-role inventories is largely defined by caring, sensitivity, and attentiveness to the needs and feelings of others, might female adolescents who adopt this orientation be more preoccupied with relationships, making opposing attributes and accompanying conflict more salient? Moreover, might it be more important for feminine girls to be consistent across relationships, a stance that may be difficult to sustain if significant others in different roles are reinforcing different characteristics? These are all new directions in which attention to gender issues should proceed.

The challenges posed by the need to create different selves are exacerbated for ethnic minority youth in this country, who must bridge "multiple worlds," as C. H. Cooper and her colleagues point out (C. H. Cooper, 2011; C. H. Cooper, Jackson, Azmitia, Lopez, & Dunbar, 1995). Minority youth must move between multiple contexts, some of which may be with members of their own ethnic group, including family and friends, and some of which may be populated by the majority culture, including teachers, classmates, and other peers who may not share the values held by their family of origin. Rather than assume that all ethnic minority youth will react similarly to the need to cope with such multiple worlds, these investigators have highlighted several different patterns of adjustment. Some youth are able to move facilely across the borders of their multiple worlds, in large part because the values of the family, teachers, and peers are relatively similar. Others, for whom there is less congruence in values across contexts, adopt a bicultural stance, adapting to the world of family as well as to that of the larger majority community, presenting different selves in each context. Others find the transition across these psychological borders more difficult, and some find it totally unmanageable. Particularly interesting is the role that certain parents play in helping adolescents navigate these transitions, leading to more successful adaptations for some than others (see Chapter 8, which addresses multicultural issues).

Self-Esteem

A major source of global self-esteem, beginning in mid- to late adolescence, is the internalization of the opinions toward the self that are communicated by significant others (see Cooley, 1902; Harter, 2006a). As observed earlier, adolescents during this period become extremely preoccupied with the opinions and expectations of significant others in different roles. As our prototypical respondent indicates with ambivalence, "I care what they [my parents] think about me"; "I don't really care what they [other kids] think. I mean I don't want to care, that is. But you have to, because what all of the other kids think of you is important"; "I want adults at work to approve of me"; that is, adolescents gaze intently into the social mirror for information about what standards and attributes to internalize, even though they would like to deny it. However, as the number of roles proliferates, leading to feedback from different significant others that are potentially contradictory, adolescents may become confused or distressed about just which characteristics to adopt. We see this in the cameo self-description with regard to scholastic performance, in that the adolescent feels she "should get better grades" to please her parents but confesses that "I'd be mortified in the eyes of my friends if I did too well."

As Higgins (1991) has observed, in their attempt to incorporate the standards and opinions of others, adolescents at this level develop conflicting "self-guides" across different relational contexts as they attempt to meet the incompatible expectations of parents and peers. He reports evidence indicating that such discrepancies have been found to produce confusion, uncertainty, and indecision, consistent with our own findings. Moreover, as M. Rosenberg (1986) notes, the serious efforts at perspective taking that emerge at this stage make one aware that no human being can have direct access to another's mind, leading to inevitable ambiguity about others' attitudes toward the self, producing yet another source of doubt and confusion.

Contradictory messages from different significant others can lead to self-volatility, what M. Rosenberg (1979) has called the "barometric self." Differential approval across roles will also lead to different levels of role-specific self-esteem in each context; what we have termed "relational self-esteem" (Harter, Waters, & Whitesell, 1998). The potential for displaying differing levels of role-specific self-esteem across relational contexts is exacerbated during this period, to the extent that significant others are providing different levels of validation for who one is as a person. For example, as the cameo adolescent explains, "How much you like yourself as a person, I back and forth on that. My self-esteem is higher with kids who know me than with my parents," a pattern that our normative findings document. M. Rosenberg's concept of the barometric self refers to volatility in the overall *level of global* self-esteem. However, because adolescents report that their self-attributes and self-esteem vary across relationships, we have coined the term "the kaleidoscopic self" to capture this greater complexity.

Relational self-esteem with *classmates* is the most predictive of *global* self-esteem (Harter, Waters, & Whitesell, 1998). As the cameo adolescent observes, "What all of the other kids think of you is so important to how much you like yourself as a person." As reported elsewhere (Harter, 1990), the approval of *close friends* is not highly related to self-esteem because there is less variability (scores are uniformly high because, by definition, a close friend is one who likes you). The perceived approval from classmates presumably reflects a more objective index of validation from those whom Mead (1934) referred to as the "generalized other."

Global self-esteem declines between early to midadolescence (Harter, 1990, 2006a). The increased penchant for introspection, given attention to one's negative attributes, is in part responsible. Experimental manipulations reveal that inducing a self-focus on one's weaknesses produces self-criticism and that introspection reduces self-enhancing tendencies (Sedikides & Herbst, 2002; Sedikides, Horton, & Gregg, 2007). Thus, the normative penchant for intense introspection during adolescence will naturally lead to more negative self-perceptions. Second, introspection can contribute to lowered self-esteem by facilitating the contrast between one's *real* and *ideal* self-concepts. This produces a heightened awareness of the *discrepancy* between the real self (I'd like to be friendly and tolerant all of the time; that's the kind of person I *want* to be, and I'm disappointed in myself when I'm not"). Thus, consistent with James's (1892) formulation, the more one's aspiration or ideal outstrips perceptions of one's actual capabilities across different domains, the lower one's self-esteem. The realm of physical appearance becomes increasingly salient in its contribution to global self-esteem.

Perceived attractiveness looms large in importance, yet most cannot meet the punishing societal standards so salient in our culture. The media demands that females be excessively thin, tall, long-legged, and with ample breasts and a pretty face framed in flattering hair, is an ideal that 95% of those in this culture cannot attain (Kilbourne, 1995). As a result, aspirations far outweigh perceived appearance, contributing to lowered self-esteem at this period (see Chapter 5). The cameo adolescent reveals that she wants to look like Beyoncé and knows that she doesn't, and this sets up a painful discrepancy. In reality, she falls far short of the cultural standards for beauty. Similar dynamics are emerging for males who attempt to emulate the cultural criteria of male attractiveness that now include muscularity, ripped abs, and great hair (see Kiang & Harter, 2006).

Adolescent Egocentrism

Perspective taking has been touted as the antidote to egocentrism and clearly perspective-taking skills improve with development (Selman, 1980). However, in his more recent theorizing, Selman (2003) presents an overly positive picture of high school students' perspective-taking abilities. He argues that, starting at age 15, the adolescent develops an appreciation for his/her own perspective in the context of the multiple perspectives of significant others. He proposes that intimate, in depth, relationships with peers allow for shared reflections and the integration of the goals of self and others that serve in collaborative endeavors. These emerging strategies supposedly allow teenagers to let go of their singular, personal pursuits in order to achieve mutually acceptable goals.

Although this is an admirable endpoint for a stage model of perspective taking, identifiable limitations in the cognitive, social, and emotional skills available to those in midadolescence preclude this level of maturity for most. The cameo adolescent expresses these weaknesses, including her admission that she is not yet ready to have a boyfriend. The adolescent is still struggling to define the self, in relation to others (Harter, 2006a). He/she still has difficulty in differentiating the self from others, as well as in clearly identifying separate, personal goals, much less clarifying *realistic* mutual goals. Moreover, the contemporary "new look" with regard to adolescent egocentrism supports such a conclusion.

Elkind's (1967) original formulation identified two egocentric processes that emerge in adolescence: the *personal fable* and the *imaginary audience*. These stemmed from the Piagetian concept of egocentrism that represented the failure to clearly distinguish between one's own perspective and that of others (see also Flavell, 1985). The personal fable includes a sense of *invulnerability* ("I am incapable of being harmed"), *omnipotence* ("I possess special attributes of influence and power"), and personal *uniqueness* ("My thoughts and feelings are unique experiences that others, particularly parents, simply cannot understand"). The last feature is exemplified by our cameo adolescent who exclaims: "They [my parents] don't understand me. What do *they* know about what it's like to be a teenager?" Her very first utterance to the interviewer ("What am I like as a person? You're probably not going to understand") also reflects the conviction that adults can't possibly fathom their uniqueness, be it either the agony or the ecstasy that they experience. The theme of invulnerability is evident in her comment about behaviors that her parents would consider risky: "I would never be the one who was hurt or got in trouble."

The *imaginary audience,* according to Elkind (1967), reflects the assumption that others, particularly peers, are as preoccupied with your behavior and appearance as you are, and that peers are constantly submitting you to scrutiny and critical evaluation. When our prototypical adolescent attempts rather unsuccessfully to act like the hot singer Beyoncé, she concludes that "Everybody, I mean *everybody* else is looking at me like they think I am totally weird!" Elkind suggested a link between these two forms of adolescent egocentrism. The belief that one is of such importance to so many others may lead to the conclusion that one is special or unique.

These two sets of perceptions reflected, for Elkind (1967), cognitive *distortions*, biased or faulty interpretations about the attitudes of significant others toward the self. Because adolescents do not yet have command of their newfound formal operational skills, they make errors in judgment. In the case of the imaginary audience, they fail to differentiate their thoughts from those of others, they overgeneralize, projecting their own concerns onto others. The opposite misrepresentation characterizes the personal fable, in that the adolescent overdifferentiates the self and others, failing to appreciate the commonality of shared experiences with peers or parents.

Although the personal fable and the imaginary audience had great appeal for over four decades, front and center in textbook treatment of adolescence, there have been critiques, focusing on several themes. First, critics have questioned the cognitive-developmental foundations of these processes, grounded in Piaget's stage of formal operations. Logically, as

Lapsley and Murphy (1985) have argued, it makes little sense to have cognitive limitations (i.e., serious distortion) arise from what is presumed to be the final, most mature, stage of cognitive development. There is also little convincing evidence that adolescent egocentrism is empirically linked to formal operational thought processes (see Frankenberger, 2000; Vartanian, 2000).

Second, evidence challenges the ages that Elkind (1967) proposed for the emergence and the subsequent diminution of these processes; namely, that the personal fable and imaginary audience arose in early adolescence and subsided in midadolescence. A more neo-Piagetian analysis suggests that it is not until the beginning of midadolescence that such processes could emerge. Moreover, there is evidence that adolescent egocentrism does not subside, even in late adolescence. P. D. Schwartz, Maynard, and Uzelac (2008) report that it persists well into late adolescence and beyond, citing similar findings by Peterson and Roscoe (1991). Frankenberger (2000) has also reported that the personal fable and imaginary audience extend into early adulthood (ages 19 to 30), with declines eventually occurring in middle and late adulthood.

A third criticism is articulated by Vartanian (2000), who questions the assumption that the personal fable and the imaginary audience reflect distortions, biases, or fundamentally flawed thinking. She argues that given the actual age-related scrutiny by one's peers (e.g., the close attention that peers pay to clothes, hair styles, activities, and interests), these perceptions may well be relatively accurate. That is, peers probably *are* observing and evaluating the self and thus the audience is not necessarily imaginary. She bolsters her point by noting that the instruments to assess these processes do *not* tap flawed or distorted thinking, per se. Vartanian raises a related point that is not a critique of Elkind's (1967) original formulation but rather the failure to appreciate the fact that for Elkind, observing others were not uniformly *critical* of the self but might, in certain circumstances, represent an *admiring* audience. While the cameo adolescent is humiliated by the negative attention she perceives by acting weird, she initially notices the admiration of guys.

A fourth critique of Elkind's (1967) original concept of adolescent egocentrism is that the presumed underlying processes were too narrowly defined as merely cognitive in nature. Others have offered alternative, functional explanations that focus on how the construction of a personal fable, as well as the belief in an imaginary audience, serve more psychosocial needs. Perhaps the most compelling alternative explanations reflecting the "new look" focus on the role of *separation–individuation* processes, considered to be the primary developmental task for adolescents, according to Lapsley (1993). Lapsley and colleagues (Lapsley, 1993; Lapsley & Murphy, 1985; Lapsley & Rice, 1988) put forth a model in which the imaginary audience and personal fable aid the adolescent in his/her separation from parents (see also Blos, 1962). The need to individuate from parents brings with it a related goal, which is to create an identity that will serve one, given the impending transition to adulthood. The challenge of this process is to remain connected while at the same time forging an independent identity (J. P. Allen, 2008; J. P. Allen, Hauser, Bell, & O'Connor, 1994; Grotevant & Cooper, 1986; Harter, 2006a; Hill & Holmbeck, 1986; Marshall, Tilton-Weaver, & Bosdet, 2005; Steinberg, 1990; Vartanian, 2000).

In the service of this challenge, adolescents become increasingly focused on their nonfamilial relationships and begin to fantasize about themselves in various interpersonal scenarios, where the self is at the center. The construction of an imaginary audience allows them to create and maintain feelings of connectedness to peers, helping them to feel important, as they renegotiate relationships with parents. The creation of a personal fable, emphasizing uniqueness, omnipotence, and invulnerability, allows the adolescent to conceive of the self as independent, apart from rigid family ties. The cameo adolescent expresses her version of separateness: "Let's face it, at my age you have to be different with your parents. You have to try things with other *kids* to see what fits who you are." Another part of distancing from parents includes a certain degree of secretiveness, in which the adolescent no longer shares certain experiences, particularly those that he/she feels will not meet with parental approval (see Marshall, Tilton-Weaver, & Bosdet, 2003). The cameo adolescent admits that "I'm still pretty secretive about some things, particularly behavior that my parents wouldn't approve of."

While this analysis is compelling, it should not replace the contribution of cognitive-developmental processes. Granted, the position that the single Piagetian stage of abstract formal operations represents the key to adolescent egocentrism is not tenable. That said, a cognitive-developmental perspective needs to incorporate an appreciation for *neo*-Piagetian thinking. Fischer's more differentiated theory of development (see Fischer, 1980; Fischer & Bidell, 2006), that identifies four substages of abstract thinking, provides a more comprehensive understanding of adolescent development, one that complements the separation–individuation motives that demand the construction of a personal identity.

Fischer (1980) observes that with the advent of any new cognitive capacities comes the difficulty in controlling and applying them effectively. In midadolescence, lack of control is reflected in all-or-none thinking at the level of abstractions (see Dawson et al., 2006). Thus, the adolescent overdifferentiates self and other, concluding that there is little overlap. This supports the construction of a personal fable in which one's own experiences are divorced from those of others, primarily parents. This observation does not preclude the functional analysis provided by Lapsley (1993) and Vartanian (2000). To the contrary, the cognitive-developmental structures during midadolescence actually *support* the psychological separation from parents.

Similarly, these structures aid in the construction of an observing audience, be it real or imagined. The lack of control over abstractions can lead to fusions or confusions in the perspectives of self and other, such that one overgeneralizes in concluding that others and self are equally concerned about or interested in one's behavior. Given this perspective, the issue of whether the audience is imagined or real, and whether the adolescent is distorting or reporting the behavior of peers, becomes semantic. It is most likely somewhere in between; that is, the heightened sensitivity to the opinions of others represents an adaptive combination of fantasy and reality that conspires with the need for connection (Lapsley, 1993; Vartanian, 2000). Should the balance tip *wildly* toward illusions of omnipotence, grandiosity, and personal uniqueness, or toward a highly unrealistic fantasy audience that idealizes one's uniqueness, then this moves into the realm of narcissistic pathology (see Lapsley & Stey, in press).

Normative Liabilities for Self-Development during Middle Adolescence

Many of the normative liabilities of this stage can be inferred from the previous discussion, and therefore will only be briefly reviewed here. The proliferation of multiple selves across multiple roles ushers in the potential for personal attributes to be viewed as contradictory. Moreover, the emergence of new cognitive processes such as abstract mappings forces the adolescent to compare and contrast different attributes, increasing the likelihood that contradictions will be detected. The ability to identify opposites becomes problematic because the individual cannot yet truly integrate such self-representations and thus resolve the contradictions. Therefore, the adolescent is likely to experience conflict, confusion, and distress. Contradictions are particularly likely to occur for attributes across different roles, rather than in the same role. Females are particularly likely to display these negative outcomes. Opposing self-attributes also lead to unstable self-representations, in addition to concern over which characteristics represent one's true self.

At a more general level, Fischer (1980) observes that movement to new skill levels of development, for example, abstractions, typically brings with it lack of *cognitive control*, in part because earlier strategies are rejected but are not yet replaced with new solutions (Dawson et al., 2006). By analogy, attempts to master new *athletic* skills, for example, hitting a tennis ball, also provokes lack of *physical* control. Sometimes one hits the ball out of the court and at other times one hits it into the net. Practice is necessary, both in the development of physical as well as cognitive skills. Kuhn and Franklin (2006) label this process as *learning to manage the mind*. The adolescent must develop a new mental executive that monitors and manages the deployment of cognitive resources, given situational demands. One function of this metacognitive awareness is to "bracket" the personal perspective dictated by one's belief systems, extracting more decontextualized representations about the situation or the self. The development of this process is not immediate or automatic, it requires scaffolding.

As adolescents gaze intently into the social mirror, contradictory messages from different significant others can lead to confusion about just what characteristics to adopt. Differences in approval or validation will also lead to differing levels of self-worth across relational contexts. The contradictory feedback that adolescents may receive from different sources will, therefore, lead to self-esteem volatility across interpersonal contexts.

Contradictory standards and feedback can also contribute to a lowering of global self-esteem between early and midadolescence if one cannot meet the expectations of everyone in each relational context. To the extent that the adolescent does not meet the standards of others, he/she is likely to experience less approval, which in turn will lead to lower global self-esteem. Moreover, the abstract mapping structure, coupled with the increase penchant for *introspection*, may also contribute to lowered self-esteem in that it facilitates the comparison of one's *ideal* and *real* self-concepts. Such a focus can lead to a heightened awareness of the discrepancy between ideal conceptualizations and how one perceives the self to be in reality.

Cognitive-developmental advances during mid-adolescence also represent limitations that can lead to distortions in the interpretation of the opinions of significant others. As observed earlier, with the advent of any new cognitive capacities comes difficulty in controlling and applying them effectively. For example, teenagers have difficulty differentiating their own mental preoccupations from what others are thinking, leading to two forms of adolescent egocentrism (Elkind, 1967). The "imaginary audience" reflects assumptions that others are as preoccupied with their behavior and appearance as they themselves are, an overgeneralization (or failure to differentiate) in that adolescents project their own concerns onto others. The "personal fable" leads to the creation of narratives in which the adolescent asserts that his/her thoughts and feelings are uniquely experienced. This construction reflects an overdifferentiation between self and other.

The liabilities of this period, therefore, are legion with regard to potential conflict and confusion over contradictory attributes and messages, concern over which characteristics define the true self, and distortions in the perception of self versus others, as well as a preoccupation with discrepancies between the real and ideal self-concepts, which can lead to lowered self-worth. Some of these processes would appear to be problematic for particular subgroups of adolescents, for example, females who adopt a feminine gender orientation, as well as ethnic minority youth who are challenged by the need to create selves that bridge "multiple worlds" across one's own ethnic group and those within the mainstream majority culture (Cooper, 2011).

An appreciation for the ramifications of these normative processes is critical in interpreting the unpredictable behaviors, shifting self-evaluations, and mood swings that are observed in many adolescents during this age period. Such displays are less likely to be viewed as intentional or pathological, and more likely to meet with empathy and understanding to the extent that normative cognitive-development changes can be invoked as partly responsible. For many parents, as well as other adults working closely with teenagers, these seemingly inexplicable reactions often lead to perplexity, exasperation, and anger, provoking power struggles and altercations that strain the adolescent–adult relationship. The realization that this is a normative part of development that should not persist forever may provide temporary comfort to adults who feel beleaguered and ineffectual in dealing with adolescents of this age. Indeed, this framework provided gives a more charitable rendering of this period of development.

The Accuracy of Self-Appraisals

Many of the processes identified above will compromise the accuracy of self-appraisals at this stage of development. The obdurate view of one's characteristics and even early adolescence become challenged in mid-adolescence, in part, due to the confusion produced by the differing opinions of the self by others in different roles that can now be detected and compared. Thus, accuracy is threatened. In addition, the adolescent at this stage becomes preoccupied with the discrepancy between his/her *real* self and the *ideal* self. Given abstract constructions of the self, it becomes more difficult to ground the real self in actual behaviors that justify conclusions about domain-specific competencies as well as global self-esteem. Moreover, as implied in the preceding discussion, adolescent egocentrism and the personal fable can clearly lead to distortions in the evaluation of one's self-attributes.

The school system itself may encourage unrealistic self-perceptions, as some have argued about the self-esteem movement. This extravagant initiative to enhance the self-esteem of Californians became a subtext in the playbook of many educators across the country who sought to raise students' self-esteem and perceptions of competence. Despite claims that raising self-esteem would produce higher levels of achievement, critics have vociferously argued that such efforts are misguided, at best, and destructive, at worst (see Chapter 7). Damon (1995) has argued that the attempts to inflate students' perceptions of their competence and self-esteem lead to unrealistic self-views that are detrimental, particularly if students have not earned the right to feel good about themselves (see Cote, 2009, and Covington, 2009, who have decried the "cult of self-esteem" that has gripped schools in this country).

Self-Enhancement and Self-Serving Strategies

Our developmental analysis has focused on several themes, including the needs or motives fueling attempts to protect and enhance the self and, second, the skills to enact the various strategies that have been identified in adulthood. Certain skills are in place (e.g., the ability to engage in downward social comparisons). In addition, as can be observed in Figure 3.2, adolescents place their most *positive* attributes (e.g., understanding, nice, caring, smart) in the small core circle labeled "most important." In contrast, the most *negative* characteristics (e.g., lazy, depressed, nervous, confused) are relegated to the periphery of the self, as the "least important" attributes. This pattern is consistent with Greenwald's (1980) concept of "beneffectance," in which favorable attributes are highlighted, whereas less desirable characteristics are minimized.

However, contradictions between multiple selves may preclude a thoughtful consideration of just which selves should be protected or enhanced. As such, the adolescent may be overwhelmed with the enormity of this challenge. Given that the adolescent at this stage is ill equipped to resolve the various contradictions in his/her self-portrait (Harter, Bresnick, et al., 1997), it is unlikely that he/she will be very effective in employing self-protective or self-enhancing strategies. The cameo adolescent expresses this distress. When she puts on her extroverted face, she asks "Am I just trying to impress the other kids, when really I'm an introvert?" Thus, there would appear to be a motive to engage in self-enhancement, although her efforts are not that successful. Therefore, the need to enhance the self is powerful at this age level, although the skills may not be readily accessible.

Paradoxically, certain features of adolescent egocentrism may come to the rescue. For example, the personal fable involves a sense of personal uniqueness. This perception may aid those at this stage to engage in the "false-uniqueness" strategy identified in adults, where perceptions of being special can serve self-protective and self-enhancing functions. The cameo adolescent entertains the fantasy that she is the most attractive girl in the room and that, as a result, the guys will treat her like she is special. The second form of adolescent egocentrism, the imaginary audience, may also provide self-protective and self-enhancing assistance, but only if such an audience includes *admiring*, not just critical, observers.

These processes will only be self-protective to the extent that they are not employed in excess. That is, some have argued that there is an optimal level of positive illusions about the self that may be adaptive, a bandwidth, as it were (see Baumeister, 1987; Leary & Baumeister, 2000). Moderate biases may enhance and protect the self; however, if one strays beyond this optimal level, into overly inflated or grandiose self-views that are clearly unrealistic, then negative social consequences may ensue. Conversely, self-perceptions that are overly negative may undermine a sense of confidence and motivation that are compromising and can lead to depressive symptoms.

Pathological Self-Processes and Outcomes during Middle Adolescence

In trying to meet cultural standards of appearance, females are much more likely to suffer from pathological processes including depression as well as eventual eating disorders. Our own model of the causes and correlates of self-esteem indicates that an intense preoccupation with attempts to meeting the impossible standards of beauty, coupled with very negative perceptions of one's body image, can lead to extremely low self-esteem, depression, and in the extreme, eating-disordered behaviors. We have documented the links between high discrepancies between the high importance attached to physical appearance and negative perceptions of one's body image, leading to extremely negative reports of self-esteem and depression, among those in mid-adolescence (Harter, 2006a). In a subsequent section on later adolescence, we provide further documentation about how these processes can lead to pathological eating-disordered behaviors.

However, numerous findings (Harter, 2006a; Harter & Marold, 1993; see also Nolen-Hoeksema, 2000; Nolen-Hoeksema & Girus, 1994) reveal that dramatic gender differences in depression emerge in middle adolescence. The discrepancy between impossible ideals for appearance and perceptions of one's own body image contributes to very low self-esteem for some, particularly those who are overweight, that in turn leads to profound depression that can require clinical intervention. In addition, Nolen-Hoeksema and Girus present considerable evidence that females, beginning in this age range, are much more prone to *rumination*. The focus of these thoughts can be turned toward perceived inadequacies such as appearance. They can also lead to a preoccupation with the social dilemmas of the day such as lack of popularity or being overlooked when it comes to affronts such as not being invited to parties. Concerns over perceived lack of romantic appeal may come to the fore at this developmental juncture. The ruminative beacon can shift to other arenas such as academic difficulties that seem insurmountable if they threaten one's future goals for success.

Girls, much more than boys, also engage in corumination with their close girlfriends. This results in both positive and negative consequences. It can cement connectedness with close friends in whom one confides. However, it can also lead to communal wallowing in perceived problems, exacerbating negative thoughts about oneself and one's life, leading to feelings of hopelessness. Thus, the potential for such internalizing symptoms looms large for females during middle adolescence.

Suicidal Manifestations

The incidence of suicide among adolescents has tripled in recent decades, leading to the identification of the determinants of this major mental health threat to our youth (see Alcohol, Drug Abuse, and Mental Health Administration's Report of the Secretary's Task Force on Youth Suicide, 1989; Noam & Borst, 1994; Pfeffer, 1988). In addition to biological precursors, evidence has revealed a constellation of social/psychological correlates that are predictive of suicidal behaviors. These include depressed affect, poor self-concept in particular domains such as physical appearance, real–ideal discrepancies, low self-worth, hopelessness, and lack of social support.

From a developmental perspective, these particular risk factors become increasingly salient, particularly in mid-adolescence and beyond into emerging adulthood. Self-awareness, self-consciousness, introspectiveness, and preoccupation with one's self-image dramatically increase, and self-worth becomes more vulnerable. Depressive symptomatology increases, and certain associated features such as hopelessness take on increasing importance, as they require a level of cognitive functioning that is not completely developed at earlier stages (see Harter, 2006a). As we have argued, movement to a new stage of cognitive development brings with it costs and hazards, particularly when adolescents are not yet capable of controlling these new acquisitions.

M. J. Chandler et al. (2003) have applied the notion that higher stages of development are not invariably adaptive to their own framework on the challenges provoked by justifying self-continuity in the face of developmental change. They provide findings indicating that those adolescents who fail to develop a strategic justification of the continuity of the self are more prone to suicidal behavior. They may be dismissive of earlier developmental solutions but cannot create a new workable rationale, which brings with it a lack of personal connectedness to one's current and future self, leading to a sense of futility. Thus, those who "lose the thread of their own personal persistence are at special risk for suicide" (p. 116).

M. J. Chandler et al. (2003) fall short of providing compelling reasons why some adolescents fail to cope with developmental challenges in the face of the discontinuities (biological, social, cognitive) that are ushered in at this particular period. Our own perspective offers suggestions for why some adolescents are derailed at this developmental juncture, where, as Erikson (1968) has argued, the task is to construct a coherent and continuous sense of one's personal identity. As pointed out in the previous chapter, an important developmental task in childhood is the creation of an autobiographical account, a narrative, that links one's past, present, and future selves. The role of supportive parents in co-creating such a narrative is critical. Those who lack such support are subject to what we have labeled an "impoverished self." Such children are particularly vulnerable during middle adolescence when developmental demands require that they now create a self-identity that is coherent and continuous.

Further support from significant others is also highly relevant during adolescence. As Fischer and colleagues (Fischer, 1980; Fischer & Bidell, 2006) have convincingly and perhaps paradoxically argued, higher levels of cognitive development requires sustaining support and scaffolding. In the absence of such support, adolescents will have difficulty coping with the curve balls that new developmental demands have thrown them. Assertions from benevolent adults that one is still the same person whose past self is meaningfully connected to one's present and future selves can provide understanding that will serve to propel them forward.

The challenge to establishing a coherent identity becomes particularly problematic at adolescence because the analytical beacon turns on the self, which becomes grist for the introspective mill. Adolescents are now confronted with the need to actively wrestle with issues of self-coherence and continuity, but do not have the cognitive abilities to resolve contradictions and perplexities. For some, consternation leads to depression and to suicidal thinking and behaviors.

For males in particular, there is also the potential for the escalation of violence, as observed in the high-profile cases of school shootings carried out by White, male, middle-class adolescents. Intense rejection by peers, at a time when self-consciousness and the need for approval are so salient, sets the stage for violent ideation that can turn into action. The fragile and vacillating self-structures of this particular period can, in the face of humiliation, result in a lack of control, both over cognitions about the self (Harter, 1998) as well as behaviors that these cognitions may drive. Given the lack of cognitive control (Fischer, 1980), the male adolescent during this period may act more impulsively on his thoughts. Recent work on the adolescent brain demonstrates that the frontal cortex is not yet completely developed, leading to gaps in executive functions that, if mature, could serve to curb such impulsive, violent intentions and behaviors (Dahl, 2004).

While the fragmented self is a normative liability of this period of middle adolescence, a history of severe and chronic physical and sexual abuse may lead to pathological outcomes. The effects of abuse on the self-system are legion (see review in Harter, 1998). From a developmental perspective, a history of abuse can lead to dissociative symptoms that serve to further fragment the fragile multiple selves in the process of psychological construction (see also Putnum, 1993; Westen, 1993). As a result, there is no core self at the helm, there is little communication between multiple selves that can become "alters," compromising the ability to construct an integrated self. As a result, there is the risk for dissociative identity disorders that represent severe pathological conditions that may require years of treatment.

True- versus False-Self Behavior

The creation of multiple selves, coupled with the emerging ability to detect potential contradictions between self-attributes displayed in different roles, naturally ushers in concern over which characteristics define the true self, as our studies have demonstrated (Harter, Bresnick, et al., 1997). Participants would spontaneously agonize over which was their true self, the real me. References to this preoccupation are legion in the cameo. When she switches to being cheerful with friends to being nasty with parents, she asks: "Which one is the real me?" When she agonizes over being both an extrovert and an introvert, she laments that "I don't know who I really am!" When she reflects upon the fact that she is both irresponsible with friends but responsible on the job, she queries: "So which am I, responsible or irresponsible? How can the same person be both?" She further reveals that she can be her true self with her close friends, but not with her parents. At the end of her self-reflection, she reveals that she thinks a lot about "who is the real me, and sometimes I try to figure it out when I write in my diary, but I can't resolve it." Thus, from a normative perspective, the adolescent at this age level is ill equipped to solve these dilemmas.

The issue of true- versus false-self behavior also plays out in the school setting, which represents a microcosm of society at large. Gilligan and colleagues (Gilligan, 1993; Gilligan, Lyons, & Hanmer, 1989) have argued that one form of false-self behavior, the inability to voice one's thoughts and feelings, declines, for females, in midadolescence. She attributes this loss of voice to the demands, for pubertal girls approaching impending womanhood, to adhere to the feminine stereotype. Other motives include the realization that the public expression of female opinions is not valued in our patriarchal society, and that to express one's true feelings will alienate others in relationships. Despite these provocative claims, our own research (Harter, Waters, & Whitesell, 1998; Harter, Waters, Whitesell, & Kastelic, 1998) reveals no decline in voice among females during midadolescence. Rather, our findings indicate that there are enormous individual differences in self-reported voice and that this form of false-self behavior is highly related to the amount of support for voice from significant others within each specific relational context (e.g., with parents, teachers, male classmates, female classmates, and close friends). Moreover, females with a self-reported feminine gender orientation report lower levels of voice in the more public context of school than do those with an androgynous orientation.

Narcissism

As has been argued, it is important to distinguish between the typical crises of adolescence, the *normative liabilities*, and the pathological manifestations of disturbed youth. Nowhere is this more evident than with narcissism (Bleiberg, 1994; Lapsley & Stey, in press). These theorists discuss this distinction with the context of a major developmental challenge during midadolescence, namely, the need to begin the process of separating from parents, to individuate, while at the same time remaining appropriately connected. This demand further requires that one develop a sense of personal identity, finding an independent niche in the world. In healthy adolescent development, teenagers maintain basically good relationships with parents, despite the squabbles and normative conflicts (Bleiberg, 1994). They build and strive toward an ideal self as they explore their expanding world. They struggle with the construction of realistic self-images, in their pursuit of future goals, and in the process create their own personal fable. This narrative contains feelings of *omnipotence*, a perception of *uniqueness*, and a sense of *invulnerability*. How, then, do these presumed normative characteristics differ from pathological manifestations of narcissism?

Bleiberg (1994) offers several contrasts, as do Lapsley and Stey (in press). For Bleiberg, feelings of excessive omnipotence among pathological narcissists interfere with their ability to achieve realistic competence goals or to be effective. Omnipotence defensively expands into even more extreme grandiosity that provokes desperate maneuvers to protect very precarious self-esteem and an illusory sense of control. Thus, they fail to construct an ideal self that approximates their talents and opportunities. Unlike healthy adolescents, who maintain a reasonably positive relationship with their parents, the pathological adolescent narcissist devalues or mercilessly denigrates parents. Attempts to protect the self from a sense of personal failures are unsuccessful, provoking shame and humiliation. Separation from family threatens their sense of invulnerability, in part because they have no realistic road map guiding them toward adulthood. This psychological scenario precludes their capacity for love and intimacy.

Lapsley and Stey (in press) argue that narcissistic dysfunction is defined by excessive forms of the omnipotence, uniqueness, and vulnerability expressed in the typical adolescent personal fact that reflects "normal narcissism." They offer several contrasts between normal narcissism and pathological narcissism. These include (1) grandiosity without the exploitation of others; (2) illusions without a sense of entitlement; (3) expressions of invulnerability without shame; (4) a sense of omnipotence that does not risk the isolation from others; (5) the desire for the realistic admiration of others versus the unrealistic demands for attention associated with preening self-preoccupation; and (6) positive affect and warm relationships with others versus derision, lack of empathy, and envy. Thus, these distinctions mark the boundaries between normal and dysfunction narcissism.

Barry and Malkin (2010) provide a complementary analysis of how peer problems contribute to pathological manifestations of narcissism during adolescence. Grandiosity may mask a very fragile sense of self as well as vulnerability. Peer rejection may defensively trigger the presentation of an inflated self-portrait that reflects unrealistic bravado that, in turn, provokes negative social feedback. This further rejection propels a vicious cycle in which the narcissistic individual blames others for his/her misfortune and engages in aggression and other antisocial behaviors in order to restore damaged self-esteem and sense of power. For Barry and Malkin, this not only perpetuates peer problems but also provokes *internalizing* symptoms such as feelings of depression and anxiety that they observe in narcissistic adolescents with a strong sense of entitlement and an excessive need for attention and admiration. With these general characteristics as a backdrop, we turn to Bleiberg's (1994) distinction among three variations of pathological narcissism to emerge in adolescence that have identifiable child-rearing precursors: (1) histrionic exhibitionism, (2) ruthless psychopathy, and (3) self-serving masochism.

Those adolescents displaying *histrionic exhibitionism* organize their sense of self around presumed talents such as their competences, charm, and physical attractiveness that are dramatically on display. They seek an inordinate amount of admiration by others in their dependence upon social feedback to confirm their fragile self-perceptions. They feel exhilarated when they receive confirmation but feel devastated and become spiteful if their bids for attention are ignored. Their excessive dependence can be traced, developmentally, to child-rearing experiences in which their parents rewarded passive dependent, clinging behavior and punished their children if they actively strived for separation or autonomy. Such parents also fostered any signs of uniqueness and exhibitionistic displays of talent.

Ruthless psychopathic adolescents deny pain, helplessness, and vulnerability. They rigidly attempt to maintain an illusion of control. They ruthlessly exploit, intimidate, and manipulate others. In addition, they vigilantly scan their social environment for threats to the self and are preoccupied with the expectation that they will be attacked. These youth harbor deep-seated rage, display disdain for their victims, and are indifferent to human warmth. The child rearing of these adolescents is characterized by early parental rebuffs, neglect, and abuse. Many develop self-numbing strategies in the face of inflicted pain. Bleiberg (1994) also observes that chronically abused children can come to actively evoke abuse from others, as a form of control, in that it is better to provoke abuse rather than to wait passively for it to occur.

Self-serving, masochistic adolescents organize their sense of self around the experienced of being victimized. However, they manifest helplessness, anxiety, and dependence, but maintain and fuel a secret conviction of power, control, and superiority. Their rage toward those who victimized them eventually gives way to depression and self-pity. Many have histories of chronic illness or physical handicaps, leaving them with a warped sense of entitlement, namely, that the world owes them something. Such a history leads them to feel unique, because of their suffering, and thus they are entitled to special treatment.

Late Adolescence: Ages 17 to 19

Normative Self-Representations and Self-Evaluations during Late Adolescence

VERBAL CAMEO

"I'm a pretty conscientious person, particularly when it comes to things like doing my homework. It's important to me because I plan to go to college next year. Eventually I want to go to law school, so developing good study habits and getting top grades are critical. I'm going to be one of those famous defense lawyers that you see on TV! Every now and then I get a little lackadaisical and don't complete an assignment, particularly if our high school has a big football game that I want to go to with my friends. But that's normal, I mean, you can't just be a total 'grind.' You'd be pretty boring if you were. You have to be flexible. I'm also sort of religious, not that I am a saint or anything. Religion provides me with personal guidelines for the kind of adult I'd like to be. I hope to be an ethical person who treats other people fairly; that's why I want to be a lawyer. Sometimes I do something that doesn't feel that ethical. When that happens, I get a little depressed because I don't like myself as a person. But I tell myself that it's natural to make mistakes, so I don't really question the fact that deep down inside, the real me is a moral person, more moral than the average person my age, which makes me kind of special. Basically, I like who I am, so I don't stay depressed for long. Usually, I am pretty upbeat and optimistic. I guess you could say that I'm a moody person. I'm not as popular as a lot of other kids. To be really popular, you have to look a certain way, have the right body image, and wear the right clothes to be accepted. At our school, it's the jocks who are looked up to. I've never been very athletic, but you can't be good at everything, let's face it. Being athletic isn't that high on my own list of what is important, even though it is for a lot of kids in our school. I don't really care what they think anymore, at least I try to convince myself that I don't. I try to believe that what *I* think is what counts. After all, I have to live with myself as a person and to respect that person, which I do now, more than a few years ago. I'm pretty much being the kind of person I want to be, at least here in high school. I'm doing well at things that are important to me like getting good grades. That's what is probably most important to me right now. Having a lot of friends isn't that important to me. I wouldn't say I was unpopular, though. While I am basically an introvert, especially on a date when I get pretty self-conscious, in the right social situation, like watching a ball game with my friends, I can be pretty extroverted. You have to be adaptive around other people. It would be weird to be the same kind of person on a date and with my friends at a football game! For example, when our team has a winning season and goes to the playoffs, everyone in the whole school is proud; what the team does reflects on all of us. On a date, the feelings are much more intimate, just between you and the other person. I sort of have a girlfriend, but we aren't super serious. We talk a lot about our dreams for the future. As much as I try, I don't always understand her perspective. For example, she wants to be a hairstylist, which I don't get, but I do listen. As much as I enjoy my high school friends and activities, I'm looking forward to leaving home and going to college, where I can be more independent, although I'm a little ambivalent. I love my parents, and really want to stay connected to them, plus, what they think about me is still important to how I feel about myself as a person. So leaving home will be bittersweet. But sometimes it's hard to be mature around them, particularly around my mom. I feel a lot more grown-up around my dad; he treats me more like an adult. I like that part of me because it feels more like my true self. My mom wants me to grow up, but another part of her wants me to remain 'her little baby.' I sort of understand her point of view as a mother; it's hard to let go. But she also understands how important it is for me to go to college. I'll probably always be somewhat dependent on my parents. How can you escape it? I'm a little nervous thinking about leaving home but I'm also looking forward to being on my own. Plus, I know my parents will always be there for me."

Self-Awareness, Self-Agency, Self-Coherence, and Self-Continuity

The self-representations that begin to emerge in late adolescence reflect personal beliefs, values, and moral standards that have become the internalized standards of others (Ryan & Deci, 2009). Alternatively they have been directly constructed from their own experiences (see findings by Damon & Hart, 1988). These characteristics are exemplified in the prototypical cameo. The adolescent expresses the personal desire to go to college, which requires good grades and discipline in the form of study habits. In addition, the focus on one's future selves (e.g., not only becoming a lawyer but also an ethical lawyer, as a personal goal), gives the older adolescent some sense of direction, albeit often idealist. Thus, compared to midadolescence, the teenager at this stage demonstrates a greater sense of *agency*.

Noteworthy in this narrative is the absence of an explicit reference to the potential origins of these goals; for example, parental encouragement or expectations that one pursue such a career. The failure to acknowledge the socialization influences that might have led to these choices does not necessarily indicate that significant others, particularly parents, had no impact. In fact, findings (see Steinberg, 1990) reveal that the attitudes of adolescents and their parents are quite congruent when it comes to occupational, political, and religious decisions or convictions. The failure to acknowledge the influence of significant others suggests that older adolescents and young adults have come to "own" various values as personal choices, rather than attribute them to the sources from which they may have been derived (Damon & Hart, 1988; Ryan & Deci, 2009).

In Higgins's (1991) terminology, older adolescents have gone through a process in which they have actively selected among alternative "self-guides" and are no longer merely buffeted about by the expectations of significant others. These self-guides become increasingly internalized and therefore less tied to their social origins. Ryan and Deci (2009) make the distinction between the more mature process of internalization at this stage and the developmentally earlier process of *introjection* in which the adolescent is still aware of the source of his/her attitudes and values, namely, parents and peers. This transition also supports a sense of *self*-agency. Moreover, there is a greater sense of direction as the older adolescent comes to envisage future or "possible" selves (Markus & Nurius, 1986) that function as ideals toward which one aspires. These serve one's sense of self-continuity. Chandler et al. (2003) also describe more mature justifications for self-continuity in the face of change but appealing to the fact that one is responsible for recreating the self, where one is personally at the helm (e.g., "I am steering the ship of my life").

Another feature of the self-portrait of the older adolescent can be contrasted with the period before, in that many potentially contradictory attributes are no longer described as characteristics in opposition to one another. Thus, being conscientious as a student does not appear to conflict with one's lackadaisical attitude toward schoolwork: "That's normal, I mean, you can't just be a total 'grind.' You'd be pretty boring if you were. You have to be flexible." Similarly, one's perception of the self as ethical does not conflict with the acknowledgment that one also has engaged in some unethical behaviors ("It's natural to make mistakes"). Introversion no longer conflicts with extroverted behaviors: "You have to be adaptive around other people. It would be weird to be the same kind of person on a date and with my friends at a football game!"

There are important cognitive acquisitions that allow the older adolescent to overcome some of the liabilities of the previous period, where potentially opposing attributes were viewed as contradictory and a cause of internal conflict. The general cognitive advances during late adolescence involve the construction of *higher-order abstractions* that involve the meaningful intercoordination of single abstractions (see Case, 1985; Fischer, 1980; Fischer & Canfield, 1986). For example, the fact that one is both introverted and extroverted can be integrated through the construction of a higher-order abstraction that defines the self as "adaptive." The observation that one is both depressed and cheerful or optimistic can be integrated under the personal rubric of "moody." Similarly, "flexible" can allow one to coordinate conscientiousness with the tendency to be lackadaisical. The higher-order concept of "ambivalence" integrates the desire to be independent yet still remain connected to parents. Moreover, "bittersweet" reflects a higher-order abstraction combining both excitement over going to college with sadness over leaving one's parents. Such higher-order abstractions provide self-labels that bring meaning and therefore legitimacy to what formerly appeared as troublesome contradictions within the self.

The assertions about these changing cognitive structures to emerge, ideally in late adolescence, allows for a potential reduction in the number of contradictory attributes identified in one's self-portrait, as well as diminished conflict, have found support in our own findings. For example, in one study (Harter & Monsour, 1992) in which adolescents described their attributes in four roles—with parents, friends, romantic others, and as a student—we found a dramatic rise in the number of opposites and conflicts identified at midadolescence, followed by a decline among older adolescents. Evidence that older adolescents become better able to consolidate or integrate seeming contradictions within the self-theory come from the comments they made in response to a follow-up interview. As one older adolescent explained, "Sometimes I am really happy, and sometimes I get depressed. I'm just a moody person." The cameo adolescent also acknowledges that his optimism does not conflict with his depression because it signifies that he is "moody." Extraversion and introversion are no longer viewed as contradictory but rather are integrated into a higher-order abstraction of being "adaptive." The ability to construct higher-order abstractions that resolve the many contradictions of the previous period allows for a much more integrated and *coherent* self-portrait.

Moreover, another conscious strategy employed by older adolescents is to *normalize* potentially contradictory attributes in their personality. The tendency to normalize or find value in seeming inconsistency can be observed in the comments of older adolescents in our research study (Harter & Monsour, 1992). As one participant asserted, "It wouldn't be normal to act the same way with everyone. You act one way with your friends and a different way with your parents. That's the way it should be." Others made similar comments; for example: "It's good to be able to be different with different people in your life. You'd be pretty strange and also pretty boring if you weren't. You can be outgoing with friends and then shy on a date because you are just different with different people; you can't always be the same person and probably shouldn't be." Yet another indicated that "There are situations where you are a good listener and others where you are talkative. It's good to be both." Thus, older adolescents come to the conclusion that it is desirable to be different across relational contexts, and in so doing, they would appear to be cultivating the stance that social psychologists (see Gergen, 1968; Mischel, 1973; Vallacher, 1980) identify as more the rule than the exception for adults. Self-awareness is reflected in the older adolescents' recognition of these cognitive strategies and their effectiveness.

Despite these seemingly personal convictions, neo-Piagetians (e.g., Case, 1985: Fischer, 1980; Fischer & Bidell, 2006) and contemporary cognitive developmentalists (e.g., Kuhn and Franklin, 2006) observe that developmental acquisitions at these higher levels typically require greater scaffolding by the social environment in the form of support, experiences, instruction, and so on in order for individuals to function at their optimal level. If these new skills are fostered, they will help the adolescent to integrate opposing attributes in a manner that does not produce conflict or distress. Thus, efforts to assist the adolescent in realizing that it is normal to display seemingly contradictory traits, and perhaps quite appropriate, may alleviate perceptions of conflict. Moreover, helping teenagers to provide higher-order labels that integrate opposing attributes (e.g., flexible, adaptive, moody, inconsistent) may avert some of the distress that was salient during middle adolescence.

These suggestions complement the more general observations of Fischer (1980), Case (1985), and Kuhn and Franklin (2006), who note that these cognitive solutions will not necessarily emerge automatically with development. Nor will the potential benefits of movement to late adolescence necessarily accrue. Development may be delayed or even arrested if there is not sufficient support for the transition to higher levels of conceptualization. Karcher and Fischer (2004) present compelling evidence for the role of support or scaffolding at higher levels of cognitive development (see also Fischer & Bidell, 2006). Their findings clearly reveal the role of adult support, documenting that the advantage of high versus low support conditions widens with age during late adolescence. Examples of high support include priming for the complexity of thought, encouraging the adolescent to give additional examples of concepts, and stimulating their evaluation of the intercoordination and logic of his/her responses.

Fischer (see Fischer, 1980; Fischer & Bidell, 2006) has long made the distinction between *functional* and *optimal* levels of cognitive development. Functional levels, unaided by support or scaffolding, will result in lower levels of demonstrable cognitive skills. Optimal, higher levels of manifest cognitive complexity of thought are displayed under conditions of high support. These distinctions become more apparent at the higher levels of abstract thinking.

As Kuhn and Franklin (2006) have argued, many adults fail to show any development beyond the level of the typical young adolescent (as perhaps manifest by the mentality of "reality TV," which seems to increasingly dominate the entertainment menu, apparently satisfying the appetites of both young teens and many adults, alike). Kuhn and Franklin conclude that the "good enough" intellectual environment, sufficient to support the basic cognitive transitions during childhood development, appears not to be good enough to promote higher cognitive capacities that could emerge and develop during adolescence.

This instructive lesson was recently driven home to me in the natural laboratory of the supermarket. I was standing in the checkout line and overheard a conversation between a young adolescent girl and her mother, standing close behind me. The girl was lamenting the fact that she had to type up a one-page report, using a 12-point font, about her "service learning project." She was agonizing about how she couldn't *possibly* come up with an entire page, "no way!" In addition, she complained that she did not have the requisite computer skills to complete this assignment. Rather than ask her daughter to describe the project, help her daughter to generate some ideas, or support her daughter's thinking the mother sternly, in a very authoritarian tone, asserted "Well you had better do it!" In what she felt was a charitable gesture, the mother added "I'll type it up for you." Not only did this parent fail to support her daughter's intellectual development, given this obvious opportunity, but she undermined the daughter's ability to master the needed computer skills that are essential in this day and age, for middle and high school students.

EGOCENTRISM

The antithesis of egocentrism is perspective taking, a theme that has been traced through the stages that define childhood and adolescence. Although Selman's (2003) developmental perspective-taking formulation has limitations for midadolescence, it does speak to advances for the older teenager. He suggests that older high school students should, in close relationships, be able to compare and contrast their own perspective to that of another, appreciating multiple viewpoints. Many are more attuned to the need to take the perspective of significant others. The cameo adolescent attempts to listen to his girlfriend although he doesn't completely understand her perspective. He seems to comprehend that his mother will have a hard time letting him go although she knows how important it is to him to go to college. These perspective-taking skills, however, depend upon the quality of the relationship and the extent to which members of the dyad appropriately share their perspectives and respect the viewpoint of the other (Selman,

2003). These skills do not automatically emerge at late adolescence, where there is considerable variability in the ability to understand the perspective of others.

Finally, specific forms of adolescent egocentrism, namely, the construction of a personal fable and an imaginary (peer) audience (Elkind, 1967), formerly thought to emerge in early adolescence and abate in late adolescence, have been found to continue into the high school years and emerging adulthood (see Peterson & Roscoe, 1991; P. D. Schwartz et al., 2008). Thus, the narratives that are observed will still contain some elements of omnipotence or grandiosity, uniqueness, and invulnerability. The cameo adolescent is going to be a famous defense lawyer, and also considers himself to be more moral than most. Moreover, there is still a concern with what others think of the self, although the cameo adolescent admits that he tries to convince himself that he doesn't really care about their opinions.

THE ACCURACY OF SELF-APPRAISALS

Certain higher-order cognitive skills allow the adolescent to become more realistic in evaluating the self and to bring evidence to bear on self-appraisals. For example, the ability to resolve contradictions about the self, by integrating what were contradictions during midadolescence, leads to greater realism (Fischer, 1980; Harter, 2006a; Harter & Monsour, 1992). For example, the cameo adolescent justifies the observation that he is both an introvert, on a date where he is self-conscious, but an extrovert with friends at a football game. The older adolescent is also better able to appreciate weaknesses as well as strengths, presenting a more balanced self-portrait. In the cameo self-description our older teenager acknowledges that he is not that athletic nor terribly popular. This would appear to be offset by the fact that he gets top grades and is a moral person, both of which are critical to his future occupational aspirations. That said, his goal of being a famous defense attorney and his supposition that lawyers are ethical people concerned with fairness may require a bit more reality testing as he moves toward emerging adulthood.

GLOBAL SELF-ESTEEM

The recognition of one's weaknesses need not take its toll on global self-esteem. As James (1892) argued, and our research has demonstrated (Harter, 2006a), high self-esteem is dependent upon being able to tout one's strengths as important, simultaneously discounting the importance of domains in which one is not successful. The cameo older adolescent admits that he is not athletic, but quickly adds that "Being athletic isn't that high on my list of what is important."

Evidence (reviewed in Harter, 1990) reveals that self-esteem improves as one moves into late adolescence (see also Harter & Whitesell, 2003). Several interpretations have been offered. As just noted, the older adolescent becomes more adept at discounting the importance of success in domains where he does not feel adequate. This, in turn, may reduce the discrepancy between one's ideal and real self-image. In late adolescence there are more opportunities to select performance domains in which one does have demonstrated competence, as one find's one's niche. Gains in autonomy and greater freedom of choice (e.g., elective courses at school, extracurricular activities) also contribute. Greater freedom may also provide the older adolescent with more opportunity to select those support groups that will provide the positive regard necessary to promote or enhance self-esteem. Increased perspective-taking skills may also lead older teenagers to behave in more socially acceptable ways that enhance the evaluation of the self by others.

In addition, there is movement toward the establishment of more true or optimal self-esteem that is less contingent upon the need to meet the external demands of significant others (see J. Crocker, 2006a, 2006b; Deci & Ryan, 2000; Ryan & Brown, 2006; Ryan & Deci, 2000). The cameo older adolescent likes who he is as a person, more than a few years ago, and is less directly dependent upon the opinions of others: "I try to believe that what *I* think is what counts. After all, I have to live with myself as a person and to respect that person."

Although it has been common in treatments of adolescent development to suggest that the influence of peers increases, whereas the impact of parental opinion declines, findings do not support the latter contention. As our cameo subject indicates, "What they [my parents] think about me is still important to how I feel about myself as a person." Our own findings reveal that the correlation between classmate approval and global self-esteem does increase between childhood and adolescence; however, the correlation between parental approval and global self-esteem, which is high in childhood, does not decline during adolescence (Harter, 1990). The latter correlation does decline, however, during the college years among students who are away from home, as will be discussed in the description of emerging adulthood, in the following chapter.

SELF-ENHANCEMENT STRATEGIES AND SELF-SERVING BIASES

Clearly, in late adolescence, cognitive advances in the form of higher-order abstractions and efforts to *normalize* potential contradictions serve to reduce distressing conflict and negative self-appraisals. In addition, efforts to discount lack of success in domains that are deemed unimportant reflects another strategic attempt to maintain high self-esteem. In discounting the importance of athletic competence and popularity, the older cameo adolescent displays a strategy that Greenwald (1980) labeled as "beneffectance." Other strategies, identified in the adult literature, become even more available to the older adolescent who is no longer overwhelmed with the contradictions and confusion that were experienced in midadolescence. For example, the "better than average effect" can be observed in the cameo adolescent's declaration that "the real me is a moral person, more moral than the average person my age" and requires downward social comparison. Thus, the majority of self-protective and self-enhancing strategies exhibited by adults are in the repertoire of older adolescents and can continue into adulthood.

Normative Liabilities for Self-Development during Late Adolescence

It should be noted that although there are definite psychological gains during late adolescence, the world of the older teenager is still rather limited and primarily defined by the parochial contexts of school and home. Doing homework, getting good grades, going to high school events, taking pride in going to the playoffs, worrying about being self-conscious on a date, enjoying high school friends and activities, experiencing concerns, who and what one is around parents (e.g., feeling more mature with one parent than the other), pretty much define the psychological landscape. As in the cameo description, there has not yet been any real thoughtful exploration of potential occupational roles, just an ideal, to be a lawyer, about which he has little knowledge. Religious and moral values are expressed, but not questioned, and thus serious identity exploration has not yet begun. We will see how the world stage broadens for emerging adults who face an ever-widening set of personal challenges, the need to make life choices, and to take the perspective of a much wider and more diverse audience (Arnett, 2000).

A critical cognitive advance can be observed in the ability to construct higher-order abstractions that involve the meaningful integration of single abstractions that represent potential contradictions in the self-portrait (e.g., depressed and cheerful do not conflict because they are both part of being moody). Moreover, older adolescents are more likely to normalize potential contradictions, asserting that it is desirable to be different across relational contexts. However, conflict between role-related attributes does not totally abate in later adolescence. Conflict will be more likely to occur if the new skills that allow for an integration of seeming contradictions are not fostered by the socializing environment. Furthermore, opposing attributes across particular role combinations, notably self with mother versus self with father, continue to be problematic in late adolescence, especially for girls (Harter, Bresnick, et al., 1997). To the extent that one's mother and father elicit or reinforce opposing attributes, cognitive solutions for integrating seeming contradictions would appear to be more difficult to invoke.

Pathological Self-Processes and Outcomes during Late Adolescence

Many of the pathological processes that have been described in the earlier periods of adolescence can be observed, albeit in a somewhat different form, due to developmental advances. Those in late adolescence are *less* likely to report the vacillations that are observed during middle adolescence, making their negativity more stable, because they have become entrenched in these views as a core belief system.

True- versus False-Self Behavior

The issue of authenticity remains on the personal radar screen of older adolescents, although they are less likely to agonize about it, nor are they as preoccupied with whether they or their parents are phony or hypocritical. That said, given cognitive and linguistic advances, their vocabulary also expands to include such terms as "charlatan," "chameleon," "imposter," "evasive," and "two-faced." Manifestations primarily refer to verbal expression in which one's true beliefs and attitudes are suppressed and in their place, false opinions are endorsed. However, as a strategy to gain or maintain approval, from both peers and parents, these strategies ultimately backfire. Our findings reveal that those who display higher selves of false-self behavior within a given relational context (suppressing their voice) report lower levels of approval from relevant others (Harter, Waters, Whitesell, & Kastelic, 1998). Our cameo adolescent expresses some awareness of issues involving authenticity. He likes parts of himself that are more like his true self, consistent with our research revealing that greater true-self behavior is related to high self-esteem (see also Ryan & Brown, 2006). Those admitting to false-self behavior devalue their worth as a person, raising another causal question for further research. Do adolescents not like themselves as a person because they do not voice their true opinions, or do they not express themselves because they devalue the self?

Risk Factors for Females and Males

Preoccupation with impossible cultural standards of attractiveness looms even larger as the older adolescent anticipates emerging adulthood, making it even more critical to attain these standards in order to be socially acceptable and successful in the new adult world order. For females, failure to meet these standards can lead to more pathological processes that may include eating disorders. In one of our studies (Kiang & Harter, 2006), it was observed that those females who endorsed the link between meeting cultural standards of attractiveness and outcomes such as popularity and love reported markedly lower self-esteem, depression, and eating-disordered symptoms.

Male adolescents are clearly at continued risk for violence, particularly the type of violence that emanates from peer rejection and humiliation. Chronic rejection and humiliation are likely culprits for violent ideation (Harter, 2006a) and for violent action, as in the case of the school shooters. Unlike the impulsive acts of the school shooters in middle adolescence, the violent killings of older teenagers (e.g., Eric Harris and Dylan Kleibold from Columbine), are likely to be far more *planful*. For over a year, they had plotted their revenge, some of which was revealed in Harris's written manifesto. As noted in the description of middle adolescence, in examining the media accounts of the 11 high-profile school shooting cases, it would appear that the dynamics may be different from what we normally consider to be delinquent, conduct-disordered behavior that typically comes to the attention of teachers, school officials, school psychologists, peers, and parents. In most of these cases, there had been few warning signs with regard to the male shooters having been in trouble with the law, having been identified as troublemakers in the school, having clinical diagnoses, or being placed in special classes for students with a penchant for acting out. In one normative study that we conducted on violent ideation (Harter & McCarley, 2004), we found that 33% of middle school students reporting to us that they had serious thoughts of harming others who humiliated them went undetected by their classroom teachers who were given parallel rating forms. This issue may become more serious among older teenagers who are likely to be more planful, secretive, and resourceful.

Thus, there is a need to discriminate the form of violence that has recently emerged from the high-profile killings from acts that have been committed by known delinquents and conduct-disordered youth who have come to the attention of school and mental health professionals. This latter group commits different types of crimes, for example, drive-by shootings to target one individual versus the random shooting of as many classmates as possible. The dynamics would appear to be different and deserve our attention.

Risks Associated with Multiple Selves and Abuse

The construction of multiple selves, while a normative process, can also have pathological implications. It was pointed out in the section on middle adolescence that the effects of abuse can lead to dissociative symptoms that prevent one's multiple selves from being integrated. In the severest cases, this can lead to dissociative identity disorder (what used to be termed multiple personality disorder). Abuse has also been found to impact the valence (positive or negative) of those attributes judged to be one's core self (vs. more peripheral attributes). Normatively, we have asked older adolescents to rate their attributes across multiple relational contexts with regard to whether they are central core characteristics or more peripheral, less important attributes that define the self. Adolescents will define their most important attributes as *positive* and assign their more negative characteristics to the periphery of the self; namely, they are reported to be less important attributes (Harter & Monsour, 1992). This self-protective strategy has been labeled "beneffectance" by Greenwald (1980), namely, seeing one's positive attributes as central to the self and one's negative attributes as more peripheral.

Colleagues Fischer and Ayoub (1994) employed our multiple-selves procedure with an inpatient sample of seriously abused older adolescent girls and found just the opposite pattern. Compared to a normative sample, the abused patients identified *negative* attributes as their core self, labeling the few positive characteristics they could identify as peripheral. Herein, we can detect another deleterious effect of abuse on self-processes in later adolescence, leading to potential pathological outcomes requiring clinical interventions that can hopefully restore a more positive balance of self perceptions.

Narcissism

Characteristics of both normative and pathological narcissism emerge as salient during the previous period of midadolescence (Bleiberg, 1994; Lapsley & Stey, in press) where a major developmental challenge is to begin, in earnest, to separate from the family, to individuate. This theme can be activated or exacerbated for those in late adolescence when the end of high school looms large and separation issues come to the fore if one is college bound or moving out of the home given job or new age-appropriate relationship demands (e.g., marriage). Leaving home can trigger excessive separation anxiety that, for those whose upbringing has put them on a path to maladaptive narcissism, can provoke rage at parents who are perceived as the perpetrators.

Those who fit Bleiberg's (1994) description of the *histrionic exhibitionism* type of narcissism may become especially troubled over separation issues provoked by impending adulthood. Their excessive dependency upon parents and their inordinate need for admiration, which may not be forthcoming in their new environment, will not bode well at this developmental juncture. A healthier reaction to these new demands (Bleiberg, 1994; Lapsley & Stey, in press) can be observed in our prototypical older adolescent. He admits to being "ambivalent" about going off to college and that leaving home will be "bittersweet." While he is looking forward to leaving home and going to college, "I'm a little nervous," and that "I'll probably always be somewhat dependent upon my parents," reassuring himself that "my parents will always be there for me."

Healthy reactions notwithstanding, Twenge, Konrath, Foster, Campbell, and Bushman (2008) review convincing evidence that narcissism has been on the rise over the past few decades. Other findings reveal that contemporary youth in this country display narcissistic overconfidence. W. K. Campbell, Goodie, and Foster (2004) report findings indicating that today's students have markedly higher and more unrealistic educational expectations and aspirations for success. By way of illustration, slightly more than half of recent high school students predicted that they would earn graduate or professional degrees, even though only 9% of 25- to 35-year-old high school graduates actually obtain such credentials. Similar findings have been reported by Ruthig, Haynes, Perry, and Chipperfield (2007). (This does not bode well for our cameo adolescent who has aspirations, with his law degree in hand, to become a famous criminal defense attorney!)

Chapter 4

Self-Processes during
Emerging Adulthood

Arnett (2000, 2007, 2010) introduced the term "emerging adulthood," bringing credibility to a new and distinct transitional period of development. This stage is applicable for those between ages 18, when most youth in the United States graduate from high school, and 25, before they officially enter true adulthood as we know it. Individuals in this age range are supposedly no longer as dependent upon the preceding generation of adults (typically parents) as they were during childhood and adolescence. However, they have not yet taken on the more enduring responsibilities of adulthood (e.g., career, financial independence, marriage, and parenting). A wall plaque I recently discovered sums it up succinctly: "She isn't where she has been, she isn't where she is going, but she is on her way." Scholars in this subfield have now articulated the criteria that define this developmental period and its psychological boundaries.

Normative Self-Representations
and Self-Evaluations during Emerging Adulthood

VERBAL CAMEO

"It's been challenging to get a life after high school where we knew what we had to do, where there were teachers and coaches and counselors to guide us, and where we had a lot of support from friends who we saw every day. I've put off some major life decisions. I was trying to figure out whether to go to college or some type of trade school or whether I should just get a job to support myself. I finally decided to try a 2-year community college, to start with. It's a lot harder than high school. I'm doing OK and have made some new friends but they're not like my old friends who I don't see much any more. Many have gone their separate ways. I really miss the social life that I had in high school. In fact, to tell the truth, I'm often kind of lonely. I stayed with my parents for a while. I was working part-time to save some money for what to do next. I am trying to decide whether to go to a 4-year college after I finish at the community college. I'm still not sure what I want to major in; I've already changed my mind several times. As a result, I don't yet have a clear occupation in mind. There are so many possibilities! It's exciting but also a little scary because I know that someday soon I'll be entirely on my own so I have to start making my own decisions about a job or career, but what if I fail? I could go into my father's business, he'd like that. But I'm not really cut out for his line of work. My brother decided to work for my father but he has more aptitude for business than I do. Plus, I just don't want that kind of pressure or responsibility right now. I'm sure I'll settle on something in a couple of years, I just need more time to explore my options. (I guess you could say that I don't know what I want to be when I grow up!) My fantasy is to become rich, have an extravagant home, and famous friends! Dream on, right? I finally moved out of my parents' house and got an apartment with a new friend from the community college where I am trying to fit in. I have learned to pay a lot more attention to how I look and dress now compared to when I was in high school; you have to at my age. I feel better about myself as a person when I go along with today's standards of appearance, even though it's tough to meet them. It can be very discouraging. But you need to measure up otherwise you won't be accepted by peers and then you will get down on yourself and become depressed. It was great that my parents allowed me to stay at home until I got my feet on the ground. But it was also confining, if you know what I mean. I felt stifled, I couldn't really be myself. They felt that if I lived under their roof they could still set some rules, like curfews and demands that I do chores around the house and in the yard, and contribute to meals. They also wanted me to go to church with them, but I no longer can accept their religious values; I need to develop my own. Living at home also cramped my style when it came to dating. I'm not serious about anyone in particular right now. I'm not ready to get married any time soon. I don't really have a clear idea right now of what type of person I would want to marry. Then I wonder if it's OK to live with someone if you are not married. I'll try to figure that out once I get the rest of my life more settled. I didn't realize how many decisions there were to make after high school! Becoming an adult is challenging, but I'll figure it out when I'm a little older. I've become closer to my two older siblings, my brother and sister, well, more close to one than the other. They are a little more mature than I am and they can give me good advice. They help me keep my head on straight and keep me from making risky decisions, without thinking things through, things like unprotected sex or drugs or drinking too much if I have to drive. They remind me that I have to be financially responsible, particularly since I am no longer primarily dependent on my parents. My brother and sister have taught me about credit card debt and credit scores, something I never before really considered seriously. I'd rather turn to them, at this point, than to my parents who tend to preach a little bit too much. Don't get me wrong, I love my parents and they have been generous and it was hard to move out and separate myself from them. I hope I can still be close to them as I become an adult. But our relationship is different now, particularly since I am no longer that financially dependent on my parents, well still some. So it's time to move on and get a life of my own."

Research reveals that most 18- to 25-year-olds do not consider themselves to be adults (Arnett, 1997). They realize that they are no longer adolescents, but have yet to embrace adult roles and responsibilities. Studies have examined how those in this age group define adulthood (see Arnett, 1997, 2000, 2001, 2010; L. J. Nelson & Barry, 2005). There is agreement among emerging adults that, unlike previous eras, today they no longer consider external criteria such as marriage, completion of their education, or career attainment to be critical markers of adulthood. Rather, youth in the United States today use more internal and individualistic characteristics to define adulthood. These include (1) taking personal responsibility for their actions, (2) making their own independent decisions, and (3) obtaining financial independence from their parents.

In the three cameos describing childhood and the three periods of adolescence, the gender of the speaker was apparent and therefore, the discussion touched on how the cameo might be different for the other gender. In contrast, the cameo for emerging adulthood could apply to males or females. Fivush and Buckner (2003) have presented evidence that the autobiographical narratives of college students describe desired goals, plans for the future, and social relationships; however, gender differences are much less marked among this population. They conclude that college students, who are living away from home for the first time, are surrounded by others of a similar age, with similar goals. They face the fundamental challenge of creating their self-identity. As Erikson (1959, 1968) observed, this period is rife with doubts about whom one is, about one's belief systems, and about how one should live one's life. Fivush and Buckner have argued that as young adults in college begin to think about long-term goals, gender may not be very relevant. Gender, they suggest, may be "backgrounded." Academic achievement, concerns about a future career, and professional aspirations are paramount for both males and females and therefore come to the forefront. In the same vein, Shulman, Feldman, Blatt, Cohen, and Mahler (2005) speculate that emerging males and females today face similar dilemmas and developmental tasks.

Fivush and Buckner (2003) have urged that more research attention be devoted to *non-college* populations, in which different life goals, such as marriage and family, may be salient at earlier ages. Others (e.g., Arnett, 2000; L. J. Nelson & Barry, 2005; Shulman et al., 2005) make similar arguments. Shulman et al. suggest that economic pressures may expose noncollege youth to different challenges leading to alternative life choices. More recently, Arnett and Tanner (2011) have addressed the issue of social class, arguing that the defining features of emerging adulthood apply primarily to those middle class youth who attend a college or university. Such individuals typically have enough financial support from parents, allowing them the personal freedom and leisure to explore occupational options and potential relationships. Arnett and Tanner point out that the majority of those in the lower social class do not have the luxury of such exploration but instead must "struggle to enter an uncompromising and unwelcome labor market." They are much less likely to experience these years as an optimistic *age of* possibilities. Arnett and Tanner urge that those in the field direct greater attention to what they term the "forgotten half" of working class young people who do not attend a college or university after high school.

It should also be noted that from a research perspective, college students have been, for many years, largely "convenience" samples and thought to represent proxies for adults. However, with Arnett's (2000, 2007, 2010) focus on a new, transitional stage of "emerging adulthood," one needs to question whether the large body of past psychological research that has been conducted with college students is truly representative of more mature individuals who have supposedly met the requisite criteria for adulthood.

In addition to the three primary criteria for adulthood identified above (personal responsibility, independent decision making, and financial independence), there are specific developmental tasks and related issues during the period of emerging adulthood. These center on experimentation in several domains. For example, those in this period experiment with various vocational and occupational possibilities, the development of new friendships, intimate (but typically nonmarital) relationships, the renegotiation of the parent–child bond, and belief systems (e.g., religious, moral, and political identifications).

Tanner (2006) introduced the term "recentering" to describe a three-stage process that captures the transition from adolescence (Stage 1) into emerging adulthood (Stage 2), followed by an exit from this transitional period, entering into young adulthood (Stage 3). Emerging adulthood, the focus of this chapter, is marked by a recentering process in which individuals make serial and therefore *temporary* role commitments that serve the purpose of exploring potential identities in the domains mentioned above. During this active phase of identity exploration, the emerging adult typically attempts to match his/her changing sense of self with socially sanctioned adult roles (see also Arnett, Kloep, Hendry, & Tanner, 2011).

Moreover, in exploring these issues, emerging adults engage in considerable *risk taking* as they navigate these treacherous psychological waters (Arnett, 2000, 2010; Arnett et al., 2011). L. J. Nelson & Barry, 2005; Shulman et al., 2005). Risky behaviors include unprotected sex, substance abuse, driving at high speeds while intoxicated, and binge drinking. While risk taking has been, in past developmental analyses, primarily associated with adolescence, the authors above have observed that it is even more prevalent in emerging adulthood as young people typically have less adult supervision or monitoring. In addition, L. J. Nelson and Barry point out that the cessation of risk-taking behaviors is not, in the eyes of emerging adults, a necessary criterion for admission into adulthood. Finally, as is discussed in the section below on normative liabilities, those researching brain development have now established that the frontal lobes, responsible for planning, sound judgment, and the curtailment of risk taking, are not fully developed until age 25 (see Dahl, 2004). In the cameo description, our emerging adult prototype realizes that he/she makes risky decisions and turns to siblings for guidance and advice, to help curtail such behaviors.

The period of emerging adulthood also makes one vulnerable to *depression*. Research (see Arnett, 2000; L. J. Nelson & Barry, 2005) points to four possible sources of such psychological dejection that represent normative manifestations during emerging adulthood. *Separation* issues represent one source of vulnerability to depression, as emerging adults attempt to establish some degree of autonomy from parents. What makes this period particularly conflictual is that the urge to become autonomous is juxtaposed to the desire to remain connected. In the cameo, there is the observation that "It was hard to move out and separate myself from them [my parents]. I hope I can still be close to them as I become an adult."

There is also the potential for depression as emerging adults seriously explore the realm of dating and intimate relationships, prior to eventual commitments, that may involve cohabitation and eventually the consideration of marriage. The formation of romantic relationships, while exciting, can also come to cause ambivalence and indecision. Breakups can be traumatic, leading to depression. Feelings of loneliness can also arise with the scattering of high school friends, who provided support and companionship. Added to this is the challenge of making new friends and forming new support systems. The exploration of educational and occupational realms also brings normative challenges that will understandably provoke concerns about one's *competence*. Fears of failure are inevitable, and can contribute to depression, particularly if one treads a path that requires the development of new, and therefore unpracticed, skills. As the cameo emerging adult questions, "What if I fail?"

Unlike previous periods of development, there is a heightened *awareness*, sometimes painful, of the challenges associated with growing up (see Arnett, 2010; L. J. Nelson & Barry, 2005; Shulman et al., 2005). No longer is the question of "What do I want to be when I grow up?" the earlier frivolous query of children, where answers range from outlandishly unrealistic to endearing. In emerging adulthood it represents a nagging question where answers are imperative and require immediate attention. Our cameo prototype is well aware of the dilemma in discussing occupational decisions: "I'm sure I'll settle on something in a couple of years, I just need more time to explore my options. I guess you could say that I don't know what I want to be when I grow up!"

The task at this stage is not only to explore and experiment with possible life choices in the realms of occupational and educational options, social and romantic decisions, and belief systems (e.g., moral, religious, political). One must also *integrate* the outcomes of such explorations in a manner that brings meaning and coherence to one's identity. During the process of reappraising previous life patterns and experimenting with new possibilities for personal growth, the emerging adult becomes aware of the social and historical context of his/her life (Shulman et al., 2005). These authors observe that the ability to become *aware* of one's aspirations, qualities of character, and the role of one's torments, as well as an appreciation for fulfillments, will facilitate the individual's capacity to deal with the demanding developmental tasks that require attention (see also Levinson, 1978). Awareness heightens the sense of *uncertainty*, which is decidedly different from the confusion that freezes midadolescents in their psychological tracks. The emerging adult in our cameo is well aware of the decisions that must be made, although he/she is awed by the many possibilities and expresses uncertainty about just how to proceed. An awareness of the need to integrate one's "possible selves" (Markus & Nurius, 1986) turns the psychological spotlight on this daunting developmental task.

What do we know about the relevant cognitive-developmental advances and/or limitations that characterize emerging adulthood? Fischer (1980) acknowledges that the ability to truly integrate one's different identities across these realms requires the development of what he has labeled "an abstract system of systems." More specifically, the individual must construct a conceptual self-system that cognitively combines the previous single and higher-order abstractions that became available during the substages of adolescence. This is a lengthy process that requires extensive life experiences, considerable reflection, the support of more mature individuals, and the cooperation of neurological development, in order to reach such a teleological end state. Many adults never achieve this cognitive-developmental nirvana.

Discordant compromises may well be required, as one is forced to make realistic decisions given pragmatic life constraints that may not reflect one's idealized goals and aspirations. Thus, many life dreams must necessarily be abandoned or substantially revised (see also Levinson, 1978). Arnett (2010) observes that the age period of 17 to 22 represents a time of "grand dreams" such as being wealthy or landing a glamorous job. This is reflected in the cameo: "My fantasy is to become rich, have an extravagant home, and famous friends! Dream on, right?" Beyond the period of emerging adulthood, the visions of one's possible selves narrow as realism comes to take precedence.

As noted earlier in this volume, Fischer (1980) has cogently argued that, with increasing cognitive development to more advanced stages, there is a greater need for support or scaffolding from mature adults, if one is to achieve the potential for optimal development. However, unlike earlier stages, life for the emerging adult is less structured, there may be less social support, and there are fewer unambiguous societal norms or rules to guide one's behavior (Buchmann, 1989). Shulman et al. (2005) concur, pointing out that young people find less direction, in the form of traditions or customs, and therefore may find themselves rudderless and alone in the search for their appropriate social role in contemporary society. The prototypic cameo description begins with the observation that "It's been challenging to get a life after high school where we knew what we had to do, where there were teachers and coaches and counselors to guide us."

Vocational and Occupational Exploration

For many theorists of this period, *identity achievement* is the hallmark of the transition to adulthood (see S. J. Schwartz, 2001). Vocational or occupational identity represents center stage for the drama of exploration. Serious choices must be in place before the final curtain call. In American society, the emerging adult is given a reprieve in the form of a protracted decision-making time frame. Such a deferment is most obvious in the case of attendance at college. From one perspective, these college youth have been afforded the luxury of assisted exploration through the exposure to different ideas, belief systems, competencies conveyed in coursework, and higher-order thinking skills (Cote, 1996; Kitchner et al., 2006). Thus, they have an extended period of time to explore and adopt, as well as shed, various possible selves. They may find a job, decide on an occupation, later leave it in order to return to some other kind of training, and then pursue a different occupational path. Others may vacillate between periods of work and nonemployment. Some may remain in the parental home during this period or leave, only to return to live with their parents (Shulman et al., 2005). Thus, emerging adulthood is characterized by "fluctuations, discontinuities, reversals, and uncertainties" (p. 579). L. J. Nelson and Barry

(2005) note that two such educational manifestations are changes in majors (the average at my university is four to five) and the decision to attend graduate school, which further prolongs many of the decisions demanded of adulthood, proper.

I have personally observed this phenomenon in the life of a very bright and talented Yale undergraduate who was in my senior honors seminar. He had decided to pursue graduate school in psychology and asked if I would write a letter of recommendation, which I readily agreed to do. He was accepted into a prestigious graduate program and was on the path to his chosen profession (I assumed). One year later, he wrote to tell me that he had changed his mind and now wanted to attend law school, which he thought was a better match for his interests and capabilities. I felt I could alter my letter, adapting it to the demands and skills needed to succeed in law school. He was accepted into an excellent program and I wished him well. One year later, I received another letter indicating that law school was not his "thing," he had learned. He feared that he didn't have the flexibility needed to arbitrarily argue either side of a debate. He required an occupation where the decision-making process was clearer and had more integrity. (I could muster some empathy for his conclusion.) Thus, he had now banked his future on becoming an architect and was applying to appropriate training programs. However, this latest decision on his part began to strain the credulity of my recommendation, as I had little evidence that he had the requisite talents for this new occupational choice. (My letters were getting shorter and shorter!) A year later I received a communication, thanking me for my continued support, given the fluctuations that defined his occupational quest. He had dropped out of architectural school for the time being ("I'm afraid I just didn't have the visual aptitude needed for architectural design"), and was doing local construction work, having returned to live with his parents, until he could "get his act together." This young man always "wore his heart on his sleeve" and was frank and honest about his professional aspirations and dreams as well as his fears and failures. That awareness gave me hope that someday he would successfully find his final chosen profession.

Many theorists and researchers who address issues of identity have accepted the framework provided by Marcia (1980, 1988), who built upon the seminal writings of Erikson (1963, 1968). Erikson focused on two processes, exploration and commitment, that would lead to *identity achievement*. After an appropriate period of exploration, individuals would eventually commit to a vocational or occupational choice, and pursue that path.

Marcia (1980, 1988) elaborated on Erikson's (1963, 1968) model by proposing a typology of four identity statuses that represented combinations of exploration and commitment. The ideal resolution of the identity dilemma is (1) *identity achievement*, in which explorations of various options have resulted in a reasoned commitment to the occupation that is deemed most suitable. Those in (2) *foreclosure* have not engaged in extensive exploration but rather have had an identity "conferred" upon them by others (e.g., going into the family business, pursuing the career that their parents have designated as their professional aspiration for their son or daughter), or going into the military where choices in this country, contrary to the advertisements ("Be all that you can be"), are actually quite limited. Thus, there is commitment without exploration. The status of (3) *moratorium* represents an extended period of exploration, postponing commitment, and is most evident for emerging adults who attend college. In (4) *diffusion*, the individual flounders, neither exploring an occupational identity in a thoughtful or productive manner nor displaying the ability to commit to a realistic occupational choice. (My Yale undergraduate student, who initially displayed some level of commitment to chosen professions, was eventually teetering on the brink of a shift from moratorium to diffusion.)

My student illustrates an important point about this conceptual framework. Marcia's (1980, 1988) statuses implied a static conceptualization of identity formation. However, later theorists and researchers (e.g., Waterman, 1992) concluded, more appropriately, that there could be tremendous psychological movement across these statuses. For example, increases in social support, planned or unexpected, and personal determination can each serve to aid emerging adults to eventually attain identity achievement. Their absence can also cause regression to less desirable statuses. In the cameo, our emerging adult is struggling with the choice of striking out on his/her own or choosing the default option of simply going into the family business. His/her father would prefer this option (although it would vault our young adult into the foreclosure status). The conflict is exemplified by the reflection that "I'm not really cut out for his [my father's] line of work, [I don't have the] aptitude for business. Plus, I just don't want that kind of pressure or responsibility right now. I'm sure I'll settle on something in a couple of years, I just need more time to explore my options." This best characterizes the status of moratorium.

Arnett (2000, 2010) finds that the majority of youth in the United States has not reached the status of identity achievement by the age of 21. Consistent with these findings, Cote (2009) reports that by the end of adolescence, approximately 50% are still in either the foreclosure or diffusion identity statuses. In the United States, as well as other developed Western countries where many attend colleges and universities, identity achievement is normatively delayed. Although college education provides certain conceptual tools for making more informed occupational decisions, there are tradeoffs. Emerging adults who prolong their education (attendance at college, graduate school, or other professional schools) are given societal permission to defer major life decisions such as occupational commitment, marriage, parenting, and the consolidation of a belief system. To a certain extent, this is clearly a luxury. However, from the point of view of identity formation, this extends exploration that characterizes the period of moratorium and provokes a potential shift into the dynamics of diffusion. Thus, these latter processes prolong and threaten the type of commitment that leads to mature forms of identity achievement.

Romantic Relationships

It was Sigmund Freud (1952) who asserted that maturity requires the capacity both to work and to love. Emerging adulthood, therefore, involves not only occupational experimentation but explorations in love (Arnett, 2000, 2010). L. J. Nelson and Barry (2005) observe that romantic relationships are more enduring than in adolescence. They are likely to involve sexual intercourse and may include cohabitation but typically not with the explicit intent of marriage. Marriage is not one of the criteria that defines adulthood, in contemporary society. However, the issue prompts reflection about making eventual decisions such as the type of person one would want to marry. The cameo description reflects that mentality: "I'm not serious about anyone in particular right now. I'm not ready to get married any time soon. I don't really have a clear idea right now of what type of person I would want to marry. Then I wonder if it's OK to live with someone if you are not married. I'll try to figure that out once I get the rest of my life more settled."

It would appear that making a commitment to marriage is premature, until one resolves other challenges such as educational and occupational choices, financial independence, and the establishment of one's personal religious and political beliefs. From my own clinical experience, uncertainty about the type of marriage partner is not the only reason young people delay their decision; there is also a lack of clarity about the type of partner that he/she might aspire to be. Dating and serial romantic relationships, therefore, provoke not only experimentation with potential partner characteristics but soul searching about the self.

Social Support

Support from parents as well as peers will necessarily undergo transformations during emerging adulthood. The transition to college or to entry into the workforce requires the renegotiation of relationships with parents, particularly if it involves leaving home. Their previous forms of parental support may no longer be appropriate, given one's new, though tenuous, maturational status. As revealed in the cameo, "My parents tend to preach a little bit too much. Our relationship is different now, particularly since I am no longer that financially dependent upon my parents." Tanner (2006) reiterates a conclusion previously drawn by other scholars (see Harter, 1998); namely, that the goal of this period is not simply the separation from parents. Rather, the parent–child relationship needs to be psychologically *restructured* such that emerging adults gain more autonomy while at the same time maintaining parental support and mutual closeness (see Arnett et al., 2011; Swartz & O'Brien, 2009).

Going to college or obtaining a job will undoubtedly disrupt previous patterns of peer support, as well. Many high school friends may go their separate ways, requiring that one make new friends and establish new social relationships for needed support. These new friends can serve as a sounding board as one faces challenging life decisions and will hopefully bolster one's sense of self. Our prototypical emerging adult contrasts high school, in which there was a lively and supportive social environment, to community college where he/she is still trying to fit in and make friends: "To tell the truth, I'm often kind of lonely." Later, there is the admission that "I've become closer to my two older siblings. They are a little more mature than I am and they can give me good advice."

My colleagues and I have studied the role of support among students making the transition from high school to university life (Harter, 1990, 2006a). In particular, we have been interested in the role of social support, as it might change or maintain self-esteem. Students who accepted offers to attend our university were first administered questionnaires before they matriculated. After two quarters of attending classes and living on campus, we readministered the battery of instruments. In such a pre–post design, we rejected the strategy of merely examining mean differences in self-esteem at the two time periods, for the group as a whole. Of course, initially we calculated these two mean scores, which were identical, namely, 3.4 on a 4-point scale. However, the data-analytic strategy that we felt would be more revealing involved the identification of three subgroups, those whose self-esteem significantly *increased* over their first 6 months of college, those whose self-esteem significantly *decreased*, and those who reported *no change* in their self-esteem.

We next examined factors that were associated with membership in these three subgroups. Those students whose self-esteem increased dramatically, from scores below the midpoint to scores above the midpoint, reported correspondingly dramatic gains in social support in the new university environment compared to their high school experience. In addition to increases in social support from friends and classmates, they reported supportive relationships with adults such as faculty, coaches, clergy, counselors, drama teachers, and so forth. The large majority had also established connections with social groups and campus organizations providing support from like-minded peers from whom they could garner acceptance and foster new friendships.

Those in the subgroup who maintained their level of self-esteem during their first year in college were students who began with high self-esteem. Through their new experiences on campus, they were able to sustain the high personal regard that they brought from their high school days where they had considerable support. Like the subgroup whose self-esteem dramatically improved, these students quickly made connections within campus organizations and social groups with interests they shared. Thus, they were able to form socially supportive relationships among group members, classmates, dorm-mates, or fraternity brothers and sorority sisters.

Those whose self-esteem dropped precipitously, from high self-worth in high school to extremely low self-esteem 6 months into college, had been unable to garner support or make social connections in the new university environment. Not only did these students report a substantial drop in self-esteem but also an increase in feelings of depression, consistent with our model (see Figure 3.1). Thus, the ability to establish new support systems during the transition to college bore psychological fruit by increasing, or maintaining, a high level of self-esteem.

Interestingly, correlations between self-esteem and support from different sources, notably peers and parents, across the two time periods revealed differences. Support from new university peers; namely, classmates and those with whom they shared campus activities (e.g., organizations, sports, drama, political involvement) remained highly predictive of self-esteem. However, the correlation between parental approval support and self-esteem, while moderately strong in high school, declined significantly during the first year of college. This should not be interpreted as a decrease in the mean *level* of parental approval or other types of support. For example, instrumental support (translate as "financial" for students attending an expensive private university such as ours), as well as emotional support from parents, typically remained high. Parental support from all three sources (approval, instrumental, emotional), while performing important functions, was no longer predictive of global self-esteem at this particular developmental juncture.

Approval from those in the more public peer domain, where support has to be earned, not assumed, represents the primary type and source of self-esteem. Moreover, public peer support in the form of earned approval is the most critical to self-esteem across the lifespan (Harter, 1990, 2006a). The term "public support" is employed to distinguish it from the acceptance that one receives from close friends, where the correlation with self-esteem is negligible. As has been argued elsewhere, close friends, by definition, are accepting and there is much less variability in support scores from this source (Harter, 1990).

This pattern of findings is more consistent with Mead's (1934) concept of feedback from the "generalized other" than with Cooley's (1902) reflections on the role of the "particular significant other." That is, the evaluations of the larger audience with whom one interacts are considered to be a more credible index of one's worth as a person. Particular others, namely, close friends, parents, and family are more likely to bestow unconditional positive regard because this constitutes part of their social role definition.

Individual and Cross-Cultural Differences

Although the majority of individuals between the ages of 18 and 25 do not yet consider themselves to be adults, L. J. Nelson and Barry (2005) have identified a small subset (25%) who feel that they *do* meet the definition of an adult (see also Arnett, 2001; K. Nelson, 2003). This subgroup employs the same criteria, namely, taking responsibility for their actions, making their own independent decisions, and achieving financial independence from their parents.

The minority who felt that they *had* reached adulthood reported a more mature sense of their identity; that is, they were more likely to be in the identity achievement status. Second, they reported less depression, which is understandable due to their more mature sense of identity. (Depression is one of the "side effects" of emerging adulthood for those who have not yet made clear occupational commitments.) Finally, those who felt that they had achieved adulthood engaged in fewer high-risk behaviors (e.g., illegal substance abuse and drunken driving), compared to the emerging adult majority.

Shulman et al. (2005) have also employed an individual difference approach, documenting three distinctive types of emerging adults. Cluster analyses were employed, tapping various dimensions of *love* and *work,* the criteria Freud (1952) first identified as critical to the mental health of adults. The most adaptive pattern was labeled "authentic and competent." These emerging adults voiced clear occupational goals and a sense of direction with regard to where they were going in life. They were also likely to be involved in a mature romantic relationship. Their portrayal of self was integrated, cohesive, and coherent. Moreover, they displayed high levels of thoughtfulness and the self that they displayed was characterized by authenticity.

Two other identified patterns were less adaptive. One was labeled "low integrated." Members of this subgroup shared several characteristics. First, they lacked clarity of purpose in the pursuit of occupational goals. They expressed little sense of direction in terms of career or educational options. The findings also revealed difficulties in relationships; they either had no romantic partner or were involved in immature relationships. Rather than an integrated self, their self-portrait was fragmented and lacked coherence. They also expressed confusion about the future and displayed a low level of reflectivity.

Another less adaptive pattern rounded out the typology. These emerging adults were labeled as "acting competently but with low authenticity." This third subgroup intended to pursue occupational aspirations, although they did not display the clarity or sense of purpose that characterized the first subgroup. Nor did they possess the reflectivity. Such individuals also lacked a sense of authenticity and displayed limited self-awareness. Because they were less likely to reveal their true selves, and were also somewhat mistrustful, their attempts to establish close and meaningful relationships with others were often compromised. They made efforts to establish committed romantic partnerships but because they could not be open with themselves, their ability to be open with others was compromised.

To summarize, competent and authentic emerging adults fare better in achieving some degree of balance in their lives, as they approach true adulthood. Their self-awareness, reflectivity, and authenticity better equip them to succeed at requisite developmental challenges. In contrast, those with a poorly integrated self that lacked coherence were less clear about potential professional goals, less likely to be involved in a mature romantic relationship, and more likely to be defensive and confused. The third group believed that they should become more responsible and pursue occupational as well as personal relationship goals and thus adopted a competent guise characterized by a lack of authenticity. They questioned what they really wanted to do with their lives, as well as whether their decisions really reflected their true, inner self. There are normative manifestations of emerging adulthood; however, the studies just reviewed reveal that there are individual differences in how young adults cope with the developmental challenges that face them. Such differences have implications for self-related forms of psychopathology, a topic to which we shall return.

In addition to individual differences within a given society, there are also *cross-cultural* differences in how youth adapt to the demands of emerging adulthood. Theory and research suggest that the period of emerging adulthood may be a cultural construction. Arnett (2000) has proposed that emerging adulthood is not a universally experienced stage of development. Rather, it constitutes a period that only exists in those cultures that postpone entry into adult roles and responsibilities until young people are well into their 20s. More traditional non-Western cultures have a narrower band of time in which youth experience emerging adulthood because they are more quickly thrust into the roles of mature adults, as has been conventionally defined. Dahl (2004) describes how in traditional societies, childhood is clearly demarcated by rituals or rites of passage. The onset of adulthood quickly follows, and is defined in terms of marriage, appropriate work roles, owning property, and becoming a parent. In most traditional (non-Western) societies, the interval between puberty and achieving adult status is relatively brief. On average, females are married within 2 years after puberty and males within 4. Currently, the age of marriage in American society is 26 for females and 27 for males (see Dahl, 2004).

L. J. Nelson, Badger, and Wu (2004) have addressed the dynamics of emerging adulthood among Chinese youth. Participants were students at Beijing University. As described earlier, emerging adults in the United States agree on the three criteria defining adulthood: (1) accepting responsibility for one's actions, (2) making independent decisions, and (3) becoming financially independent (Arnett, 2003; L. J. Nelson & Barry, 2005). In contemporary American society, self-reliance and self-sufficiency have also become paramount.

However, in contrast to the individualism of American culture, the Chinese people value group- or other-oriented goals and is notably more collectivistic (see Chapter 8). In keeping with Confucian dogma, Chinese youth place greater emphasis on constraining the personal self, including emotions. More emphasis is placed on obligations to others, such as marriage, becoming a parent, and caring for one's elders. Moreover, risky behaviors (e.g., substance abuse) are avoided, lest they incur embarrassment and cast shame on the family. As a culture, Chinese values caution against, rather than condone, risk taking. In addition, there are far fewer opportunities for identity exploration in China, compared to the United States. By their early 20s, Chinese youth have been forced to make their occupational or career choices, and are well on their way to achieving other-oriented goals.

L. J. Nelson et al. (2004) report that the majority (59%) of Chinese youth in their sample (mean age 20) believed that they had reached adulthood, whereas only a third expressed a sense of uncertainty about their adult status. The four criteria that were most highly endorsed by over 90% of the Chinese participants were (1) accepting responsibility for one's personal actions, (2) being in good control of one's emotions, (3) becoming financially independent from parents, and (4) becoming less self-oriented, developing greater consideration for others. Of particular interest was the finding that in this Chinese sample, 89% endorsed the importance of being capable of supporting one's parents financially, compared to only 16% of youth in the United States (reported by Arnett, 2003). For Chinese young adults, criteria such as marriage or full-time employment ranked much lower on the list (below 40%). However, obligations to significant familial others, rather than self-centeredness, are key values in this collectivistic culture, and come to be important dimensions that define the self. Moreover, the period of emerging adulthood, itself, is truncated as other constraints, demands, and values come into play in the early 20s.

The distinction between the typical patterns for U.S. and Chinese youth is but one example of cross-cultural differences during emerging adulthood. Hendry and Kloep (2011) present a much more comprehensive analysis of the dimensions that differentiate emerging adulthood for many cultures around the globe. They provide a compelling account of how differences in societal values, economic conditions, technological advances, political forces, educational expectations, and prevailing parental styles have come to impact the particular characteristics of the youth experience in any given culture. They are particularly sensitive to how these dimensions have been subject to change over historical time into the present.

The analysis of Hendry and Kloep (2011) is not merely a fascinating description of changing cultural differences in emerging adulthood. It also serves as a springboard for their contention that stage models of this period of development are obsolete. The artificial construction of stages, including the invention of a new stage, they argue, does not provide a powerful instrument for understanding developmental change or differences across cultures. Creating the stage of emerging adulthood, in particular, is not viable because it is simply irrelevant to most Third World youth. In addition, manifestations in industrialized nations vary wildly, giving this new stage designation little explanatory clout.

A detailed analysis of their argument, complete with rejoinders (see the recent edited volume by Arnett et al., 2011) is beyond the scope of this chapter. However, the spirited debate between emerging adulthood as a "stage" versus a "process" is well worth the attention of the interested reader. As with many such debates that have dominated our field over the years (e.g., nature vs. nurture), the truth would appear to lie somewhere in between.

Normative Liabilities for
Self-Development during Emerging Adulthood

The importance of Arnett's (1997) original identification of this transitional period alerts us to previously unchartered conceptual waters and the psychological pieces that complete the mosaic of adult development. For society at large, an understanding of this stage can provide an awareness of the challenges that define emerging adulthood. It can normalize features that cause parents considerable consternation, expressed, for example, in the following: "Why can't you grow up? You're 21!" "Why aren't you more responsible for what you do? How could you be so stupid?" "What do you mean you want to continue to live with us?" "When are you going to get a life?" "You need to get a real job, not just work part-time for your father, and regardless of what you do, if you continue to live here, you have to contribute by paying some rent!" "It would be great if you went to college, but remember what we told you some years ago about all of the effort and preparation it would take, on your part, in order to be accepted? Did you listen? No." "Your mother says you should go clean your room."

These parental complaints and directives are startling to many graduates who are still trying to process their senior prom and graduation. The transition can seem abrupt and daunting, bringing challenges for which many have not prepared. As a result, the features of emerging adulthood that have been previously described loom large on the impending screen of life, where one must now take center stage. The decision and opportunity to attend college may seem like a mature choice, a luxury that facilitates adult choices but will simultaneously prolong life decisions. These seem like speed bumps for some and resemble a minefield for others. L. J. Nelson and Barry (2005) have concluded that this is a normative period of instability and uncertainty. The emerging adult in the cameo, who poignantly expresses these feelings, comes across as emotionally vulnerable, all the more so because of his/her honesty, self-awareness, and openness. That said, it is critical *not* to interpret these manifestations as pathological, unless they become extreme. Emerging adulthood in our culture is a necessary developmental phase, a journey that most will eventually navigate with relative success.

Along the way, struggles with identity crowd the landscape. Decisions about occupational identity are paramount. The status of *moratorium* is common, where explorations of "what to be when one grows up" are often confusing and painful. The status of *foreclosure* can seem like a blessing in disguise, in the short run because one's identity is *conferred* with no need for exploration. For example, the emerging adult can follow his/her parents' choice for his/her career such as going into the family business. In the long run, this can lead to dissatisfaction for some who come to resist the shackles of someone else's choice.

Exploration in the realm of romantic relationships can take tortuous twists and turns before one is mature enough to settle on meaningful criteria for the choice of a partner that will dictate commitment. Relationship decisions do not only apply to romantic others. As our own study on the transition to college revealed (Harter, 1990, 2006a), it is critical to search for, and find, supportive networks of peers and friends not only to provide companionship but to also share in the various explorations that define this phase of life.

Depression is a normative liability during this period. As noted earlier, there is a need to forge new social relationships and feeling lonely, in the process, can lead one to feel dejected. Serial and unsatisfying romantic explorations are also cause for depression. If one has left home, the loss of daily support from parents can also contribute to depressed affect stemming from this form of separation. Fear of failure, both in the occupational and social realms, constitutes another determinant.

Risk taking is another liability, not always obvious at this age level. As discussed earlier, emerging adults are at heightened risk for substance abuse, unprotected sex, and drunken driving, to name three prevalent examples. A. E. Kelly, Schochet, and Landry (2004) observe that risk taking is one of the biggest behavioral changes to emerge at adolescence but it continues well into emerging adulthood. Less adult monitoring or guidance was cited earlier as one cause. In the case of college students, the influence of so many other same-age peers may also well contribute. Steinberg (2004) alerts us to the fact that most risk taking is a group activity, for example, driving while drinking. As noted in the previous discussion, the *cessation* of risk taking is *not* a criterion that defines adulthood proper for most youth. Thus, youth see no compelling reason to avoid risks and reckless behavior and thus sensation-seeking persists. Moreover, Elkind (1967) has contributed to our understanding of risk taking in his identification of the "personal fable" in which youth proclaim their uniqueness (see Chapter 3). One form of this fable is to claim their invincibility in the face of potential danger. A final contributor to continued risk taking and other liabilities can be related to the still unfinished normative hormonal and neurological development that began with puberty.

Hormonal and Neurological Development

Beginning in adolescence and continuing into the period of emerging adulthood, a variety of sources of injury and death are related to normative difficulties in the control of emotions and behavior (Dahl, 2004; A. E. Kelly et al., 2004). These include reckless behavior, risky sexual behaviors, alcohol and substance abuse, accidents, and depression. Dahl explores these issues within the context of a broadened definition of adolescence that encompasses the period of emerging adulthood. He provisionally defines adolescence as "that awkward period between sexual maturation and the attainment of adult roles and responsibilities" (p. 9). To become an adult requires more than the hormonal and sexual maturity that emerges at puberty. Adulthood demands a broader set of skills, knowledge, and experience. Moreover, considerably more neurological development is necessary.

Increasingly, puberty is occurring at younger and younger ages (see Dahl, 2004; Rutter, 1993). The recent evidence shows that puberty now begins with a cascade of hormonal changes between the ages of 9 and 12. For females, Dahl notes that the average age of menarche for females in the United States is now 12. Hormonal changes at puberty exacerbate strong drives, emotional intensity, and sensation seeking associated with reckless behavior. Most risk taking occurs under conditions of high emotional arousal (see also Steinberg, 2004). Moreover, the lack of affective regulation stems from the fact that the amygdala, a brain center that involves the expression of emotion, becomes more activated beginning in adolescence. Cognitive development, however, has *not* kept pace with these changes in pubertal development. As Dahl points out, cognitive acquisitions such as advanced reasoning, problem solving, decision making, and judgment, as well as the ability to regulate one's emotions, do *not* emerge with the advent of puberty. These skills are more highly related to age, experience, and later neurological development rather than to pubertal changes, themselves.

One implication, according to Dahl (2004), is that adolescents and young adults have not developed the skills to harness intense emotional reactions. Skills in the self-regulation of affect await further neurological development as well as social experiences that profit from scaffolding by mature adults. Dahl's conclusion is that self-regulatory processes involve the development of complex neurobehavioral systems that are the last regions of the brain to fully mature. There is considerable evidence for the continued development in many neurological structures during adolescence and early adulthood (A. E. Kelly et al., 2004). For example, it is now accepted that the frontal lobes, primarily responsible for judgment, reasoning, planning, inhibitory control, and anticipation of consequences, are not completely developed until age 25. Thus, as Dahl astutely observes, the intense affects that *are* associated with puberty can hijack responsible decision making from adolescence into emerging adulthood. This mismatch can compromise the ability to make the kind of reasonable independent choices that society seems to expect if not demand of emerging adults.

Steinberg (2004) concurs, observing that two contributors to risk taking operate in tandem. There are hormonal factors that drive adolescents to seek higher levels of novelty and stimulation than they did in childhood but also neurological regulatory mechanisms that would curb risk-taking behaviors mature more slowly. Together, these lead to the vulnerability of this period of youth development.

Dahl's (2004) argument leads to the conclusion that it is crucial for adolescents and young adults to have access to social *scaffolding* from parents and other responsible adults such as teachers, coaches, ministers, and extended family. Biological or pubertal immaturity without a corresponding shift toward cognitive-emotional maturity, given a sometimes unsupportive social environment with minimal adult supervision and guidance, contributes to the vulnerability of our youth in contemporary society.

It may be instructive to surmise that were it not for the risk-taking predilections of those in the period of emerging adulthood, particularly for males, our all-volunteer army would not be sustainable. Male youth are often eager to sign up for military service and some harbor visions of becoming decorated heroes. Their risk-taking propensities on the battlefield often lead to their taking dangerous risks that would be judged unwise, foolhardy, and life threatening in civilian contexts. For those who survive such risks and whose actions are deemed heroic, a Purple Heart may well be a potential reward for a few. For others, it may be awarded posthumously.

Fortunately, the psychological picture that Dahl (2004) paints of risk taking is not categorically bleak. The passions that adolescents and emerging adults experience are not restricted to sex, drugs, loud music, and reckless behaviors. Rather, they can also ignite fervor about more adaptive pursuits, such as music, art, literature, hobbies, sports, science, and a passionate commitment to idealistic, political, and humanistic causes. Here, responsible adult role models can be of tremendous value in channeling intense interests in adaptive directions. From a historical perspective, many of the intellectual, scientific, technological, and artistic achievements and inventions that we have witnessed over the centuries, and across diverse cultures, could not have been possible, were it not for risk taking that eventually proved creative and productive.

Pathological Self-Processes and Outcomes during Emerging Adulthood

The more public *context* of the social and societal environment in which emerging adults find themselves has implications for how various forms of psychopathology might be manifest differently compare to previous stages of development. Against the backdrop of cultural expectations that one should be developing occupational goals, moving into more mature intimate relationships, and becoming financially independent of parents, failure to meet these goals may provoke symptoms that come to be viewed as pathological. Identity diffusion, failure to develop meaningful and longer-lasting relationships, severe depression and hopelessness, dissociative identity disorders, extreme lack of authenticity, and eating disorders are all potential forms of psychopathology that can emerge during this stage of development.

Pathology of mental health proportions can also result when normative liabilities are exacerbated (Dahl, 2004). For those who have extreme difficulties in controlling their behavior and related emotions, much higher levels of risk taking are observed (see also Steinberg, 2004). Acts of homicide, suicide, other forms of violence, and eating disorders are literally leading to the death of many youth in our contemporary society.

Dahl (2004) also includes clinical manifestations of depression in this list. Some level of dejection is normal during emerging adulthood, given concerns over occupational choices and relationship issues. However, when the pressures, either external or internal, become overwhelming, depressive disorders can ensue. During my own college years, the "sophomore slump" was a popular term. Many of us experienced it, but most of us who had adequate support systems moved through this period to make appropriate life decisions. Some did not cope as well and fell into deep depression that required counseling and, in some cases, students dropped out of college because the psychological demands were overwhelming.

I would conjecture that another factor contributing to pathological processes among both college youth and those in the workforce (particularly those who cannot obtain a satisfying job), is that one's deficiencies are now on public display. That is, there are new societal expectations that one act like an adult and be able to obtain and hold down a job. For those in college, there is the pressure of performing well scholastically, and of choosing a major that will shape one's career decisions. Moreover, depressive reactions in college can seriously interfere with the rigorous academic demands, leading students to compromised performance, lack of motivation, poor grades, and the possibility that one will be asked, or choose, to leave their collegiate life. Regardless of whether depression occurs in the context of college or the labor force, it is all the more debilitating because it is highly associated with hopelessness about the future (see Harter, 2006a). College counselors should be sensitive to the dynamics of student depression in order to distinguish between normative liabilities and more severe pathology that would dictate a different, more aggressive, intervention approach.

Another red flag concerns problematic identity development. The emerging adult could be mired in the throes of identity *diffusion* (Erikson, 1968; Marcia, 1988). This status is characterized by floundering, the inability to appropriately explore options. Failure to make decisions, and therefore to commit to a life path, is crippling psychologically. It can provoke criticism from one's family as well as society at large, given that normative expectations of maturity, now observed by a larger audience on the stage of one's life, are not met.

Self-awareness, including the need to develop an integrated, coherent self in an age-appropriate manner, represents a critical challenge during emerging adulthood (see also Shulman et al., 2005). Failure to meet this challenge can also result in various forms of pathology, including the perpetuation of false-self behavior that can compromise the formation of meaningful, intimate relationships. The lack of an ability to develop an integrated, coherent self that also possesses a sense of *continuity over time* will also compromise the goal of identity development. The establishment of a core identity in various spheres (e.g., occupational, moral/spiritual, marriage) also requires an adaptive projection of the self into the future, a significant developmental task. Thus, although the disruptions in I-self processes have meaning at every developmental level, they represent unique manifestations during emerging adulthood. The fact that this is a transitional period requires that issues must be resolved in order to advance to true adulthood. Progress disrupted by earlier negative socialization experiences will become more evident and reveal signs of pathology, in part because one is now on the public stage of societal expectations and therefore under more scrutiny. No longer is one sequestered in the safe haven of the high school environment or the bosom of one's family.

The broader public stage also has implications for pathological eating-disordered behaviors. If that platform is college, the audience includes classmates, other peers on campus, and those in dormitories and sororities, in the case of females. For those in the labor force, others include coworkers and superiors. From a symbolic–interactionist perspective, particularly as articulated by Mead (1934) who alerted us to the "generalized other," there are now many more potential observers of one's behavior and one's outward appearance. In our own research, we became particularly interested in the pathological manifestations of eating-disordered behaviors among college women who were living on campus, in either sorority houses or dormitories. In a thesis conducted by Danis and Harter (1996), two eating-disordered groups were identified, those with symptoms of anorexia and those with symptoms of bulimia, both of clinical significance. These two groups were compared to a control sample that did not display such symptoms.

We applied a Jamesian (1892) analysis to the dynamics of each group. Both the anorexic and bulimic group reported that appearance was markedly more important, compared to the normative sample. In evaluating their physical appearance very negatively, they created a large discrepancy, between the excessive importance of appearance and the vastly lower perceptions of their attractiveness. This discrepancy clearly predicted the very low self-esteem scores for the two eating-disordered groups compared to the normal sample. These low self-esteem scores, in turn, were predictive of extremely high levels of self-reported depression. Of particular interest were the findings that although both eating-disordered groups reported this negative constellation of symptoms, those in the bulimic group were most at risk given the lowest ratings of perceived physical appearance, self-esteem, and the highest levels of depression.

We interpreted this difference between the two eating-disordered groups in terms of perceptions of control. We argued that because those with symptoms of anorexia were objectively thinner, they would feel more successful in terms of their weight control. The bulimics, who by definition binge and purge, reported that they felt less in control; moreover, and on average, this group was heavier. We also addressed the role of *social comparison,* finding that the living circumstances of these college women, in sorority houses or dormitories, enhanced the salience of societal standards of appearance, scrutiny, and evaluation by others.

Mental health will also be compromised to the extent that in certain relationships one has developed an *insecure attachment style* in certain relationships. This observation raises a controversial issue in the field of developmental psychology, namely, whether one's attachment style can, in fact, differ across relationships. Classic attachment theory (see Bowlby, 1979) postulates that self-representations, or working models of self, develop in early interactions with caregivers, typically parents, that then generalize to subsequent relationships, for example, with peers and romantic others. Thus, those children and adolescents who are securely attached to caregivers and who feel lovable and capable (defining predictors of high self-esteem) should transfer these representations to relationships with significant others in later stages of development. However, there is some tension between classic attachment theory and more contemporary perspectives about the stability, consistency, and continuity of these working models and attachment styles across relationships, over the course of development. More contemporary theoretical accounts of working models of the self, based on attachment status, posit that individuals may simultaneously manifest different attachment styles across different relationships (see Cozzarelli, Hoekstra, & Bylsma, 2000; Ross & Spinner, 2001). According to neo-attachment theorists, the development of different attachment styles across relationship contexts may well represent more realistic adaptations (see Baldwin, Keelan, Fehr, Enns, & Koh-Rangarajoo, 1996; Bridges, Connell, & Belsky, 1988).

We sought to investigate this issue among a sample of emerging adults in college, ranging in age from 18 to 25, with a mean age of 20.1 (Badanes & Harter, 2007b). We examined three attachment styles, secure and two insecure styles, anxious–ambivalent and anxious–avoidant, across four relationship contexts, with mother, father, close friends, and a romantic other. We adapted our multiple-selves procedure (Harter, Bresnick, et al., 1997), which requires participants to provide their own six prototypical self-descriptive adjectives for each of the six relationships. In our adaptation, we first generated a list of descriptive attributes for each attachment style and asked participants to select the six most self-descriptive.

One advantage of this procedure was that participants had the option of describing the *same attachment style* (be it secure or one of the two insecure styles) but with different self-descriptors appropriate to a given relationship. For example, securely attached young adults might describe themselves as "understood" and "supported" by a parent, "open" and "valued" by close friends, and "intimate" and "warm" with a romantic other. Possible examples selected by an anxious–avoidant individual might be "distant" and "reserved" with one's father, "self-focused" and "unmindful" in relationships with friends, and "dismissing" and "unemotional" in a romantic relationship. Those displaying an anxious–ambivalent style across relationships could feel "vulnerable" and "unloved" with one's mother, "guarded" and "worried" in relationships with friends, and "reserved" and "shy" in a romantic relationship. Thus, to reiterate the advantages of this procedure, one could describe the self as different with regard to the specific attributes displayed in a given relationship but maintain the same attachment style, be it secure or insecure.

The findings revealed that attachment style consistency across dyads (e.g., mother and close friends, mother and father, father and romantic other) was only 58%, ranging from a high of 63% for the mother–close friend dyad to a low of 31% for the father–romantic other dyad. The degree of overlap for the mother–father dyad fell in between; namely, 40% for these emerging adults. Thus, overall, an average of 42% of the sample reported *different attachment styles* across relationships. These values support the conclusion that for many, there is no one single attachment style that unilaterally generalizes to all relationships, at this developmental level.

Experiences and socialization history, as yet to be fully explored, lead to different attachment styles for many, across particular relationship contexts.

We further explored the correlation between secure and insecure attachment styles within each relationship and both self-esteem and reported true-self attributes (Badanes & Harter, 2007a). Securely attached emerging adults reported more true-self behavior and higher levels of relational self-esteem within each relational context, compared to insecurely attached individuals. Furthermore, the more positive attributes reported by participants, the higher their self-esteem ($r = .54$). In addition, the greater the number of positive attributes, the more one reported true-self behavior ($r = .51$). Finally, positive attribute selection was strongly related to the number of secure relationships ($r = .59$).

Thus, attachment styles for many differ across relationships during emerging adulthood. Those more securely attached within a given relationship were more likely to express higher self-esteem and to view their attributes as true-self behavior. Those with insecure attachment styles were more at risk for pathological-self symptoms; namely, low self-esteem and false-self behavior. How the various pathological manifestations that can be documented during emerging adulthood carry over into "true" adulthood, as defined by the criteria that have been agreed upon for our culture, is as yet undetermined. Longitudinal studies are therefore much needed, in order to further our understanding of the continuity of all of the pathological indices described in this chapter.

The Popular Press Weighs In

The period of emerging adulthood is no longer merely the construction of academics. The concept has filtered down to the lay person. In the *Denver Post* (June 25, 2010) there appeared an article by Mike Littleton titled "Parents Face New Stage in Child's Life." It begins with the following observation: "In the glow of the college graduation season across America, many a proud tuition-paying parent sighs with relief and thinks 'My work here is done.' Well, think again, Mom and Dad." (p. 2A). Tell-tale signs of this period follow. There is constant flux and uncertainty about the purpose and direction of one's life, in that emerging adults are unsettled about some of life's most fundamental issues, including their individual identity and moral and religious values. The article insightfully highlights the challenge of renegotiating the relationship with parents. Emerging adults prize their freedom and autonomy, but their parents may not recognize that they still long for a sense of direction and guidance. I would add that many emerging adults may not fully recognize this need, either.

The media is rife with such articles. A recent *New York Times* piece

(August 18, 2010) asked the question "Why are so many people in their 20s taking so long to grow up?" It makes reference to two new sitcoms that feature grown children moving back in with their parents. The cover of the May 24, 2010, issue of *The New Yorker* depicts a scenario in which a young man, having just completed his doctorate, hangs up his PhD diploma in his boyhood bedroom, as he moves back home because he cannot find a job to his liking. *The New Yorker* cover points out how the traditional cycle, in which one finishes school, grows up, begins a career, and marries and starts a family, has gone off course. The article continues in observing that young people remain untethered to romantic partners and avoid other serious life commitments. They choose instead to travel, opt for more schooling, accept temporary internships, and so on, forestalling their entry into adulthood. Thus, for many, the lockstep march is no longer the preferred path.

Another pair of articles in the *Denver Post* (August 22, 2010) recently described the "millennials" (ages 18 to 29) as uninterested in finding a job, citing their weak work ethic. Titles, degrees, years of service, and climbing the corporate ladder no longer hold any appeal for many of today's emerging adults. But neither do they want to spin their wheels in a dead-end job. Thus, many opt to live with mom and dad, leading to a new sociological phenomenon of stay-at-home youth. Thus, the academic community and the media both agree that emerging adulthood is a palpable new period of development, and many parents would appear to concur.

Concluding Comments: Is Emerging Adulthood a Legitimate Stage or a Process?

This issue has recently led to a spirited debate, played out in an edited volume by Arnett et al. (2011). Arnett (2007) and Arnett and Tanner (2011) have forcefully argued that the prototype of the emerging adult best applies to a certain segment of youth. These include those in the affluent middle class who can afford the luxury of an extended moratorium to explore their life choices and associated identities.

In contrast, there are those, notably Hendry and Kloep (2011), who adamantly reject the idea that emerging adulthood is a legitimate stage. They suggest that the concept merely defines a "lifestyle, limited to a certain age-cohort in certain societies at a certain historical time within particular socioeconomic conditions" (p. 110). Currently, privileged middle-class youth in the United States and certain other Western youth (e.g., those attending a university), qualify. The experiences of most others around the globe, particularly those in Third World countries, do not meet the criteria for emerging adulthood. Hendry and Kloep cite the obvious mediators such as social class, gender, culture, ethnicity, income, educational environment, and the particular point in historical time. However, they observe that there are also numerous more idiosyncratic factors (e.g., parenting, labor market opportunities, individual skills) than can color the experiences during this age period. Hendry and Kloep conclude, therefore, that the concept of a *stage* of emerging adulthood is untenable, with little explanatory power. The very heterogeneous nature of how this transition is experienced argues against a stage interpretation. Hendry and Kloep also contest Arnett's (2007) claim that the moratorium associated with this stage is necessarily a period of an optimistic exploration of life options.

The alternative, argued by Hendry and Kloep (2011), is to focus on a *systems* analysis that includes *process* variables. This age period is conceptualized as an *open system* without rigid boundaries where there is continual heterogeneous, but nonlinear, movement. Their theoretical framework identifies two primary process variables, *resources* and *challenges*. Resources consist of an individual's potential to cope with various changing life challenges. Resources vary over time, as some are added whereas others are lost, making this an open system. It is the *balance* between resources and challenges that shapes development. New challenges can disrupt the equilibrium of the system, requiring the individual to acquire new resources to cope with a given situation. Hendry and Kloep observe that a challenge that "disturbs" the system can be both exciting and anxiety provoking; for example, the transition to college.

Hendry and Kloep (2011) liken these challenging experiences to the "perturbations" that disturb the equilibrium, in Piaget's (1960) theory, or the *crises* in Erikson's (1968) developmental theory. These challenges represent the mechanism of developmental change in that new resources and coping mechanisms are required. In the absence of new challenges, the individual may experience psychological *stagnation*. Certain normative challenges are culture bound, such as the age of starting school, achieving legal status, and so on. However, important to their argument is the vast, if not infinite, number of non-normative challenges that may be unique to a small segment of the population. Their conclusion is that "We develop by meeting and coping with a myriad of challenges from day to day—and not by moving through age-bound stages" (p. 74).

Arnett and Tanner (2011) offer a rejoinder to Hendry and Kloep's (2011) critique of their stage conceptualization of emerging adulthood. They view this critique as one reflection of the general backlash against historical stage models of development. The grand theories of Freud (1952), Piaget (1960), and Erikson (1968) have clearly fallen out of favor in the 21st century. In part, they fell from grace because they did not take into account individual differences or the various contexts of development, for example, social class and culture. However, Arnett and colleagues (Arnett et al., 2011) have never claimed that the stage of emerging adulthood was a universal period of development, applicable across cultures or social class within a culture. They have acknowledged such variation and have urged that those interested in this transition period directly study such differences. They have hoped that the construct of emerging adulthood would inspire new knowledge and research that, in the last decade, it clearly has stimulated. Many of the parameters of emerging adulthood have now been addressed in a burgeoning literature on this transition period.

Arnett and Tanner (2011) further point out that the abstract *process* language employed by Hendry and Kloep (2011) (e.g., the relationship between resources and challenges) is disconnected from the reality of how people live their lives. Moreover, it is never directly or comprehensively applied to the period of emerging adulthood. Rather, only a few isolated examples are provided. Arnett and Tanner argue that "Without an anchor in specific life stages, statements about systems and processes have limited usefulness in understanding human development" (p. 126).

Arnett and Tanner (2011) acknowledge that emerging adulthood is perhaps the most diverse of all life stages and that this heterogeneity must be respected. They conclude that emerging adulthood represents a single stage, but with multiple pathways. Cultural differences and socio-economic variations within a given culture reflect but two examples of heterogeneous paths. There are many patterns that characterize emerging adulthood (Arnett, 2010). Arnett and Tanner conclude that the two perspectives (theirs and the views of Hendry and Kloep, 2011) both have merit and that stage and systems/process models can, with some tension, coexist.

Chapter 5

The Inextricable Link between Perceived Physical Appearance and Self-Esteem

The identification of different domains of the self-concept raises an interesting question: Are some domains of the self-concept more predictive of global self-esteem than others? One domain consistently and robustly heads the list, namely, perceived physical appearance (see Harter, 2000), leading us to ponder whether self-esteem is literally only skin-deep. The literature clearly reveals that the *inner self* (one's global esteem) is highly correlated with an evaluation of the *outer self* (perceptions of one's physical appearance, attractiveness, or body image). Those who positively evaluate their looks report correspondingly high global self-esteem. Conversely, those who view their appearance negatively report low self-esteem.

At every developmental level we have addressed (i.e., young children, older children, adolescents, college students, and adults in the world of work and family, as well as senior citizens), the self-evaluation of appearance is highly predictive of global self-esteem (Harter, 2000). In other studies with special groups of children, we initially speculated that domains that we assumed to be of greater relevance would be more highly related to global self-esteem (Harter, 2000). For example, we reasoned that for gifted as well as learning disabled students, scholastic competence should bear the strongest relationship to self-esteem, as presumably academic performance is very salient for these two groups. Contrary to our expectations, perceived physical appearance was the best predictor of self-esteem.

In a second study of conduct-disordered youth (Harter, Whitesell, & Junkin, 1998), we reasoned that because the domain of behavioral conduct should be very salient, perceptions of conduct should best predict self-esteem. Contrary to expectations, this hypothesis was not supported. Rather, perceived appearance was the domain most highly correlated with self-esteem. Finally, in a third study with older disabled children who competed in the Special Olympics, conducted at the time of the games, we predicted that perceptions of *athletic competence* would be most highly correlated with self-esteem, given the salience of athletic ability. Once again, the findings failed to confirm our expectations. Perceptions of appearance best predicted self-esteem! We have yet to find a group for whom physical appearance is *not* the best predictor of one's overall sense of worth as a person. This raises the question of why the *outer self*, the perceptions of one's appearance, should be so intimately tied to the *inner*, psychological self.

We suggest two possible post hoc explanations for this robust relationship that are understandably related. First, the domain of physical appearance is qualitatively different from the other self-concept domains. Appearance is an omnipresent feature of the self, it is always on display for others, or for the self, to observe, scrutinize, and judge. We gaze at ourselves in real mirrors and we anticipate the evaluations of others, as social mirrors. This was the crux of Cooley's (1902) looking-glass-self formulation. In contrast to appearance, adequacy in domains such as scholastic and athletic competence, peer likeability, and behavioral conduct or morality, is not constantly on display for the evaluative scrutiny of others; it is more context specific. Moreover, one has more control over if and when adequacy in these domains will be revealed.

A second interpretation lies in the societal emphasis of appearance in the media. Contemporary culture highlights appearance and the need to adhere to strict standards of attractiveness, for every age, across the lifespan (reviewed in Harter, 2000). The media (e.g., movies, television, magazines, rock videos, and advertising), put forth powerful and pervasive messages about the standards of appearance to which one must adhere. The literature has burgeoned in the last decade, with very persuasive evidence that is reviewed in this chapter.

The range of instruments demonstrating the inextricable link between appearance and global self-esteem has been broadened. Our original measure (Harter, 1985) yielded a single subscale score that tapped perceived physical appearance (defined as a composite of satisfaction with one's looks, the judgment that one is attractive, positive acceptance of one's appearance, and so forth). Newer instruments have focused on discrete indices such as satisfaction with one's weight, shape, bodily self-esteem, facial features, and in one study, penis size (see Stewart & Williamson, 2004). Other researchers have yoked an objective measure, the Body Mass Index (BMI; a ratio of the individual's height to weight) to body satisfaction and global self-esteem. This measure serves as a proxy for obesity, which has become a major contemporary health concern in our culture for children, adolescents, and adults, alike (McCabe & Ricciardelli, 2004).

Across different measures, the pattern of results is extremely robust. Consistently, negative perceptions of physical appearance are highly correlated with global self-esteem. Across 13 different U.S. samples (that have included older children, adolescents, and college students), our findings have revealed an average correlation of .65, with a range from .52 to .80. Moreover, this same pattern has been duplicated in 12 other countries, including *England* (K. Fox, Page, Armstrong, & Kirby, 1994), *Ireland* (Granlese & Joseph, 1993), *Scotland* (J. Williams & Currie, 2000), *Australia* (Trent, Russell, & Cooney, 1994), *Canada* (P. R. E. Crocker & Ellsworth, 1990), *Germany* (Asendorpf & van Aken, 1993), *Italy* (Pedrabissi, Santinello, & Scarpazza (1988), *Greece* (Makris-Botsaris & Robinson, 1991), *France* (Bolognini, Plancheral, Bettschart, & Halfon, 1996), *Holland* (Van Dongen-Melman, Koot, & Verhulst, 1993), *Japan* (Maeda, 1997), and *Korea* (J. Kim, Kim, Kam, & Shin, 2003). The average correlation between perceived physical appearance and global self-esteem across the studies in these 12 countries is .64, with a range of .54 to .70.

In a meta-analysis of the relationship between weight and self-esteem (C. Miller & Downey, 1999), lower self-esteem was consistently related to heavier weight. Interestingly, the correlations were higher in those studies of *perceived* weight than of *actual* weight. Effect sizes were larger for females than for males, which was interpreted as a consequence of overweight females who felt that they had violated cultural standards dictating appropriate body weight.

It is noteworthy that in our society, the domains of physical *appearance* and *athletic* skills are very distinct. In contrast to physical appearance, the correlations between perceived athletic competence and global self-esteem range from .23 to .40, with an average of .33. The pattern is similar in other countries (identified above) where the range is .24 to .38, with an average of .30. The obvious conclusion is that there is a clear distinction between these two "physical" domains, and that perceptions of appearance are far more important to the evaluation of global self-esteem than are athletic skills.

Recent findings add a new twist on the lack of a strong link between physical fitness and body esteem. Duncan, Al-Nakeeb, Jones, and Nevill (2007) found that perceptions of *fatness* were predictive of body image, but there was no relationship between fitness and body image. In a related study, Duncan, Al-Nakeeb, and Woodfield (2008) found that for females, body image was related to body fatness and waist circumference but not to physical activity.

Within the last decade, many more studies have reported a strong correlation between perceived physical appearance and global self-esteem. However, these more recent studies go beyond the mere demonstration of a correlation. They include other variables that may serve as predictors, correlates, or consequences. For example, more contemporary investigations have included indices of depression or negative affect, as have we. Considerable evidence has documented the strong relationship between global self-esteem and depression.

More recent research has identified depressed affect as another major consequence of the dissatisfaction with one's appearance. These studies highlight how negative attitudes about one's looks not only predict a *cognitive* evaluation, namely, global self-esteem, but an *emotion,* in the form of depressed affect or mood.

We have conducted two studies (Kiang & Harter, 2006; Lancelotta, 1999) demonstrating that body satisfaction among college students predicted both self-esteem and depressed affect. In addition, Boyes, Fletcher, and Latner (2007) have reported that among adult women, those with higher self-esteem and fewer depressed symptoms were more satisfied with their body. In a related study, K. Allen, Byrne, Blair, and Davis (2006) found that children (ages 7–13) with weight and shape concerns reported greater body satisfaction, lower self-esteem, and depression, compared to a control group. Blond, Whitaker, Lorenz, Nieto, and Pinto-Martin (2008) have also reported that weight concerns among low-birth weight adolescent boys predicted low self-esteem and clinical depression. Many of the studies to be reviewed will further document the relationship among perceived appearance, self-esteem, and depressed affect, asking more complex substantive research questions, employing more sophisticated designs.

These more recent studies have added features that reveal the numerous complex causes underlying the relationship between body satisfaction and self-esteem. Certain studies have included an objective measure such as the BMI. This index is of increasing importance because it has been the primary measure of the dramatic rise in obesity among adults in this country since 1980. More recently, children and adolescents have been a major focus of the obesity epidemic. Statistics for 2003–2006 indicate that 32% of children and adolescents are at or above the 85th percentile for dimensions that define obesity (Ogden, Carroll, & Flegal, 2008).

Many recent studies have incorporated a longitudinal component, a gratifying new trend, because it can bear upon the *directionality* of the link between perceived physical appearance and global self-esteem. That is, which comes first? Do children and adolescents base their self-esteem upon the perceptions of their physical appearance or do they first make a judgment about their global self-esteem that, in turn, impacts their perception of their appearance? Research bearing upon this issue is presented shortly.

There has also been a major upsurge in the number of studies that address the impact of the media upon perceptions of attractiveness. Still others address the *salience* of physical appearance as a personal attribute, and are directed at cognitive *self-schemas* that involve appearance, *rumination* over appearance, *body fixation*, and the perceived *importance* of appearance. The impact of peers' evaluations of one's appearance and resulting global self-esteem has now also been documented. Studies that have examined gender differences in the level of perceived appearance and its relationship to self-esteem have escalated, as we shall come to see. Another recent trend has been the importance of the bodily self in the lives of males, in contrast to previous research that primarily dealt with the media's impact on females' perceptions of their appearance. The literature on the relationship among perceived appearance, self-esteem, and eating disorders has also received increasing attention. In a number of other studies, race has been the focus. Finally, those investigators concerned with applied issues have put forth intervention efforts to enhance self-esteem and its relationship to appearance-related issues. All of these more recent themes are next addressed.

Longitudinal Investigations and the Directionality of the Appearance–Self-Esteem Link

One example of the inclusion of the BMI is represented in research by O'Dea (2006) who conducted a longitudinal study of 13-year-old girls. The results revealed that higher BMI scores at age 13 predicted more negative evaluations of perceived physical appearance, global self-esteem, and close friendships 3 years later indicating that being overweight is a liability. In another investigation, McCabe, Ricciardelli, and Holt (2005) employed the BMI with 9-year-old girls and boys, finding that overweight children of both genders were more likely (compared to a normal-weight comparison group) to be dissatisfied with their weight, placed more *importance* on their weight, and felt more pressure from peers to lose weight. In addition, these overweight 9-year-olds reported lower levels of self-esteem and more negative affect than normal-weight children. Furthermore, 16 months later, overweight girls as well as boys reported a reduction in their self-esteem.

Another longitudinal study (Paxton, Neumark-Sztainer, Hannan, & Eisenberg, 2006) included early and midadolescent youth of both genders. Time 1 dissatisfaction predicted Time 2 low self-esteem and depressive mood, 5 years later, for *young* adolescent *females*. For boys, this relationship only held for those in midadolescence. The previously documented effects of appearance on self-esteem and depressed mood were obtained; however, they were observed at different periods of adolescence, for females compared to males. One may conjecture that because girls physically mature at earlier ages than boys, girls' sensitivity to cultural messages occurs at earlier ages and has a negative effect, accordingly. For boys, these effects are observed later in adolescence.

Tiggemann's (2005) longitudinal research (over a period of 2 years) with female high school students, specifically addressed the issue of directionality, as a function of time. It was determined that the Time 1 objective measure (BMI) and personal evaluation of weight and body dissatisfaction both predicted global self-esteem, but not vice versa. Tiggemann concluded that heavier *actual* weight, as well as perceptions of being overweight, made adolescent females particularly vulnerable to low self-esteem.

Taken together, these longitudinal studies reveal that both objective indices of being overweight coupled with negative perceptions of one's physical appearance are precursors of later negative global self-esteem. Such findings have implications for interventions designed to impact self-esteem in our youth. Yet there is more to be considered. First, researchers need to address whether *all* adolescents show the same pattern of directionality in which perceived physical appearance determines level of self-esteem. Might there be some whose level of self-esteem precedes their evaluations of their attractiveness? The mere demonstration of a robust correlation between perceived appearance and global self-esteem cannot answer these questions. Longitudinal models, while a great improvement, do not address the *perceptions of the directionality* of the link. Second, the *causes* of the relationship between physical appearance and attractiveness need to be examined. We now turn to these topics.

Subjective Reports of the Directionality of the Link between Appearance and Self-Esteem

In exploring the link between appearance and self-esteem, we chose a methodology different from a longitudinal approach (Harter, 2000). We asked adolescents about this relationship directly. That is, we asked them to endorse one of two possible directionalities. Is it that (1) you first don't like the way you look and then that makes you not like the kind of person you are, *or* is it that (2) you first don't like the kind of person you are and then that makes you not like the way you look?

Sixty percent of adolescents opted for the first choice, indicating that perceptions of their appearance precede their self-esteem. Those in this group also reported that appearance is more *important*, they are more preoccupied with their appearance, and they *worry* more about how they look, compared to those who feel that how they look precedes or determines judgments of their appearance (see also a dissertation by Lancelotta, 1999).

Moreover, there is a particularly distressing pattern for *females* who endorsed the first directionality orientation in which they base their self-esteem on their appearance (Harter, 2000). These females (1) felt more negatively about their appearance, (2) reported lower global self-esteem, and (3) indicated that they were more affectively depressed, compared to females for whom self-esteem precedes judgments of their appearance. The first directionality orientation, therefore, is a pernicious liability for adolescent females in our society, undermining their evaluation of both their outer and inner selves. When these studies were conducted, over a decade ago, adolescent males who bought into this orientation did not show the same pattern of negative correlates, presumably because male adolescents reported that they feel reasonably attractive and therefore their self-esteem was not compromised. Given cultural changes in the expectations that men now adhere to more stringent standards that define male attractiveness, a topic to be dealt with shortly, it will be of interest to determine whether contemporary boys and men who base their self-esteem on their attractiveness manifest these liabilities, as well.

The Impact of the Media on Standards of Appearance

Direct and indirect evidence reviewed earlier in this section demonstrates that the emphasis that our culture places on appearance at every age is primarily responsible for judgments of personal attractiveness (see Hatfield & Sprecher, 1986). Movies, television, magazines, rock videos, and advertising relentlessly promote the importance of physical attractiveness, glamorizing the popular role models who should be emulated. Desirable bodily features such as thinness have become increasingly demanding and unrealistic within the past decades. For example, the Playboy centerfold models and the Miss America contestants have become increasingly thinner over the years (Garner & Garfinkel, 1980). The bar has been raised even higher in that women are not only supposed to be strikingly slim, with long shapely legs, but must have ample breasts, a virtually impossible feat for most females to achieve, as Kilbourne (1995, 1999) has cogently observed in her analyses of magazine advertisements. Kilbourne points out that many of today's models are fabrications, images that are subject to major retouching, are computer generated, or are composites of the bodies of other women. Standards of female attractiveness have become increasingly punishing in that they are unattainable by the vast majority of girls and women in our culture.

Furthermore, articles and ads specifically preach to women that they should alter their appearance through cosmetics, trips to the salon or spa, and, in the extreme, invasive procedures, through plastic surgery. The goal of these personal alterations is to approximate the narrowly defined cultural stereotypes of attractiveness. Meeting these standards will, in turn, presumably enhance self-esteem and garner the favors of others, particularly men, and intimidate women rivals.

Magazines for adolescent females are particularly relentless in their message. Any teen magazine, such as *Seventeen* (increasingly read by preteens) assaults its readers with an outrageous number of ads for make-up, perfume, skin cream, hair products, tips on dieting, provocative clothing, and other glamour items. Adherence will ostensibly enhance appearance, leading, it is purported, to romance, popularity, and high self-esteem. As a result of this barrage of media messages, most adolescent females feel that they fall far short of the ideals of beauty, leading many to feel very unattractive. These perceptions, in turn, take their toll on self-esteem. What are the indirect and direct findings in support of such contentions? We turn next to several sources of evidence.

Indirect Evidence: Gender Differences in Perceived Appearance

Gender differences represent an indirect index of media influences, given that women have by far been the bigger targets of advertising that dictates the cultural standards of attractiveness. Although men have been subjected to media messages that define what constitutes male attractiveness, there has been more latitude in the standards for men, until recently. There has not been the singular focus on physical appearance, the primary criterion for women. For men, intelligence, athletic ability, job competence, wealth, status, and power have all been routes to success, as well as signs of attractiveness. For example, a magazine poll of women, after the end of the 1990 Gulf War, revealed that General Norman Schwartzkopf was judged to be the sexiest man in America! As we shall soon discover, within the last two decades the ground rules have changed for males in our society.

Evidence from a decade ago clearly revealed that males felt better about their appearance, beginning in late childhood and continuing into adulthood (see Harter, 2000). Averaging across numerous developmental studies we found that the mean perceived physical appearance scores for females systematically declined, on a four-point scale, from 3.0 (in third grade) to 2.4 (in eleventh grade), whereas for males the scores remained high at 2.9 to 3.3. Thus, in middle childhood, beginning in third grade, boys and girls feel equally good about their looks. However, by the end of high school, females report dramatically more negative perceptions of their attractiveness than do males. We have further demonstrated this gender difference among college students and adults in the world of work and family.

Moreover, this difference has been found to be highly robust across different countries, where differences between males and females are similar in magnitude and highly significant. These differences have been documented in English-speaking countries, namely, England, Australia, and Ireland, as well as non-English speaking countries, including Switzerland, Italy, the Netherlands, Japan, and Korea (all of which have been referenced at the outset of this chapter).

In recent years, gender differences continue to be documented. For example, Davison and McCabe (2006) have reported that in eighth and ninth grades, girls reported a more negative body image than did males. A similar pattern was obtained in a Korean sample of adolescents, where a higher percentage of girls were dissatisfied with their body, and reported lower self-esteem, than did the boys (J. Kim et al., 2003). In a college sample, Lowery et al. (2005) found that women consistently reported a more negative body image than did men. Other studies, employing more complex designs, continue to document gender differences, and will be reviewed. To date, the literature review has revealed no study in which males reported more negative views of their appearance, compared to females.

In addition to comparisons of gender, research has also examined *gender orientation*. We (see Harter, 2000) determined that older adolescence females who reported a feminine gender orientation, as compared to an androgynous orientation, reported more negative perceptions of their appearance (2.3 and 2.9, respectively). Attentiveness to appearance (as judged by ratings of its importance to their feminine agenda) may well highlight the difficulty of meeting the impossible standards of beauty that are touted by our culture, leading to unfavorable judgments of attractiveness. Masculine males judged their appearance more favorably than androgynous males, although the scores of androgynous males were higher than either androgynous or feminine females. In another study on gender orientation (Forbes, Adams-Curtis, Rade, & Jaberg, 2001), women classified as having a feminine gender orientation were more dissatisfied with their bodies and reported lower self-esteem than women with either an androgynous or masculine orientation. Thus, if a focus on femininity requires adherence to largely unattainable cultural standards of appearance, more negative judgments of the outer and the inner self will prevail for those with a feminine orientation.

The Role of the Media: Direct Effects

Within the past decade, scholars have continued to expand upon the detrimental role of the media. As Levine and Harrison (2004) cogently observe, it is indisputable that media content is rife with unhealthy messages about attractiveness and ideal body sizes and shapes, as well as food and weight management. The thinness mandate for females includes clear directives that beauty is a woman's principle project in life and that slenderness is crucial for success and to attract the interest of males. From a biological growth perspective, the cultural ideal of long legs, thinness, and a low percentage of body fat is closer to the first stages of puberty than to the shape girls should naturally attain at the end of puberty, bringing wider hips and more body fat. Attempts to adhere to the cultural ideal of beauty, therefore, derails adolescent girls from normal, healthy development (Smolak & Murnen, 2004).

For females, internalization of standards of attractiveness begins at an early age (Smolak & Murnen, 2004). (I was dumbfounded when our teenage daughter babysat for an 8-year-old girl who told our daughter that she, the 8-year-old, needed a tummy tuck!) In this internalization process, females are viewed as objects that bear the scrutiny of others. On their path to womanhood, adolescent girls are treated as commodities to be looked at and evaluated, particularly by boys and men. In internalizing the gaze of others, females also treat *themselves* as a commodity or object to be viewed and evaluated, a phenomenon that has been labeled as "self-objectification" (see Tiggemann & Lynch, 2001). In the extreme, sexual harassment makes females feel as if their bodies are no longer their own. This loss of control represents a stressor that eventually results in body dissatisfaction, low self-esteem, and eating-disordered behavior.

Moreover, the internalization process can lead to bodily shame (Smolak & Murnen, 2004; Tiggemann & Lynch, 2001). As clinicians working with women in therapy, Roberts and Waters (2004) argue that in a culture obsessed with women's attractiveness, media messages preach to women that their corporeal bodies are unacceptable. Women's bodies need sanitizing, deodorizing, exfoliating, and denuding. The authors observe that female clients must cope with self-loathing about their bodily selves, including reactions of shame and disgust. These emotions target such bodily issues as menstrual periods and vaginal cleanliness, with which women should ideally be preoccupied.

The "tyranny of slenderness" and the culturally manufactured need to make one's body more acceptable stoke the industries of diet, exercise, make-up, hair coloring, personal hygiene products, and cosmetic surgery. Women can be trapped in an ever-escalating expenditure of money, time, and effort, often gaining them little but ill health (Smolak & Murnen, 2004). Sarwer, Magee, and Crevand (2004) document the explosion of cosmetic medical treatments. Heightened body dissatisfaction, frequently accompanied by low self-esteem, is the primary motivation for seeking cosmetic surgery. Sarwer et al. reviewed 30 different procedures over a several year period in the last decade, comparing their frequency. For women, these include breast augmentation, tummy tucks, and face-lifts, and for men, nose alternations, abs construction, and muscle augmentation. They documented a dramatic increase in such procedures from approximately 2 million in 1997, to 5.5 million in 2000, and almost 8.5 million in the year 2001.

Data from the American Society for Aesthetic Plastic Surgery (2008) charts changes from 2001 to 2007. The 2001 data match those reported by Sarwer et al. (2004). The incidence of plastic surgery remained about the same until 2004 when it rose to over 11 million procedures and remained constant at that level through 2007. When broken down by gender, 90% of these procedures are performed on women (Botox, face-lifts, tummy tucks, and breast augmentation are popular). Moreover, women account for the sharp rise in 2004. Procedures performed on men (e.g., to enhance muscles) have remained relatively constant from 2001 to 2007, hovering around 1 million per year. Clearly this is a powerful index of the impact of the media, particularly for females.

From a developmental perspective, media messages are targeting young girls. In March 2011, Abercrombie and Fitch made the headlines by introducing padded bikini tops for girls as young as 7. Outrage by many parents erupted. But the point was not lost on young girls. Large breasts are a major asset to social success.

The previous analyses have made general references to the media. However, what are the specific dimensions that define cultural attitudes about appearance? To address this issue, we (Kiang & Harter, 2006) developed a questionnaire to capture several themes that have appeared in the literature and the popular press. We identified five themes that reflected separate factors, statistically (in an oblique rotation), although the factors were moderately correlated. The first factor was labeled attractiveness and self-esteem, tapping the link. The second factor was labeled attractiveness and happiness, stressing attractiveness as the pathway to a happy life. A third factor emphasized the importance of being thin, like media models. A fourth factor, attractiveness and social acceptance, causally links good looks to acceptance by others. A final, fifth factor, attractiveness and job success, stresses the important of meeting standards of attractiveness in order to ensure occupational success. Items were scored on a 4-point scale. Means for the all-female sample hovered around 3 for all subscales, revealing awareness of the cultural stereotypes that pertain to appearance. Interestingly, the correlation of perceived appearance and global self-esteem was stronger for those high in sociocultural awareness ($r = .64$) than for those low in awareness ($r = .30$).

Studies Examining Exposure to Visual Representations of Appearance Ideals

Several researchers have either presented visual representations of standards of attractiveness in a laboratory setting or assessed natural indices (e.g., TV viewing) of exposure to cultural stereotypes. One study (Bell, Lawton, & Dittmar, 2007) addressed the effect of music videos that depicted scantily clad female models whose bodies epitomize the ultrathin sociocultural ideal for young women. The target participants, older teenage females (16 to 19), watched three music videos while the control group was presented with a word-learning task. In this pre–post design, measures of body dissatisfaction were administered before and after the two conditions. Only those females who were exposed to the music videos reported increased body dissatisfaction at the posttest.

Studies reviewed by Levine and Harrison (2004) have revealed that elementary and middle school girls, as well as college women, who devour fashion magazines, typically compare themselves to the models. They reported greater body dissatisfaction, as well as higher levels of disordered eating, compared to those less likely to consume such magazines. In a similar vein, Hargreaves and Tiggemann (2002) found that females, 15 to 18, were more negatively affected by the thin-beauty ideal on television if appearance was judged to be highly important.

In a subsequent study (Dohnt & Tiggemann, 2006), the investigators demonstrated the negative impact of appearance-focused television programs at even earlier ages, namely, 5- to 8-year-olds. Girls who witnessed the thin ideal on television expressed dissatisfaction with their appearance, 1 year later. Moreover, the desire for thinness was found to temporally precede low self-esteem. The authors concluded that as early as school entry, girls are already aware of the thin ideal in a way that negatively impacts the development of body image and self-esteem.

In another study with adolescent females as well as males, Harrison (2001) demonstrated that greater exposure to the television exposure of media images of attractiveness. This increased the discrepancies between peoples' perception of their actual body (which became more negative) and their ideal body (to match the media images). These discrepancies led to greater body dissatisfaction, the drive for thinness, and eating-disordered symptomatology. Barlett and Harris (2008) have also studied both female and male college students, to determine whether playing a video game that emphasized cultural ideals of attractiveness would impact body image. Female characters embodied the thin ideal, whereas for males the ideal was muscular. For both genders, more negative body esteem was reported after the video exposure. In a different experiment, men who viewed ideal body images reported more negative perceptions of their body and lower global self-esteem than men presented with neutral images (Hobza, Walker, Yakushko, & Peugh, 2007). These studies provide more direct evidence demonstrating the pernicious effects that media images of idealized standards of attractiveness can produce in both females and males.

The continuing preoccupation with women's thinness, weight, and physical appearance could recently be observed in a February 2011 *New York Times Book Review*, in the section on "Advice, How-To, and Miscellaneous" new offerings. Fourteen of the 20 books listed were insistent on particular diets. These included "the lean belly prescription," "the crazy sexy diet," "the carb lover's diet," and "eat this, not that." Thus, women continue to be assaulted with messages emphasizing the need to meet unrelenting cultural standards of thinness.

The Role of Social Comparison

Exposure to idealized media images of attractiveness is assumed to stimulate social comparison whereby individuals compare themselves to media images and to others of their gender. For most American females, the results of such comparisons are unfavorable, because it is virtually impossible for most women to emulate the punishing standards of beauty (see Levine & Harrison, 2004). In an interesting historical analysis, Anderson-Fye and Becker (2004) observe that the early 20th century brought with it the introduction of ready-to-wear clothing that came in standardized sizes. The awareness of such sizes, in combination with advertising, encouraged if not forced women to compare themselves to one another, often negatively.

An empirical study of teenage girls by Clay, Vignoles, and Dittmar (2005), found that older, compared to younger, adolescents reported lower self-esteem that was predicted by a corresponding difference in body dissatisfaction. The pattern paralleled the internalization of sociocultural attitudes toward appearance as well as social comparison with media models. In another investigation, Lennon, Lillethun, and Buckland (1999) determined that women with high self-esteem reported less social comparison when presented with fashion advertisements, and less dissatisfaction with their appearance, than low self-esteem participants. Moreover, those who reported less social comparison were found to use various strategies, such as merely scanning rather than scrutinizing the ads, in order to distance themselves from the idealized images. Thus, both sociocultural analysis and empirical evidence document the detrimental effects of the social comparison process for women. For those who compare their appearance to either media models or to other women, in general, the preoccupation inherent in subjecting themselves to such comparisons provokes negative evaluations of their attractiveness.

The Impact of Peers on Perceived Appearance and Self-Esteem

Cooley's (1902) looking-glass-self formulation has clear implications for the potential impact of peers upon perceptions of appearance and self-esteem. For Cooley, significant others are the social mirrors into which we gaze for feedback about the self. These processes clearly apply to the arena of physical appearance where the judgments of others can have a dramatic impact on one's self-perceptions. As noted earlier in the chapter, the "outer self" is always on display for others to evaluate. Peers constitute an important and very prevalent class of others who can be relentless and sometimes cruel, in their evaluations of attractiveness.

One study (Dohnt & Tiggemann, 2006) has revealed that the peer expression of ideals for attractiveness (e.g., thinness for females) begins at very early ages. In their sample of 5- to 8-year-old girls, peers' idealization of thinness predicted young children's desire for thinness, even 1 year later. Despite the fact that most children are raised within the crucible of the family, findings demonstrate that peer and media influences are greater than the impact of parents (see McCabe & Ricciardelli, 2004).

A major focus in research on the impact of peer attitudes has been peer reactions to others' weight. These effects, which begin in childhood, can be seen in several studies conducted during the last decade. Findings with 9-year-olds (McCabe et al., 2005) demonstrated that both overweight girls and boys were more likely, than a normal-weight comparison group, to place importance on their weight, perceive more peer pressure to lose weight, and be dissatisfied with their weight. In addition, these overweight 9-year olds reported lower levels of self-esteem and more negative affect than normal-weight children. Over time, both overweight girls and boys reported a reduction in their self-esteem, 16 months later. In a related study (J. Thompson et al., 2007), overweight and at risk for overweight adolescent girls reported greater body dissatisfaction than average-weight girls. The overweight groups also reported that they encountered more negative comments by peers about their appearance.

Wertheim, Paxton, and Blancy (2004) have pointed out that friendship groups exhibiting relatively high body dissatisfaction are more likely to talk to each other about weight, shape, and diet. This style of talk (e.g., "I'm so fat," "No, you're not" conversations) has been described as "fat talk" (Nichter, 2000). One consequence of "fat talk" may be to set up norms about acceptable body shape, size, and appropriate behaviors to maintain or achieve the ideal.

A number of studies have investigated the impact of teasing by peers on self-perceptions of appearance. In a recent longitudinal study by M. Eisenberg, Neumark-Sztainer, Haines, and Wall (2006), adolescents who were teased about their weight at Time 1 in early adolescence reported lower self-esteem, a more negative body image, and greater depression at Time 2, 5 years later. These adolescents experienced continual teasing over the 5-year period.

In addressing a similar issue, Adams and Bukowski (2008) found that obese female adolescents (unlike those who were nonobese) experienced peer victimization about being overweight. Moreover, peer victimization predicted more negative perceptions of appearance that, in turn, predicted depression and an increase in the BMI, 4 years later. For males, victimization by peers also predicted more negative appearance self-evaluations. Interestingly, however, the males manifest *decreases* in BMI. One possible explanation is that males take a more proactive approach to losing weight. Studies have found that males are more prone to exercise in response to negative perceptions of their weight. For example, as McCabe and Ricciardelli (2004) note, exercise is a more likely strategy for males than females, in order to avoid fat and build a muscular physique.

Finally, one study indicates that the effects of peer teasing can have long-lasting effects (Gleason, Alexander, & Somers, 2000). Among 20-year-old college students, retrospective memories of childhood teasing about their physical appearance was still significantly predictive of poor body image and lower self-esteem, for both genders. Across all of these studies, it is clear that peer feedback about appearance can have a resounding impact on negative self-evaluations of unacceptable appearance that, in turn, will produce feelings of low self-esteem.

The Role of Appearance Schemas

Appearance schemas refer to several phenomena including cognitive filters, making appearance highly salient, the fixation on appearance, rumination about appearance, emphasis on the importance of appearance, and an orientation in which appearance is perceived to determine self-esteem. The research consistently demonstrates that a preoccupation with appearance, as manifested by these phenomena, leads to more negative evaluations of one's attractiveness.

Certain studies combine a focus on appearance schemas with media exposure to ideal body images. For example, Ip and Jarry (2008) classified women as high versus low with regard to their investment in their appearance as a salient self-evaluative dimension. Those identified as highly invested reported more negative evaluations of their appearance as well as lower self-esteem when exposed to advertisements portraying today's thin media ideal, revealing how such schemas can make one vulnerable to media messages. In a related laboratory investigation, J. Jung and Lennon (2003) noted that women vary in their appearance schemas, defined as a cognitive representation of the self in relation to appearance. As in the previous study, women (of college age) were divided into two groups: highly schematic and those for whom appearance schemas were not that salient. Half of the women in each group were exposed to photos of attractive female images, culturally defined. The other half was not exposed to such images. Among those presented with photos, the women who were schematic for appearance exhibited a more negative body image, lower self-esteem, and more depressed mood than those who were aschematic.

Clark and Tiggermann (2008) examined these appearance schema processes in a 12-month longitudinal study of 9- to 12-year-old girls. Those with more pronounced appearance schemas, greater internalization of appearance ideals, and a higher BMI reported a more negative body image, 1 year later. In a cross-cultural study, J. Jung and Lee (2006) compared American and Korean college women, each group divided into those with high and with low appearance schemas. Those in the first group, for whom appearance was a very salient feature of their self-evaluation, were less satisfied with their bodies and reported lower self-esteem than those in the second group, with low appearance schemas. Interestingly, Korean women placed greater importance on appearance, were more critical of their bodies, and reported lower self-esteem than American women. One can conjecture that Western ideals of attractiveness (e.g., height, breasts, and features such as eye shape), which are difficult for Asian women to attain, may be responsible for the more negative evaluation of their appearance.

Other research has directly assessed the role of the *importance* attributed to physical appearance. Mendelson, Mendelson, and Andrews (2000) conducted a study of participants, ages 16 to 21, who rated their weight as important, compared to those for whom weight was not that important. Women in the first target group gave low ratings of their appearance, weight satisfaction, and self-esteem. In addition, for those who regarded weight as important, a higher BMI also predicted negative evaluations of appearance, as well as perceptions of the negative judgments of self by others. Positive evaluations of appearance, in contrast, predicted higher self-esteem. In an interesting twist, Tiggemann (2001) addressed adolescent life concerns in several domains. Although academic success and intelligence were rated as major personal goals, it was the importance of appearance and the emphasis on slimness that most strongly predicted global self-esteem, as well as body dissatisfaction and disordered eating behaviors.

A variant of this theme can be seen in a study by Verplanken and Velsvik (2008), who addressed chronic negative body image thinking among adolescents (ages 12 to 15). Such rumination was found to contribute to low self-esteem, over and above mere body dissatisfaction. The authors indicate that a negative body image as a "mental habit" contributes to greater body dissatisfaction and may have implications for intervention to alter attitudes and their potentially harmful consequences. In a similar vein, Wrench and Knapp (2008) examined the effects of body image *fixation* among gays and lesbians. Image fixation was related to lower self-esteem and depression. Moreover, gay/bisexual males had significantly higher levels of image fixation, antifat attitudes, and depression than did lesbian/bisexual females.

Other studies have examined appearance-related cognitions in the form of directionality orientation, asking which comes first, perceived appearance or self-esteem. We have found that those who base their self-esteem on perceptions of how they look, compared to those who report that self-esteem precedes their evaluation of their appearance, report more negative perceptions of their appearance, lower self-esteem, and more depressed affect (Harter, 2000). In an interesting outcome study, Park and Manor (2009) demonstrated that *high*-self-esteem adults who based their self-esteem on appearance sought to connect with others following a threat to their physical attractiveness. In contrast, *low*-self-esteem adults who staked their self-esteem on appearance wanted to avoid social contact, viewing it as risky. Thus, coping strategies for those who base their self-esteem on their appearance interact with one's initial level of self-esteem.

The two studies summarized above addressed the directionality between appearance and self-esteem. However, a sociocultural approach must also contend with perceived *consequences* of adherence to societal norms of attractiveness, other than self-esteem. As Kiang and Harter (2006) documented, one belief is that attractiveness will promote social acceptance. In a dissertation, Lancelotta (1994) built upon this perceived link. He constructed two types of questions designed to assess young adolescents' perception of the strength of this perceived relationship. Link questions asked if respondents felt that how they look affects whether their classmates accept them, thus reflecting sociocultural values that emphasize the importance of appearance. Nonlink items assessed the perception that how one looks does not affect whether peers accept them. Adolescents were divided into two groups: those who endorsed the link statements and those who selected the nonlink statements.

There were several interesting outcomes predicted by these two types of orientations. Link adolescents (63% of the sample) reported (1) more attunement to media messages emphasizing the importance of appearance in garnering peer approval, (2) greater preoccupation with their appearance, (3) less satisfaction with their appearance, (4) lower levels of peer support, and (5) lower self-esteem, compared to their nonlink counterparts. Thus, endorsement of links, be they between appearance and self-esteem or appearance and peer approval, has demonstrable negative psychological consequences for the individual.

Interlude on the Impact of Female Media Icons on Women's Changing Hairstyles

The preceding discussion of media influences on standards of beauty has drawn upon sociocultural commentary and research investigations. What else might we learn to enhance our understanding of these phenomena, from women working in the beauty trenches, namely, experienced hairstylists? To address this question, I interviewed my hairstylist, Darlene Stuart, who owns Salon Marquis in Lakewood, Colorado. Her experience and knowledge tells a story of how for decades, women in our society have flocked to salons trying to emulate the hairstyles of the media icons of their day (D. Stuart, personal communication, September 18, 2009). Stuart further observed, insightfully, that those popular media role models who have frequently changed their hairstyles triggered a correspondingly immediate, if not frantic, shift to attain the latest hairdo of their idol.

Examples of women in the limelight who have maintained a relatively *constant* hairstyle can be traced back to Mamie Eisenhower, whose ever-present bangs were cherished and emulated by women of her generation. From some years later, we recall an indelible image of Jackie Kennedy's sophisticated cut, for her day, a look that women implored their hairdressers to duplicate. My interviewee went on to identify other role models.

The ice-skater Dorothy Hamill sported a trademark "bob-wedge" cut that became extremely popular and a necessity for many admiring women. Marilyn Monroe, one of the greatest movie icons of her day, spawned the brassy, blonde look that soon became the favored hairstyle of that era. Moving forward in time, model and actress Farrah Fawcett, originally of *Charlie's Angels* fame, flaunted a hairstyle to die for, long, rather unruly locks that women desperately desired to copy. Popular singer Barbra Streisand donned a different look, popularizing the corkscrew or "tootsie-roll" curls framing the sides of her face, another hairstyle to emulate.

Among the more chameleonlike characters on the hairstyle stage, England's Princess Diana qualified for the most awards. Constantly donning a different look, women scrambled to keep up with Diana's latest "do" (much to the delight of hairstylists whose coffers soared)! Two decades ago, another political wife, Hillary Clinton, admittedly less flamboyant, had her fans among a certain segment of the population, who tried to first duplicate her "bob" cut, only to implore their hairdressers to change their style when Hillary went to a more layered look. Oprah Winfrey is another icon who alters her hairstyle as frequently as the wind changes, requiring some women to make yet another hair appointment to keep up with the latest style that graces numerous magazine covers.

Those on the contemporary movie scene, such as actress Jennifer Aniston, popularized the "Rachel" look on the TV show *Friends*. My hairstylist expert also noted that actress Demi Moore made the shift from long locks to a severely short hairstyle for her role in the film *Ghost*, and many fans dutifully followed, in an attempt to replicate the look. Katie Holmes, wife of Tom Cruise and an actress in her own right, also shifted to the very short, but sophisticated cut. So did model and actress Halle Berry. Another media role model, Victoria Beckham, once a Spice Girl and now the glamourous wife of soccer star David Beckham, is another hair Houdini of change. Frequently, she alters her hair length, color, or cut, representing a challenge for her younger female audiences who struggle to keep up with her latest "in" look.

On the current political front, first lady Michelle Obama has already, at the time of this writing, changed her hairstyle three times. It will be interesting to see whether there will be a difference in whether African American women will be more likely to attempt to emulate these changes than European American White women. Finally, although no one has apparently sought to emulate her hairstyle (other than actress-comedian Tina Fey), vice presidential candidate Sarah Palin has popularized the rimless glasses look that seems to be emerging on the societal scene. That said, starting in March 2010, I have observed, in several optical showrooms, that the fashion is now shifting to darker, heavier rims and wider lenses, for women and men! No comment.

Obviously not all women flock like social sheep to achieve the latest "hairdo" of cultural icons. What might determine who is at the head of the line? The themes discussed before this interlude would certainly be critical. Here, we can speculate that (1) those with strong appearance-related schemas, (2) those who are heavily into social comparison, and (3) those who immerse themselves in media messages and the icons whose images are touted, will be the most likely to try to mirror the hairstyles on public display.

Men and Celebrity Hairstyles

But what about *men*? Are they not equally victimized? The fact that their hairstyle history is not as extensive may be a testament to the fact that males have not been as intensely subjected to the unattainable standards of attractiveness that have been the bane of women's existence. Nevertheless, those men upon whom the camera has focused over the years have included Clark Gable, with his slicked-down look, and James Dean, whose more carefree style defined sexiness in his day. Of course, we cannot ignore Elvis, a sex symbol who ascended to the media stage beginning in the 1850s.

On the more contemporary scene, my hairstylist expert pointed to David Schwimmer of *Friends*, who introduced the "comb your hair forward" look that young men began to demand upon their arrival at the salon. Moreover, my interviewees indicated that when Tom Cruise appeared in the movie *Top Gun*, with a very shorn crop of short hair, that became the latest style of choice for those requiring the most current, sexy, look. Only a few years ago, Patrick Dempsey, star of TV's *Grey's Anatomy*, inspired another style, a lush head of hair to die for. Oops, back to the salon!

To confuse men ever further, the bald look has intermittently appeared on the scene. Many will recall actor Telly Savalas, whose hairless sex appeal contributed to his powerful portrayal of a dominating detective. Tennis great Andre Agassi shifted from a fop of long, unruly hair to the bald look, and neither his appeal nor his stellar performance on the tennis court suffered. More recently, basketball star Michael Jordan not only promoted an attractive line of athletic shoes, Air Jordan, but experienced little air resistance on the court given his classy baldness. However, as my hairstyle expert was quick to point out, few men possess the head shape that makes the bald look flattering.

In summary, men have not been quite as victimized by the need to emulate the appearance of icons, compared to the media assault on women. This is changing, however, as the ensuing discussion reveals. A sociocultural analysis and supporting evidence now reveals that men have increasingly become subject to dictates of glamour, with just as negative outcomes, because they, like women, cannot attain the punishing standards of attractiveness demanded.

The Changing Cultural Expectations for Men and Boys

There is ample evidence that for years women have been victimized by culture ideals of beauty that most cannot attain. The media continues its insidious assault by keeping these ideals for women very salient in our society. As Frost (2003) argues, there are now similar concerns for males, beginning in childhood. Boys are now being pressured by societal standards of appearance that require their bodies to be muscular and athletic. As a result, boys who do not meet these new expectations may come to devalue the self and risk peer rejection. There is accumulating evidence for this contention.

Evidence that body dissatisfaction among males is occurring at early ages comes from a study by Schur, Sanders, and Steiner (2000), who found negative evaluations of physical appearance among boys in grades 3 to 6. At somewhat later ages, grades 8 to 11, Jones and Crawford (2005) provide support for the distinction between muscularity and perceived weight, each of which made a unique contribution to body dissatisfaction. They further documented that muscularity concerns were greater among those boys who acknowledged more frequent muscle-building conversations with male peers. McCabe and Ricciardelli (2004) have observed that since the 1950s, cultural icons as well as action figures, such as GI Joe, have become increasingly muscular, as have characters in violent video games who have become more human and less cartoon like. Witness male movie stars and male models who are presented in fitness magazines focusing on body building, rather than on overall health. Thus, males are now exposed, through television, movies, magazines, and video games, to an idealized body image that is far more muscular than the average man. (It is telling that in the play world of Barbie and Ken, Barbie recently ditched her previous boyfriend Ken, for an alternative more muscular specimen!)

Levine and Harrison (2004) observe that males are no longer let off of the stereotypic hook. Men must now adhere to the "masculinity-power" image that is defined by well-developed shoulder, arm, and chest muscles, coupled with a slim waist, hips, buttocks, and tight, ripped abs. Such a muscular body is promoted to be attractive to women because it symbolizes power and success. Central to the impact of media messages is the *internalization* of the ideals of attractiveness that currently emphasize muscularity for males. The image of oneself in the social mirror must become the internal image in one's mind's eye.

Our own research with middle school males (see Lancelotta, 1994) has documented male adolescents' preoccupation with muscularity. It is now widely accepted that dissatisfaction with one's body, including weight, shape, and muscularity concerns, have become more prevalent among adolescent and adult males (McCabe & Ricciardelli, 2004). The authors note that because of these concerns, many adolescent males and men frequent gyms and health clubs, in order to attain an ideal weight and muscularity.

Such male body dissatisfaction has been documented in a recent study of college men (Tiggemann, Martins, & Churchett, 2008). Employing a multifaceted approach, dissatisfaction with weight, height, muscularity, and penis size together predicted negative perceptions of physical appearance.

Experimental studies further confirm these observations. In an experimental study by Hobza et al. (2007), men who viewed ideal male body images reported more negative perceptions of their own body as well as lower global self-esteem than men who viewed neutral images. In another pre–post experimental study (Leit, Gray, & Pope, 2002), college men were presented with advertisements of muscular men. Greater levels of body dissatisfaction were reported after exposure to the ads, documenting the effects of presenting body ideals.

A trenchant sociocultural analysis of the plight of men has been offered by Faludi (1999) in her book entitled *Stiffed: The Betrayal of the American Man*. Much of her thesis still remains relevant. She contends that men seem to be in crisis, confused, and feeling diminished as they struggle to understand what it means to be masculine in today's world. She finds that men seem to find their status diminishing and feel less respected by society than in previous eras. Impotence is on the rise leading to a new genre of medical treatments, as exemplified by Viagra, Cialis, and more recent formulas designed to restore sexual performance and enhance feelings of masculinity. Divorce rates, she observes, are higher than ever with the majority of divorces now initiated by wives.

Faludi (1999) asks why now? She cites several economic factors. The women's movement has empowered many females and has contributed to the diminishment of men, as women advance in the workplace and obtain more educational degrees. She observes that for some men, their economic authority has become eroded. In times of economic hardship, such as the recession at the time of this writing, many men are at risk for losing their jobs. In fact, currently, women outnumber men in the workforce. Moreover, Faludi contends that many males are threatened by women's earning power, particularly in homes where women have become the major breadwinner.

A recent relevant study has experimentally examined what the authors label "threatened masculinity" theory (Mills & D'Alfonso, 2007). They conjectured that men have experienced an increased drive for muscularity, a defining feature of a "real" man, as a result of females' expanded competence in traditionally male-dominated domains. To examine the threatened masculinity hypothesis, the investigators constructed a competitive laboratory task in which there were two feedback conditions (failure vs. success) crossed with two opponent conditions (male vs. female). The primary finding was that men felt the worst about their muscularity, and therefore their masculinity, after failing to a female opponent.

Finally, Faludi (1999) has spoken to the recent culture of glamour, noting that women have historically been considered as sexual objects, as physical ornaments to be admired by men. She argues that this focus has recently shifted to men. Men must now meet new standards of physical attractiveness that require many to attend to their physique, including muscularity, biceps, and abs. However, like most women, most men cannot meet these punishing new standards of appearance. Faludi makes an interesting observation in commenting about how glamour or attractiveness, if it is achieved by men, does not really represent a domain of power, like politics, war, or sports. As such, it does not provide a viable path whereby they can regain their status, as professional and financial success still define a man's identity. In conclusion, Faludi's analysis complements the contentions of other scholars of the self, who have pointed to the detrimental effects of more challenging standards of appearance for men.

Appearance-Related Issues and Eating-Disordered Behavior

Although the etiology of various eating disorders is quite complex and beyond the scope of this chapter, it is clear that appearance-related issues, body dissatisfaction, and self-esteem are implicated in eating-disordered behavior. Our understanding of these processes is informed by the cognitive-behavioral therapy (CBT) model as applied to eating disorders (see Pike, Devlin, & Loeb, 2004). According to one CBT principle, the self-worth (or self-esteem) of the individual with an eating disorder is overly determined by body weight, shape, and appearance. In fact, one of the psychiatric diagnostic criteria for anorexia and bulimia is a disturbance in body image. Individuals with eating disorders imbue body weight, shape, and appearance with intense meaning and extreme importance and are acutely sensitive to minute changes in weight, shape, and appearance, according to Pike et al., in their review of the literature. Weight fluctuations imperceptible to others can dominate the experience of those with eating disorders and can have a significant effect on self-esteem and depressed mood.

Some of the processes revealed in studies with normative individuals can be found in the extreme among those with eating disorders (see Levine & Harrison, 2004). For example, the importance of weight and shape, which is correlated with eating-disordered symptomatology, reflects the internalization of societal values concerning appearance and the beauty ideal of thinness (Geller, Srikameswaran, Cockell, & Zaitsoff, 2000). Moreover, the overemphasis on weight and shape is motivated by the attempt to compensate for feelings of low self-esteem. Thus, for the individual with an eating disorder, the pursuit of thinness is the only pathway to enhanced self-esteem (see also Showers & Larson, 1999).

As Pike et al. (2004) have observed, the societal values that make thinness a holy virtue, and beauty a ticket to happiness, are fundamental to the maintenance of an eating disorder. Achieving the cultural standards of attractiveness is thought to remediate the detrimental experience of low self-esteem. Thus, the fragile victims of eating disorders cling with tenacity to the hope that attainment of the ideal bodily self will enhance their flagging self-esteem. Anderson-Fye and Becker (2004) have further observed a link between (desired) upward mobility and eating disorders, given the belief that social status will be enhanced by adhering to societal standards of beauty.

Concerns of weight and body shape continue to dominate in more recent studies of eating disorders. For example, Serpell, Neiderman, Roberts, and Lask (2007) have documented the fact that adolescent girls with eating disorders reported more negative evaluations of their weight and shape than those without such disorders. Geller, Zaitsoff, and Srikameswaran (2002) have broadened their approach. In addition to shape and weight, they found that those adolescent females who based their self-esteem on intimate relationships displayed more eating-disordered symptoms and reported greater body satisfaction and more negative global self-esteem. In a related study by Sanchez and Kwang (2007), women who derived their self-esteem from romantic relationships reported greater body shame that, in turn, predicted bulimic symptoms.

Our research has addressed the links between eating-disordered behavior and adherence to cultural ideals of beauty, body dissatisfaction, low self-esteem, and depression. Kiang and Harter (2006) developed a statistical model of the relationships among cultural awareness of appearance standards, perceived appearance, self-esteem, and eating-disorder behaviors, a model that has implications for the directionality of effects. Cultural awareness predicted perceived appearance, as anticipated. Perceived appearance, in turn, predicted both global self-esteem and eating-disordered behavior. Overall, the model confirmed the view that perceptions of the cultural standards concerning the value of appearance dictate the negative evaluation of one's own appearance. The subsequent prediction of global self-esteem and eating-disordered behavior is also consistent with the literature. Thus, there is clear evidence that appearance-related processes contribute heavily to the dynamics of eating-disordered behaviors, echoing some of the same effects demonstrated in normative samples, albeit in more extreme manifestations.

Appearance-Based Interventions

Given the prevalence of appearance concerns that are related to global self-esteem, in both normative and eating-disordered samples, interventions to directly impact negative body image have emerged in the applied literature. For example, there have been several targets of such programs. McVey,

Davis, Tweed, and Shaw (2004) have developed a life-skills intervention program designed to improve body image satisfaction and self-esteem. The intervention was found to be successful when the assessment was conducted immediately after the program was terminated. The gains, however, were not maintained at the 12-month follow-up. The investigators emphasized the need to address and assess predisposing risk factors in order to better identify the predictors of long-term gains. In so doing, the authors echo a point that I have argued, namely, that the target of any intervention should be the direct *causes* of the phenomena in question rather than proximal correlates.

A potentially interesting framework for intervening with adolescents who report body dissatisfaction involves the use of exercise. Studies, however, have *not* borne out the promise of such an approach, at least for women. Vartanian and Shaprow (2008) have reported that the experience of stigma around undesirable weight levels among college women was related to a *lower* desire or motivation to exercise. A related study by Strelan, Mehaffcy, and Tiggemann (2003) found that among women ages 16 to 25, appearance-related reasons for exercising were negatively related to body satisfaction, body esteem, and self-esteem. These findings are reminiscent of research cited earlier in this chapter revealing that fitness is unrelated to concerns about fatness. Moreover, many studies referenced have found negligible relationships between perceived appearance and athletic skills. Thus, the fitness–exercise emphasis does not appear to be a viable pathway to correct or improve upon most females' perceptions of unattractiveness.

The literature on treatment approaches to eating-disordered behavior is understandably complex, given that the pathogenic developmental trajectory is influenced by individual, familial, and cultural variables (Cook-Cottone & Phelps, 2006). Nevertheless, most recommendations for intervention include strategies that will lead to a more positive appearance self-concept. This sentiment is echoed by Read and Morris (2008). These authors have lamented the fact that specific treatments to promote body image acceptance is rarely provided in eating disorder services, leaving presumably recovered sufferers at increased risk of relapse. They urge that intervention programs also target both body image and global self-esteem.

In considering the link between perceived appearance and self-esteem, it may be informative to address the issue of the directionality of these two constructs, as a guide to the target of an intervention. As discussed earlier in this chapter, our own approach has been to ask adolescents directly "which comes first" (Harter, 2000). In this manner, we can assess adolescents' perceptions of the directionality of perceived appearance and global self-esteem in their own lives, which, in turn, may dictate which should be the initial focus of an intervention.

For example, a starting point could be to ask a given adolescent to articulate the reason for the directionality orientation that he/she has selected. In our open-ended questioning, we find that adolescents clearly express their personal theories. Responses for why perceived appearance precedes self-esteem include the following types of statements: "I look in the mirror and think I look terrible, you know, my hair, or I think I am fat, and then that makes me not like myself as a person"; "Others act like they think I'm ugly and I believe them and this colors how much I like myself, overall." Those whose self-esteem precedes perceptions of their appearance give explanations such as "I first think about how much I like myself, you know, my personality and stuff, and that tells me how attractive I should feel"; "How much I like myself overall as a person comes first and then that makes me decide how I think I look. If I don't like myself, how can I like how I look?" Thus, by taking these folk theories seriously, one can intervene at a very individualized level, attempting to decouple perceptions of appearance and self-esteem.

A very promising approach to intervention can be seen in the development of *media literacy programs*. One goal of such programs (see Wolf-Bloom, 1998) is to dissect deceptive media techniques (e.g., airbrushing, computerized refashioning of images, substitution of the body parts of another person) utilized to construct idealized images of attractiveness. As Levine and Harrison (2004) point out, the overarching purpose is ensure that students are not "totally naïve, gullible, and passive victims of an insidious, monolithic, media" (p. 708). Girls in the Wolf-Bloom program begin by watching Kilbourne's (1995) powerful *Slim Hopes* video that sensitizes people to advertisements that idealize products that promise instant beauty. The girls also discuss the implications of the predictable discrepancy between real girls' bodies and the "perfect" images in the media. Compared to those who did not participate in the program, participants reported a more positive body image at follow-up as well as reduced social comparison to media models. Levine and Harrison conclude that whereas such programs can create skepticism about the reality of the media images of beauty, the outcomes are short-lived and one-shot programs are unlikely to affect long-standing attitudes. Repeated psychological booster shots may be necessary. Another thought is to have the participants in such programs be leaders to younger groups of children, and thus pass on the message as informal teachers.

Perceptions of Appearance and Self-Esteem among Those with Medical Conditions or Disabilities

The preceding discussion has focused primarily on normative samples of children and adolescents in addition to a brief treatment of the perceptions of appearance and self-esteem among those with eating disorders. We next address the perceptions of appearance and related self-esteem among those children and adolescents who unfortunately must cope with a variety of medical conditions and/or physical disabilities. This topic is particularly worthy of exploration given explicit or implicit assumptions about the negative self-evaluations of these populations. We fell victim to this mentality in our study of youth who are severely asthmatic and who required inpatient care. Given that these children and adolescents were on medications that stunted their growth and distorted their facial features, that they experienced compromising physical limitations, and had been wrenched from their social network and friends from home, we anticipated a range of negative self-perceptions. We expected that they would report low levels of perceived appearance, athletic competence, peer likeability, and global self-esteem.

Nothing was further from the truth. In fact, there were no significant differences between these severely asthmatic children and adolescents from our normative samples. Of particular relevance to this chapter is the finding that both appearance and global self-esteem scores were equivalent to our normative samples, namely, relatively high. Our findings were consistent with a handful of studies that had also examined individuals who suffered from a variety of medical conditions and disabilities (e.g., cancer, diabetes, asthma, cerebral palsy, spina bifida). The earlier pattern seemed clear, namely, that such children and adolescents did *not* report unfavorable perceptions of their sense of adequacy, appearance, or self-esteem. In the first edition of this book, I offered five post hoc interpretations that might explain these seemingly counterintuitive findings, explanations that could serve as hypotheses for future research. In the present volume, this issue is revisited, looking to the literature during the last decade for findings with such special groups. An expanded list of potential interpretations and hypotheses is proposed.

There have been several reviews of this literature in the last 10 years, most of which focus on self-esteem but not specifically on the link between appearance and self-esteem. These are briefly reviewed here because so many of these conditions are physically and visibly compromising, even if perceptions of appearance are not directly assessed. For example, M. Fox (2002) began with the assumption that children with physical disabilities are likely to have lower self-esteem than their able-bodied peers. However, the findings reviewed did *not* support these assumptions. Across studies, children with disabilities reported levels of self-esteem that were similar to their able-bodied peers. Fox suggested that an appreciation for the psychological resilience of children with disabilities should be paramount, when considering such youth.

In an extensive review of the literature on children suffering from chronic diseases, Boekaerts and Roder (1999) compared the social and scholastic functioning, as well as the self-esteem, of such children to nor-mative peer control groups. They found no differences in scholastic func-tioning and reported that children suffering from chronic diseases report self-images that are commensurate with those of healthy children.

In a meta-analysis, LeBovidge, Lavigne, Donenberg, and Miller (2003) examined the psychological adjustment of children and adolescents with chronic arthritis. The children in these studies did *not* manifest signs of poor self-concept. They did, however, display increased risk for internal-izing problems. A separate, single study of adolescents with rheumatoid arthritis and with diabetes (Erkolahti, Ilonen, & Saarijarvi, 2003) exam-ined self-image as well as vocational and educational goals. Compared to a normative control group, the two medical groups showed well-developed self-images with no statistically significant differences.

In another meta-analysis of children with severe disabilities such as crip-pling cerebral palsy and spina bifida, Miyahara and Pick (2006) reported that such children do not have lower self-esteem compared to normative samples. Rather, they concluded that those with *minor* disabilities are more likely to express lower self-esteem. One interpretation, derived from our own work, is that those with major disabilities may elicit more sympathy and support from peers. In contrast, expectations may be higher for those with only minor impairments, expectations that they cannot meet. Thus, the latter group may garner less support or approval from peers, which, in turn, erodes their self-esteem.

Two recent studies have examined the effects of cancer on self-esteem. One such investigation (Langeveld, Grootenhuis, Voute, De Haan, & Van den Bos, 2004) identified young adult cancer survivors, comparing them to a control group with no history of cancer. The level of self-esteem for the long-term survivors was no different from their nonafflicted peers in the control group. The focus of the second study, by Fottland (2000), was the interplay among illness, self-evaluation, and academic experiences in a group of children (ages 11 to 19) who were cancer victims at the time. These children and adolescents clearly valued their own academic abil-ity, acknowledging that academic success was important and had a major impact on their self-esteem. The findings have implications for a Jamesian (1890) interpretation of the causes of self-esteem; namely, the emphasis on domains where one is successful in contrast to those areas that may have been compromised by illness.

Another study of visually impaired children (D. Shapiro, Moffett, Lie-berman, & Dummer, 2008) provided even more direct evidence for James's (1890) contentions regarding the discounting of the importance of domains in which one feels inadequate. These visually impaired children actively discounted the importance of physical appearance, athletic competence, and social acceptance. As a result, they reported moderately high levels of global self-esteem. In another examination of disfigurement, H. Snyder and Pope (2003) remind the reader that although children who suffer from craniofacial distortions are repeatedly exposed to negative social judgments and are subsequently expected to have negative self-evaluations, often they do not. Such children can emerge with an intact, multidimensional sense of self, they argue, even in a society that places considerable importance on physical appearance.

In a related study of disfigurement (Lawrence, Rosenberg, & Fauerbach, 2007), the authors addressed these issues among burn patients, ages 8 to 18. Their findings indicate that both boys and girls do not differ from normal comparison groups in their reports of body self-esteem. Potential protective processes that promote the development of positive self-evaluations are reviewed at the end of this chapter.

Finally, a heartwarming study by Tamm and Prellwitz (2001) assessed 8-year-olds' notions about physically handicapped children in wheelchairs. Most children had favorable attitudes toward wheelchair-bound peers. They expressed their belief that such disabled children would have many friends and would display high self-esteem.

Taken all together, the studies reviewed here point to an inescapable conclusion: children who suffer from a variety of disabilities and illnesses do *not* report lower self-esteem or negative self-images, despite the initial assumptions of many, to the contrary. Although only a few studies in this literature have explicitly focused on the evaluations of appearance, it seems highly likely that many of the disorders examined in this research reported on medical conditions that can negatively impact appearance. Obviously, severe physical disabilities leave children visibly crippled with related motor problems. Many cancer victims, subject to chemotherapy, lose their hair to the point that their heads are shaven. Asthmatic children are often medicated with steroids that can stunt their growth and lead to facial puffiness. Visually impaired and burn-victim children and those whose facial features are distorted present obvious physical abnormalities to their social world of observers. What might be the processes through which such groups of children are able to maintain their self-esteem, their positive sense of worth?

The following puts forth suggestions that may account for the positive self-evaluations reported by children with chronic illness, physical disabilities, and other impediments.

1. *Similar social reference group.* Children with medical conditions or physical disabilities may compare themselves to others with the same condition, rather than to nonafflicted peers in their school or neighborhood. This may be particularly relevant for those attending an inpatient program or a camp for others with the same illness or disability. As a result, self-evaluations would be more positive than if they compared themselves to others without the disorder as their reference group. Relative to others

with the same medical condition or physical disability, they may well feel that they are functioning quite adequately.

Moreover, they may be receiving positive feedback, encouragement, and support from peers confronted with similar challenges. They may also be garnering support from those who are not afflicted. As the study with a normative sample of 8-year-olds indicated (Tamm & Prellwitz, 2001), attitudes toward wheelchair-bound children were favorable, and it was anticipated that they would have friends and display high self-esteem. Extensive literature reveals that support and the approving reactions of peers is a major contributor to self-esteem, as Cooley (1902) first persuasively argued.

2. *Conscious distortion or socially desirable responding.* Another possibility for very positive scores, an interpretation that we entertained in thinking about our asthmatic sample, was that such children were purposely withholding their actual self-perceptions. They simply may not have felt comfortable expressing their true feelings to survey administrators whom they did not know or trust. As a result, they consciously chose to present themselves in the most favorable light possible. Although our question format has been found to be effective in offsetting socially desirable response tendencies in normative samples, it may well be that its effectiveness is limited for children with medical conditions or physical disabilities who need to consciously "table" any personal limitations that could lead to an underlying negative self-image.

3. *Unconscious denial.* At another psychological level, children with medical conditions or disabilities may *unconsciously* deny their inadequacies; that is, they may unwittingly distort the self-portrait that they present to the world given their defensive need to protect and/or enhance the self, in order to avoid the painful realization that they do have limitations.

4. *Confusion between the real and the ideal self.* A related explanation is that such children blur the boundaries between their actual level of competence or adequacy and their desired or ideal image of competence or adequacy. For example, with regard to the realm of physical appearance, asthmatic children present a picture of how they would *like* to look, which perhaps was how they actually did look, before they were put on medication. This psychological strategy may also apply to cancer victims who have lost their hair or those with physical disabilities who anticipate remediation. Thus, in the realm of appearance, there may be two distinct bodily self-images: the real and the ideal (which at one point in time *was* real). On self-report measures such children opt to present the idealized perception of the self.

5. *Healthy adjustment or adaptation to personal challenges and self-standards.* A more charitable interpretation is that these children have

come to grips with the limitations that their medical condition or physical disability has imposed and have adaptively adjusted their standards accordingly. That is, the portrait of the self that they present does *not* constitute distortion, denial, or confusion, but a healthy adaptation to reality and the belief that, given the constraints of their condition, they are actually doing quite well. Several specific processes that are highlighted in earlier sections of this chapter may be operative.

a. Such children may eschew the type of *social comparison* that can lead to negative evaluations of appearance and the self. Two types of social comparison can erode the self: comparisons with peers as well as with media ideals of beauty. To the extent that children can psychologically avoid such comparisons, they can maintain positive self-evaluations that are both healthy and functional as they face the challenges imposed by their condition or disability.

b. Another psychological strategy is to *discount the importance* of domains that are negatively affected by their medical condition or disability. One example can be seen in the study of children with visual impairments (Shapiro et al., 2008) that actively discounted the importance of physical appearance, athletic competence, and social acceptance. To do so is admittedly difficult given a society that so blatantly promotes the adherence to ideals of attractiveness and its link to success and high self-esteem.

c. Many families of children with medical conditions and physical disabilities go to great lengths to provide instrumental, emotional, and social support for their afflicted child. Support can come in many forms, including disabusing children of media images and of the tendency toward social comparison. From a developmental perspective, preteens and adolescents normatively begin to turn to peers as a major source of support. However, for those coping with a chronic disease or physical disability, a focus on garnering parental support may be more adaptive in maintaining a positive sense of self.

The hypotheses suggested above underscore the need to go beyond the standardized administration of self-concept instruments when dealing with children and adolescents who are victims of medical conditions and physical disabilities. That is, we cannot be content to merely ask these special populations to complete our questionnaires, in a business-as-usual fashion. For children with physical handicaps and medical conditions such as asthmas, diabetes, cancer, and obesity, the processes through which self-evaluations are formulated are undoubtedly very complex. As a result, we need to develop ancillary assessment procedures that will do justice to this complexity and that will directly address the various dynamics contained in the preceding hypotheses. We need to develop specific and sensitive techniques that will allow us to test these hypotheses, which in turn will lead to a more complete understanding of the processes underlying the positive self-evaluations of children with clear limitations. Moreover, we must develop explicit models that identify both the causes and consequences of such children's self-perceptions in order to design effective interventions that will allow them to better cope with their afflictions.

Outer Selves around the Globe

The primary focus of this chapter has been the inextricable link between perceived appearance (the outer self) and global self-esteem (a manifestation of the inner self) from a decidedly Western perspective. However, we would be remiss to ignore potential *cross-cultural* differences in how the *outer self*, the bodily self, is defined and displayed, with implications for self-esteem. Western beauty ideals for women demand that one be tall, slim, and big busted as embodied by movie idols, pop singers, television stars, cultural icons, and fashion models. The media depictions underscore the virtually unattainable standards of appearance to which American women must aspire.

What are the ideals of attractiveness for women in non-Western nations? In a recent volume entitled *The World Has Curves,* Savacool (2009) takes her readers on a fascinating global tour of form and fashion, focusing exclusively on women. Her book weaves a rich sociocultural tapestry, revealing dramatic differences across six different cultures, describing historical shifts, as well. In four of the countries that she covers—Japan, Jamaica, South Africa, and Afghanistan—contemporary beauty ideals differ considerably from the Western ideal, each in their own culturally determined manner. Two other countries—China and Fiji—have witnessed dramatic shifts toward contemporary Western standards of attractiveness.

Beauty Ideals in Japan

Savacool (2009) reports that traditional Japanese conceptualizations of the desirable body shape lie in an appreciation for the role of the kimono. This garment emphasizes modesty, communicating that a woman's body, including curves and breasts, should be tastefully concealed, rather than flagrantly displayed. In contrast to American ideals, ample-sized breasts can be an embarrassment to many Japanese women (L. Miller, 2006). Savacool observes that Japanese men have always desired the "cute girl" look, women who possess baby-doll features, instead of the physical characteristics of mature women.

Being physically fit (rather than the Western ideal of excessive thinness) is an expressed value for contemporary Japanese young women that displays the cultural ideal of a strong body combined with a strong mind. Trendy clothing has also become an important definition of beauty for the

Japanese woman. The ideal body type accentuates the adornment of fashionable clothing. Moreover, fashion consciousness is considered to be a pathway to occupational, social, and financial success.

Beauty Ideals in Jamaica

A large body size for Jamaican women is considered attractive and represents a symbol of status and wealth. It reflects the fact that one's providers can guarantee sufficient food intake to maintain their desired size. Weight loss is a sign of neglect or poverty. To be full figured, displaying breasts and curves, is to be full of vitality, to be "ripe" (Savacool, 2009). Some time after Coca-Cola was introduced into Jamaican culture, the shape of the bottle took on a new meaning; it metaphorically came to represent the idealized body type for women. The bottle had a large bottom, a slightly tapered waist, and what suggested a curvy bosom. *Proportion* is the defining factor. One's bottom must be bigger than one's bust, with the waist in between. Ample buttocks are a must. As one of Savacool's interviewees exhorted, Jamaican men always want some meat to grab on to! Anderson-Fye (2004) has cogently observed that the Coca-cola body shape is *accessible* to Jamaican women, unlike the Barbie ideal heralded in the States. Thus, because Jamaican women's actual and ideal body size and shape are closely aligned, their confidence in their appearance, and associated self-esteem, are bolstered.

Beauty Ideals in South Africa

In South Africa, ideals of female beauty can only be considered against the contemporary backdrop of the health concerns in the region. HIV (positive) and acquired immune deficiency syndrome (AIDS) are now rampant among women to the point of being pandemic. Savacool (2009) describes a 2007 United Nations report revealing that 61% of women in sub-Saharan Africa are now human immunodeficiency virus (HIV) positive, the highest proportion of infected women in the world. She attributes this crisis to several factors; namely, lack of health education, dismissive attitudes toward women (lack of respect and no compunction about sexual violation), and, at its worst, rape. Moreover, infected women are stigmatized and their condition is viewed with hostility and rejection by their families. In effect, they are orphaned. Many go into prostitution where they are likely to infect others and perpetuate the cycle. One obvious physical symptom is drastic weight loss. As a result, thinness is equated with illness. A larger figure, in contrast, is considered attractive and a sign of good health.

The cultural emphasis for women with a larger and heavier body raises different, equally serious, health concerns. Faber and Kruger (2005) alert us to the fact that 41% of women in this region are overweight and an additional 30%, by medical standards, are obese. Obesity, in turn, puts one at risk for diabetes and heart attacks. However, the vast majority of women do not view themselves as overweight nor do they express a desire to lose weight. To complicate the psychological scene, Savacool (2009) observes that men equate plumpness with good health. A full-figured wife is a sign that the husband can provide for his wife, including sufficient food to allow her to maintain weight. A plump wife represents a symbol of his economic power. The obesity crisis, therefore, will go untreated because thinness is not considered to be a physical commodity; rather, it is directly equated with illness in the form of HIV/AIDS.

Researchers Puoane et al. (2005), in their article entitled "Big Is Beautiful," elaborate on the seeming positive psychological consequences of being overweight or obese. Larger women enjoy respect and the admiration of the community. Although for a brief period these full-figured women were tempted to emulate the ideals of *white* South African women, they reverted to their desire to be "natural" and to look Black. They expressed pride in their full, curvaceous bodies, and renewed their confidence in their African heritage and identity, bolstering their sense of self-worth.

Beauty Ideals for Women in Afghanistan

An appreciation for the standards of appearance among women in Afghanistan requires that one acknowledge the political realities of that country. In 1995 the Taliban seized power from the existing regime and with it came many oppressive mandates for women. For example, women were required to wear the traditional burka, a garment that completely covered the body and head (except for the face).

Afghan women described to Savacool (2009) how they have never focused on their body or body parts as do American women whom they feel are fixated on their appearance. They are aware of Western beauty ideals, but counter that they do not possess the body image concerns that preoccupy American women. Rather, Afghan women focus on a "good package," which constitutes black hair, fair skin, and round, fleshy bodies that could be described as "chubby," a body type that their men desire. Like other Third World countries that have experienced war as well as famine and its consequences, thinness is far from an ideal. Moreover, the harsh physical demands of daily life, the challenges of childbearing and child rearing, and economic hardship, as well as safety concerns, preclude any preoccupation with appearance.

Beauty Ideals in China

In contrast to the nations described above, Savacool (2009) found that the beauty ideals in China have relatively recently undergone dramatic shifts.

They have coincided with increasing access to Western values that promote a new and different ideal of attractiveness. For centuries in China, a rounded look, including a noticeable belly, was considered feminine. After the Communist takeover in the 1960s, the leadership favored (if not demanded) a more masculine, angular body ideal that would represent revolutionary fervor. Women were forced to don gray shapeless uniforms, to bind their breasts flat to the chest, and to adopt either pigtails or very short hair, devoid of style. Individuality was not permitted.

In the 1980s, politically and economically, more latitude was introduced into the system, including beauty ideals for women. Television and magazines became available, drawing women to an awareness of the standards of beauty for American women, in particular. These sociopolitical changes provided a new ideal for Chinese women. Women were now expected to be long and graceful, tall, but not taller than men. Large eyes were admired, and fair, if not white, skin was touted. The Western cosmetic industry foresaw a vibrant new market for appearance-enhancing products. Among Chinese women under the age of 30, the new look became a necessity, not just a luxury.

These new images of beauty were not lost on young Chinese girls. Several years ago, when in Beijing, I visited a Chinese department store. There, I discovered three Chinese girls, about 8 years of age, wistfully admiring an American female manikin who was white, tall, slim, blonde, and large breasted. Our Western standards have clearly been imported to China and are now flaunted for all to witness and covet, including impressionable young children.

Savacool (2009) observes that as of 2009, the beauty industry in China is thriving. Within the past 20 years, there has been an explosion in the prevalence of plastic surgery. For working women, achieving various bodily transformations is considered an economic pathway to higher-paying positions and greater social status. However, to attain the desired look comes at a painful price, both financially and physically. Determined Chinese women must subject themselves to multiple surgeries designed to produce effects such as a higher nose bridge, bigger breasts, and rounded eyes. In order to be taller, they subject themselves to *bone breaking*. Legs are literally shattered and a metal rod is inserted in order to gain a few inches in height, which will presumably bring greater economic status and power.

Sadly, 70% of Chinese female university students contend that they are too fat. Moreover, eating-disordered behaviors are on the rise among normal-weight women, documenting one negative consequence of their adherence to media images that, for some years, has been observed among young American women. In summary, Chinese women have had to endure a roller-coaster ride during their history of changing appearance ideals. Their current fixation on Western ideals is provoking many of the same liabilities we witness in contemporary American culture.

Beauty Ideals in Fiji

A dramatic technological turn of events provoked the transformation of Fiji women's ideals of beauty within just a decade. In 1989, a researcher (Becker, 1995) visited the fishing villages of Fiji to conduct a study on body image. Becker encountered a culture of women virtually devoid of any concerns about body shape or size. A larger body was considered to be a positive attribute and they were hardly preoccupied with their weight. The women were relatively short, averaging 5'5", and would be considered fat by American standards. (Their BMI in 1989 was 29.8, Becker determined, noting that in the United States a value of 30 is considered obese.) However, Fiji women viewed heaviness as a sign of health, rather than a concern.

Becker returned to Fiji in 1998, slightly less than a decade later. What he encountered was a total reversal of ideals about women's body size. Moreover, as Savacool (2009) notes, 15% of the women displayed eating-disordered behavior. What could be the explanation for this dramatic shift in values? She and Becker (1995) tell an interesting story that begins with a single cultural event, the introduction of *television*. Television came to the fishing village and soon became available to the average Fijian. In fact, it became a household fixture, the focus of home life, the centerpiece, par-ticularly at suppertime as the family gathered around the TV set.

Women observed, as they eagerly devoured American shows such as *Friends*, *Sex and the City*, and the like, that the successful, desirable woman was skinny, by their standards. These images provoked a dramatic and instant paradigm shift in Fijian body ideals. TV women stars were held up for social comparison. Moreover, TV had a more immediate impact than the mere static images in magazines. They became more enviable. Fijian women yearned to adopt the slim look but felt like failures when they discovered that most could not even approximate the new beauty ideals that they now embraced.

Another major contributor was *tourism*, which has become Fiji's fast-est growing industry. As Savacool (2009) observes, visitors began to come in droves, mostly from New Zealand, Australia, the United States, and the United Kingdom. Fiji became, and still is, saturated with wealthy white women guests who became the embodiment of the popular TV icons they had come to admire and emulate. Many women in Fiji attempted to make a transition from the previous full-bodied norm to more Western standards of beauty that emphasized thinness, although without great success.

A research team that has studied body images among indigenous Fijian female youth (L. Williams, Ricciardelli, McCabe, Waqa, & Bavadra, 2006) discovered that the contemporary beauty ideals promoted by the media emanate from Western companies that control much of the TV produced in countries like Fiji. Exposure to American television and to Western tourists led *Fijian* women to defect to Western standards of attractiveness.

In contrast, African women have retained their preference for a rounder, heavier look, and Jamaican women have kept their focus on the desirability of curves.

Concluding Remarks

The degree to which women in these nations are successful in meeting their cultural beauty standards has implications for their feelings of self-worth as well as their life satisfaction. However, there is little empirical evidence on the relationship between perceived appearance and global feelings of esteem in these cultures. Earlier it was noted that the correlation between appearance and self-esteem is high in other Western cultures, although there is little research on the non-Western cultures described in the analysis above. Moreover, in such cultures, little is known about the directionality of this link. Nor is their knowledge about the importance of social comparison, the prevalence of appearance-related schemas, or the cultural rewards and sanctions for behaviors designed to achieve beauty ideals.

Chapter 6

Self-Conscious Emotions

In addition to the construction of cognitive concepts or self-evaluations about the self that have been described in Chapters 2–4, children, adolescents, and emerging adults come to develop *affective* reactions to the self that have been labeled "self-conscious emotions" (see M. Lewis, 2000, 2007, 2008; Tangney & Dearing, 2002; Tangney & Fischer, 1995; Tracy, Robins, & Tangney, 2007). These include pride, shame, guilt, embarrassment, and humiliation. The term "self-conscious emotions" refers to the fact that these affects require self-awareness, meaning reflection upon the self that is evaluative in nature. Thus one activates "consciousness" about personal positive and negative characteristics and attaches an affective reaction. Tracy and Robins (2004) contend that self-conscious emotions primarily arise when people fail to live up to actual or ideal *self-representations* and thus personal *identity* issues are paramount. However, these emotions are also deeply embedded in the social matrix of early relationships where the evaluative reactions of *others* are paramount. That is, the individual must remain vigilant to the manifestations of how he/she is viewed in the eyes of significant others and be keenly aware of the consequences of his/her social reactions.

Leary (2008) argues that self-conscious emotions have evolved more in response to a concern with what *other people* think of us than as a reaction to what we think of ourselves. In particular, these emotions signal fear of interpersonal rejection (Leary, Koch, & Hechenbleikner, 2001). Thus, they function to regulate our social interactions with others (see also Baumeister, Stillwell, & Heatherinton, 1994). From this perspective, self-conscious emotions serve *self-regulatory functions*, in that individuals must monitor and adjust their personal behavior in the service of sustaining positive relationships with the significant others in their social network (see Tangney, 2003). Tangney takes the argument one step further, arguing that self-conscious emotions function as a *moral barometer*, providing salient feedback about our social and moral acceptability and our basic worth as human beings. They guide and regulate our behavior, providing the motivation to adhere to social and moral standards. These motivations do not preclude a concern with violating one's ideals for the self, given that these personal goals are typically defined by the social expectations of others.

This chapter begins with an examination of pride and shame, as prototypical positive and negative self-conscious emotion, respectively. We examine the cardinal features of these two emotions, about which there is now considerable agreement (Lewis, 2000, 2007, 2008; Tangney & Fischer, 1995; Tangney, Stuewig, & Mashelk, 2007; Tracy et al., 2007). Attention then focuses on the cognitive-developmental prerequisites necessary for the *display* of these emotions in early childhood as well as the socialization experiences that nurture the emergence of these affective capabilities. The early behavioral expression of self-conscious emotions is to be distinguished from the subsequent *understanding* of these affective concepts in middle childhood, as revealed through language.

Our own research, documenting a four-stage developmental sequence of this later understanding of pride and shame in childhood, is then presented. Here, we adopt an I-self, Me-self framework in demonstrating that over the course of early development, the I-self eventually becomes "conscious" of the Me-self. That is, it comes to take the Me-self as an object of reflection and evaluation, producing an emotional reaction. Thus, the I-self develops the ability to be proud of the Me-self, or, alternatively, to be ashamed of the Me-self. The *functional* value of these two emotions is also explored, in keeping with contemporary arguments emphasizing that even the negative affects have adaptive functions of evolutionary significance (see Saarni et al., 2006).

It is perhaps telling that, in general, there are more negative than positive emotions in our culture as reflected in the English language. The same holds true for self-conscious emotions. We have one positive such affect, pride (with a less flattering version in the form of hubris). In contrast, we can linguistically identify four negative self-conscious emotions, namely, shame, guilt, embarrassment, and humiliation. It has been argued (see Elison & Dansie, in press) that these negative self-affects constitute a *family* of emotions that share certain common features while also differing in their manifestations, correlates, and consequences.

It should be noted that in both past and current explorations of this family of emotions, the primary emphasis has been on shame, guilt, and embarrassment. Humiliation has been neglected, if not virtually ignored, in the literature until very recently. This is surprising, given that every day in America children and adolescents, in schools, on playgrounds, in neighborhoods, and on the Internet, are being bullied and humiliated, in increasing numbers (Mattaini, 2008; Olweus, 2008). My own interest in this topic was stimulated by the media accounts of the now 12 high-profile cases of the school shooters whose murders of classmates were first documented in 1996. An examination of the histories of these White middle-class males, who were older children and adolescents, revealed that in every case, each had been severely and chronically humiliated by peers. These observations sparked a program of research in our laboratory to unveil the dynamics and implications of this painful emotion. These efforts will be reviewed along with the few other studies devoted to this topic.

In a comparative analysis of these four self-emotions, shame, guilt, embarrassment, and humiliation, I point out both their similarities and their differences. Six themes are addressed: (1) the *causes* of each emotion, (2) the implications for the *self*, (3) the role of *others*, (4) *emotional correlates*, (5) *behavioral consequences*, and (6) the *adaptive functions* of these presumed negative emotions. Pathological implications are also explored.

Pride and Shame as Prototypical Self-Conscious Emotions

Theoretically, an individual should be able to experience self-conscious emotions such as pride and shame in the *absence* of an observing other. That is, the individual should be able to reflect on his/her accomplishments, in the case of pride, and on his/her transgressions, in the case of shame, in situations where significant others are unaware of these causes (Harter & Whitesell, 1989). However, the ability to verbally acknowledge that one is either proud or ashamed of the self represents a developmental acquisition that is highly dependent upon cognitive-developmental skills as well as socialization experiences. In fact, it does not emerge until middle childhood.

From a historical perspective, Cooley (1902) observed that the ability to experience pride or shame in the absence of an observing other must first emerge from particular social interactions with primary caregivers, experiences that promote the internalization of these affective, evaluative judgments. For Cooley, to develop a sense of shame the child must be caught in the act, displaying behaviors that the parent has forbidden. To the extent that the parents express that they are ashamed of the child, gradually this reaction will be internalized so that eventually the child will come to experience shame in the absence of overt reactions by caregivers. A similar analysis applies to pride in that the young child must first have the opportunity for others to be expressly proud of his/her accomplishments paving the way for the internalization of pride in oneself. Thus, the capacity to experience and understand self-conscious emotions is not only dependent upon the developmental acquisition of particular cognitive structures but is also deeply embedded in the matrix of interactions with caregivers. Therefore, these two self-conscious emotions only gradually emerge during childhood.

Features of Pride

The prototypical cause of pride is a personal accomplishment, typically a specific success or achievement in which one has met or exceeded one's goals or ideals. Mascolo and Fischer (1995) have defined pride as a self-conscious emotion that reflects an appraisal that one is personally responsible for a socially valued outcome (see also Tangney, 2003). Examples from interviews with older children in our own research include "I was so proud that I got all A's on my report card," "Getting the lead in the school play made me feel proud," and "I made a bathroom shelf all by myself and was so proud." The *attributions* associated with pride are internal in that the individual takes personal responsibility for the accomplishment in the form of ability and/or effort (see Weiner, 1986). In I-self, Me-self terminology there is a focus on how the I-self, as active agent, takes credit, which in turn leads to a favorable evaluation of the Me-self as competent and worthy. Thus, the I-self is proud of the Me-self.

That pride involves perceived success for a socially valued outcome can be observed by the fact that others may be afforded a role in the self's experience. For example, our own research reveals that in experiencing a private sense of personal pride, children are likely to communicate the event to significant others, in anticipation of a positive evaluative reaction. As one older child in our sample put it, "I couldn't wait to tell my parents about jumping off the high diving board, because I knew they would be very proud of me." Pride is also accompanied by the emotions of happiness, excitement, and feelings of hopefulness.

The overt, *physical* manifestations of pride include an open stance or wide posture in which the chest is literally "puffed up," with shoulders back, a tilted head, typically accompanied by eye contact and a wide grin (Stipek, 1995; Tracy & Robins, 2007a). Research (Tracy, Robins, & Lagattuta, 2005) reveals that children as young as 4 years of age can identify the expression of pride and distinguish it from expressions of happiness and surprise. Pride differs from the latter, more basic emotions, in that it is dependent upon self-evaluations (Tracy & Robins, 2007b). Moreover, Tracy and Robins (2008) have demonstrated the *universality* of the pride expression. Their studies have revealed that individuals from a preliterate, highly isolated tribe in West Africa recognized pride, whether it was displayed by their African tribesman or by Americans.

M. Lewis (2000) was one of the first to draw the distinction between pride and *hubris*. Pride is experienced in reaction to successful achievements that are more specific, whereas hubris is expressed as a more global attribution about the self that has elements of grandiosity, if not narcissism. (Muhammed Ali's frequent self-aggrandizing statements before the public; e.g., "I am the greatest!" come to mind). Lewis has viewed hubris as largely maladaptive, noting that individuals displaying this emotion are inclined to distort or invent situations in order to enhance the self, which can provoke interpersonal problems (see also Tangney, 2003; Tracy & Robins, 2007a). Hart and Matsuba (2007) link hubris to narcissism. Individuals who feel godlike may feel boundless pride that is not tempered by an awareness of their shortcomings and personal failures. Hubris and narcissism are thus fueled by similar types of self-appraisals in that positive actions on the part of the self are magnified and considered to emanate from presumed stable, dispositional qualities. Thus, an experience of elevated hubristic pride reflects the narcissist's self-serving attributions and distortions, particularly following failures (see W. K. Campbell, Foster, & Brunell, 2004).

Tracy and Robins (2007a) distinguish between "authentic" pride and hubris, from the perspective of different attributional processes. Authentic pride focuses on the specific act ("I'm proud of what I *did*") and results from attributions to internal, unstable, and controllable causes ("I won because I practiced hard"). Hubris results from exaggerated, global perceptions about the self ("I'm always proud of *who I am*") and results from attributions to internal, stable, uncontrollable causes ("I won because I am always great"). Authentic pride is based on actual accomplishments and is typically accompanied by genuine feelings of self-worth. In contrast, hubris is fueled by a more inauthentic sense of self that involves distortion and self-aggrandizement. In studying the semantic structure of these two emotions, these researchers have demonstrated that the authentic self is associated with words such as "accomplished," "triumphant," and "confident." In contrast, hubris is linked to descriptors such as "arrogant," "cocky," and "conceited." Consistent with evidence presented by other researchers, Tracy and Robins find that hubris is positively related to narcissism, whereas authentic pride is positively related to high self-esteem.

Finally, many have addressed the *functions* of pride, consistent with the observation that self-conscious emotions motivate people to protect their social well-being and to facilitate their social interactions and relationships (Leary, 2007). Tracy and Robins (2007b) contend that pride functions to foster achievement and caregiving that, in turn, allow the individual to maintain a positive self-concept and to garner the respect and acceptance of others. Hart and Matsuba (2007) further observe that pride, when appropriately experienced, propels people to act altruistically and therefore motivates *moral action*. Motives may include image improvement in the eyes of others leading people to feel better about themselves and experience enhanced self-esteem (see also Tangney, 2003; L. Williams & Desteno, 2008). Moreover, as Tangney points out, pride encourages future behavior that conforms to social standards of merit.

Features of Shame

In contrast to pride, shame is a prototypical negative self-conscious emotion caused by transgressions that constitute moral wrongdoings that *violate* social standards, others' ideals for the self, and eventually one's own ideals as social standards that have become internalized (see Tangney & Dearing, 2002). In addition to failing to meet moral imperatives, shame can result from achievement failures associated with a lack of competence. In I self, Me-self terminology, the I-self comes to denigrate, and therefore be ashamed of, the Me-self, through a developmental progression of stages that are soon described.

Individuals make a global traitlike evaluation of the self as a bad person who is immoral or feels inadequate to the point of being fundamentally flawed. As we shall come to see, from a developmental perspective, caregivers initially shame their children for their transgressions and incompetence, a prerequisite for children's cognitive capacity to feel ashamed of themselves.

Physical manifestations include a bowed head and slumped posture, including shoulders that reflect cringing, and gaze aversion. Behaviorally, with pride, there is a desire to approach evaluating others in order to communicate success, as well as the associated emotions of happiness and excitement. In contrast, shame is accompanied by the desire to hide, avoid others, and distance oneself from those who are in a position to evaluate the self. Associated emotions of disappointment, dejection, and depression are common.

At first glance, it may not appear that shame serves any adaptive function, given the tendency for one to want to avoid immediate contact with others and shrink into oblivion. However, in the longer run, shame can have positive purposes. For example, it may serve to inhibit arrogance and to promote humility. It may provoke self-awareness in the form of soul searching that may lead to the revision of one's priorities and values. It may provide feedback about certain less desirable attributes of the Me-self, leading to greater deference to social standards that may, in turn, result in self-improvement and self-repair.

Cognitive-Developmental Prerequisites of Pride and Shame

M. Lewis (1994, 2000, 2007, 2008) was one of the first to illuminate the role of the *self* in emotions such as pride and shame, that are self-evaluative in nature. From a developmental perspective, the child must first have the concept of a Me-self, what M. Lewis labels the "idea of me." This acquisition promotes the development of *self-awareness*, namely, the ability to become the object of one's consciousness and self-evaluation. These rudimentary processes emerge during the middle of the second year of life, when toddlers can first recognize and label themselves in the mirror ("That's me, Justin!") realizing that others are labeling them, as well. As M. Lewis observes, the emergence of the Me-self allows for the representation of self that can be distinguished from others. It also helps to transform behaviors and interpersonal interactions into an appreciation for the social standards, goals, and rules. These acquisitions, in turn, pave the way for self-appraisals as the young child comes to evaluate his/her behaviors against these standards.

The toddler must first take *responsibility* for adhering to such standards (in the case of pride) or violating social prohibitions (in the case of shame). Taking responsibility, in turn, allows the toddler to engage in rudimentary forms of self-evaluation, based upon a judgment about whether he/she has performed according to these standards. Thus, as M. Lewis (2007) stresses, the child must be capable of "owning" his/her behaviors. If children are unable to perceive that they are the actors or the producers of their behavior (an I-self function), then they would have no basis for evaluating the Me-self. Thus, they must fully realize that they are responsible for their successes and failures.

Others have also articulated these processes (e.g., Hart & Matsuba, 2007; Lagattuta & Thompson, 2007; Stipek et al., 1992; Tangney & Dearing, 2002; R. A. Thompson, 2006). For example, Lagattuta and Thompson identify three cognitive capacities necessary for the emergence of self-conscious emotions. First, there must be the rudimentary sense of *self-awareness* or the basic understanding of a "conceptual" self. This ability is normatively in place toward the end of the second year of life. Verbal self-referential labels are the primary defining feature. For example, looking into the mirror, the child must say something like "That's me." Possessives come to the fore at this point in development, for example, "That's mine!" Other examples indicate that the young child is taking responsibility for his/her behavior; for example, "Look what I did!"

Second, the child must be able to *recognize an external standard* against which his/her behavior or characteristics can be evaluated. That standard may be a social rule, expectation, or goal, that in the case of shame, has not been achieved according to the evaluation of significant others. Third, the child must *adopt that standard* and be able to evaluate the degree to which he/she meets, exceeds, or fails to perform according to that standard. Toward the end of the second year, toddlers become personally sensitive to these normative standards and expectations. Kagan and Lamb (1987) have interpreted such an appreciation as an emerging *moral* sense when behaviors violate the norms that parents enforce through sanctions, for example, if the child breaks an object or hits a sibling (see also Tangney & Dearing, 2002). Thus, rudimentary signs of shame may emerge. Alternatively, when the child's successes correspond to positive social standards, pride will be expressed.

The empirical work of Stipek et al. (1992) is frequently cited as compelling evidence for a three-stage developmental sequence that documents the acquisition of the prerequisites of self-conscious emotions among American children. At the first stage, prior to age 2, older infants and toddlers experience joy in mastery, reflecting their sense of agency or causality. Thus, they will display gleeful behavior if they construct a block tower or successfully complete a simple puzzle. However, they do not call their successful mastery efforts to the attention of adults, nor do they anticipate adults' reactions, nor do they alert others to their failures.

At the second stage, beginning slightly before 2 years of age, young children begin to anticipate adult reactions, seeking positive responses to their successes while attempting to avoid negative reactions to their failures. This stage corresponds to the age at which "social referencing" is observed, where toddlers turn to caregivers and rely on their signals for feedback that may "disambiguate" uncertain events (Barrett & Campos, 1987; Campos & Sternberg, 1980). Stipek et al. (1992) have reported that toddlers now show evidence that they appreciate adult standards; for example, they will turn away from adults, hunching their shoulders in the face of failures. Kagan (1984) has pointed to similar phenomena in describing toddlers' distress reactions when they observe an adult model perform a set of acts that they subsequently cannot imitate, implying that they were aware of their lack of ability to achieve the implicit performance standard.

During the third stage, beginning at age 3, there is evidence that children begin to further incorporate adult standards, in that they appear to evaluate their performance and react emotionally to their successes and failures, independent of adult reactions. For example, frowns and verbal displays of frustration (e.g., "I can't do it!") that are not directed to adults typically accompany failure experiences. These findings have suggested to Stipek and colleagues (1992) that the young child is experiencing dissatisfaction with the *self* and not just the task.

The emergence of these rudimentary forms of self-awareness and self-evaluation pave the way for the initial experience of self-conscious emotions during the second and third year of life, as argued by M. Lewis (1994, 2000, 2007, 2008). Others, however, have taken issue with the age at which M. Lewis feels that self-conscious emotions can be experienced. For example, Buss (1980) suggests that the behavioral manifestations in toddlers reflect "pseudoshame" in the form of fear of punishment, and that self-conscious emotions such as shame do not truly emerge until the age of 5, when a cognitive sense of self is sufficiently complex. (A similar argument has been advanced about pet lovers who claim that their dog experiences shame, as manifest by the head down, slumped crouch, and gaze aversion upon violating their master's moral ground rules. It could be just as easily argued that this behavior simply reflects a reaction to the fear of anticipated punishment.)

Barrett (1995) has also challenged the analysis put forth by M. Lewis, Haviland-Jones, and Barrett (2008), questioning whether toddlers actually experience self-conscious emotions. She makes the logical argument that the cognitive prerequisites postulated (e.g., objective self-awareness, the capacity for self-evaluation) are somewhat arbitrarily assigned to a given age. That is, one can always find rudimentary forms of a given cognitive process in early childhood, in keeping with the trend over the past two decades to identify skills at younger and younger ages. Barrett considers it unlikely that self-conscious emotions are manifest in toddlers.

The approach of Mascolo and Fischer (1995) would appear to circumvent this controversy. They argue that rather than ask at what single point in development self-conscious emotions emerge, we should ask what forms these affects assume at different points in development. They perform such an analysis for pride, shame, and guilt, utilizing Fischer's (1980) skill theory. Eight levels, covering the age span of 7 months to 17 years, identify the different skills and behaviors defining the developmental emergence of increasingly complex cognitive structures that underlie self-conscious emotions and their precursors. The interested reader is referred to Mascolo and Fischer's complete analysis. Here, a few examples of their approach are offered, for the emotion of shame.

The earliest precursors of shame (Step 1 in the sequence at ages 7 to 8 months) include distress over failures to produce through sensorimotor actions (e.g., putting the peg in the hole of a toy). Consistent with the observations of Stipek et al. (1992), at Step 2, approximately 11 to 13 months, distress becomes associated with the caregiver's reactions of disappointment in his/her child. At Step 3, approximately 18 to 24 months, the toddler begins to *anticipate* the negative responses of the caregiver, showing rudimentary displays of shamelike behavior, including avoidant posture and gaze aversion. In Step 4, at approximately 2 to 3 years of age, behaviors suggest that the child is experiencing the precursors of shame caused by the self performing poorly. This conclusion is inferred from statements such as "I'm not good at throwing" or "I'm a bad boy for coloring on the wall" or "Mommy doesn't like what I did."

Their analysis continues beyond the sensorimotor tier into what Fischer (1980) labels the "representational tier" and then the "abstract tier." During the intermediate stages (at the representational tier), shame is inferred from behaviors that reflect one's comparative performance, relative to peers. At the abstract tier, beginning in adolescence, shame about a general (negative) personality characteristic is experienced, for example, not being trustworthy. In later adolescence, one can experience "collective shame," for example, if one's in-group shares attitudes of prejudice toward an ethnic minority out-group. Through such a sequential analysis, one can appreciate the cognitive building blocks upon which more mature displays and understandings of self-conscious emotions rest, rather than trying to identify a particular age at which self-conscious emotions "truly emerge."

An Empirical Developmental Acquisition Sequence of the Understanding of Pride and Shame

As noted earlier, there is a need to distinguish between the *display* of self-conscious emotions and the *understanding* of these emotions that can be verbalized. In the cameo self description during middle childhood (Chapter 2), the child not only refers to the self in terms of basic emotions such as happy and sad, but also makes reference to self-conscious emotions such as pride and shame ("I mostly got A's in these subjects [language arts and social studies] on my last report card, which makes me feel really proud of myself," "If I get in a bad mood I'll say something that can be a little mean and then I'm ashamed of myself"). It is not until this age level that self-conscious emotions appear in the child's linguistic repertoire.

Cooley's (1902) formulation spoke to this issue in that the development of the self included the internalization not only of the *opinions* of significant others but also the incorporation of their *affective* reactions to the self. He specifically identified the internalization of pride and shame, leading ultimately to the ability to feel proud of oneself as well as ashamed of oneself. Moreover, Cooley set the stage for a developmental analysis of how these emotions might emerge. Although pride and shame could clearly be experienced by adults in the absence of others, Cooley noted that "the thing that moves us to pride and shame is not the merely mechanical reflection of ourselves, but an imputed sentiment, the imagined effect of this reflection upon another's mind" (p. 153).

Cooley (1902) was clear on the point that this sentiment is social in nature, based upon social custom and opinion, although it becomes somewhat removed from these sources through an implied internalization process. Cooley wrote that the adult is "not immediately dependent upon what others think; he has worked over his reflected self in his mind until it is a steadfast portion of his thought, an idea and conviction apart, in some measure, from its external origin. Hence this sentiment requires time for its development and flourishes in mature age rather than in the open and growing period of youth" (p. 199). Thus, Cooley's views on the internalization of others' opinions about the self paved the way for a more developmental perspective on how the attitudes of others are incorporated into the self.

In our own work, we have provided documentation for a four-stage developmental sequence governing the development of the conceptual *understanding* of pride and shame. Younger children may manifest or display the emotions of pride and shame through head position and bodily posture (see review by Stipek, 1995). However, it is not until middle to late childhood that children can verbalize that they can be proud or ashamed *of oneself* and that such self-affects become part of their self-definition (as in the cameo child's description). In particular, we were interested in the substages that appeared to be precursors of the child's emerging ability to appreciate that one could be proud or ashamed of the self in the absence of any observation by others.

Focusing on the socialization component of both pride and shame, we devised a procedure that would be sensitive to the role of the observing parent; that is, we sought to determine whether parents were required to "support" the reported experience of pride and shame. Toward this end, we designed two sets of vignettes. To assess shame, we constructed a pictorial vignette with several frames and a brief story line to accompany the pictures. The story concerned a situation in which the parents have forbidden the child to take any money from a very large jar of coins in the parents' bedroom. However, the child transgresses and takes a few coins from the jar.

There are two separate story sequences. In one sequence, no one observes the act, and no one ever finds out (an outcome we attempted to ensure by pictorially depicting and describing the money jar as very large and the child took only a few coins). In the second sequence, the parent catches the child in the act. The primary dependent measures included the participant's (1) description of the emotions that the story child would feel in the first sequence (where the act is not detected), as well as a (2) description of the emotions that both child and parent would feel in the second situation, where the parent catches the child in the act.

To assess an understanding of pride, we selected a gymnastic feat as the demonstration of competence. In the first sequence, the child goes to the playground on a Saturday when no one else is there. The story child attempts a flip on the bars, one that he/she has been working on at school but has never been able to perform successfully before. On this Saturday, he/she does the flip extremely well. In the first pictorial sequence, the child leaves the bars knowing that he/she was the only one at the playground and thus no one else observed the flip. The participant is then asked what feelings he/she would have at that time, if he/she were the story child.

In the second pride sequence, the parent accompanies the child to the playground and observes the child successfully performing the flip for the first time. The participant is asked how he/she would feel, as well as how the observing parent would feel having watched the child doing the flip.

The results for both pride and shame revealed a clear age-related, four-stage sequence that is interpretable within our socialization framework. Moreover, the stages that have emerged are consistent with Selman's (1980) developmental model of self-awareness in which children gradually begin to observe and critically evaluate the self. At our first level, ages 4 to 5, there is no mention of either pride or shame by either the story child or the parent, that is, regardless of whether the story child is observed or not observed. Participants give very clear responses about their potential emotional reactions to these situations, reactions that are quite telling. In the transgression situation where the story child is not observed by the parents, participants report that the child character (with whom they are encouraged to identify) would feel scared or worried about the possibility of detection. When he/she is caught by the parent, he/she also feels extremely scared or worried about the likelihood of punishment. However, there is no acknowledgment of shame.

In the pride sequences of stories, these youngest subjects report that they would feel happy, glad, or excited in the situation where their gymnastic feat is not observed by the parent. In the story where the parent witnesses their child's performance, participants reported that the story child and parent would feel happy, glad, or excited; that is, there is no mention of pride on the part of either the story parent or the story child. Thus, children at this first level are aware that their parents have reactions to their behavior. Consistent with Selman's (1980) first level of self-awareness and with Higgins's (1991) analysis, the child is not yet aware that others are *evaluating* the self, nor can the I-self critically evaluate or affectively react to the Me-self.

Our second level at ages 5 to 6 represents a very interesting transitional period. Children now demonstrate their first use of the terms "ashamed" and "proud." However, their usage is restricted to reactions of the parents. Thus, the parental response to the child's transgression is to be ashamed of the child. However, the child does not yet acknowledge that he/she is ashamed of the self. Rather, the child is still scared or worried about the parents' reaction. Similarly, in the case of the gymnastic feat, the child participants describe how the parent is proud of the child. However, the child is not yet proud of the self. Rather, he/she is excited, happy, or glad.

This level parallels Selman's (1980) second stage of self-awareness and is consistent with Higgins's (1991) analysis; that is, the child's I-self is aware that others are observing, evaluating, and affectively reacting to his/her Me-self ("I observe you evaluating me and being proud or ashamed of me"). This second level, therefore, provides the necessary building blocks for the emergence of the looking-glass self (Cooley, 1902). That is, children must first be sensitive to the fact that they are being evaluated by others in order to direct their attention to the specific content of others' approval or criticism and emotional reactions.

At our third level (between the ages of 6 and 7), children demonstrate the first acknowledgment that shame and pride can be directed by the self, toward the self. In the situation where the act has been observed, not only will parents be ashamed or proud of the child, but children report that they, too, will feel ashamed or proud of themselves, seemingly in response to the parental reaction. However, what also places children at this level is the finding that they do not report any feelings of shame or pride in the story that specifies the *absence* of parental observation. This seems to be another critical transitional level in our socialization sequence, in that the act must be observed in the case of a transgression, in order to experience shame, and competence must be observed, in order to experience pride. In the absence of parental observation, no self-conscious emotions are acknowledged. This level parallels Selman's (1980) third stage of self-awareness in that the child begins to incorporate the observations of others into his/her own self-perceptions in order to directly evaluate the self. Thus, the I-self can now adopt an attitude toward the Me-self that parallels the attitude of significant others, although these self-attitudes and self-conscious emotions must still be scaffolded by others.

The hallmark of the fourth level (beginning at ages 7 to 8), is that in the absence of parental observation, children spontaneously acknowledge that the story children will feel ashamed or proud of themselves. (It should be noted that the stories in which the child was not observed were always presented first, so that any response of shame or pride on the part of the child was not simply a generalization from the sequence in which they were observed.) Therefore, at this level, children appear to have internalized the standards by which shame and pride can be experienced in the absence of direct, parental observation. Interestingly, the large majority of children at this level does not merely report the emotions of shame and pride, but specifically indicate that "I would feel ashamed, or proud, of myself." They appear to be at the stage where these emotions do function as self-conscious emotions in the sense that one is truly ashamed or proud of the self. This final level in our sequence is consistent with Selman's (1980) fourth stage, in which the I-self can now observe and critically evaluate the Me-self in the absence of any evaluative reactions from significant others.

In summary, this sequence not only reveals the gradual nature of the normative, developmental emergence of self-conscious emotions but also suggests that the critical, underlying processes involve parental socialization. Thus, we have inferred that children must first experience others as role models who are first proud or ashamed of *them* in order to facilitate the internalization of these functions for themselves. Even when they first develop the ability to acknowledge that they are proud or ashamed of themselves, children still need the scaffolding of parental surveillance, observation, and evaluative feedback. Thus, the final stage in the internalization process during childhood occurs when these self-affects are experienced in the absence of observations by others, when the I-self can be directly ashamed or proud of the Me-self, when one is all by oneself. (There is little evidence for adolescence or adulthood.)

Other evidence supports this sequence. For example, Lagattuta and Thompson (2007) describe how parental discipline provides a cognitive structure that explicitly links the parents' reactions to the child's violation of the external standards, in the case of shame. These parental reactions will, in turn, induce the relevant self-conscious emotion, for example, a parental exhortation in the form of "You should be ashamed of yourself." Our sequence would amend this recommendation, suggesting that the first parental responses to their young children's transgression should be "I am ashamed of you," as this lays the groundwork for the incorporation of the caregiver's message.

The same is true for situations evoking pride in children, where the parental response should emphasize the child's responsibility for creating a desirable, personal, outcome that will come to elicit the relevant positive self-conscious emotion. We would argue that in the earlier stages of our sequence, the message to the young child should be that "I'm proud of you for figuring that out by yourself." However, toward the end of our sequence parents should shift to feedback in the form of "You must really feel proud of yourself for doing that all on your own."

With regard to the ages at which an understanding of self-conscious emotions is truly appreciated, other findings are quite consistent with our own. Lagattuta and Thompson (2007) report that it is not until age 8 that children, presented with hypothetical situations, could reliably differentiate pride from happiness (see also Kornilaki & Chloverakis, 2004). Other researchers have demonstrated that it is not until this age that children attribute pride to personal (internal) effort or control (see Graham, 1988). Harris, Olthof, Meerum Terwogt, and Hardman (1987) have also reported that children, age 7 and younger, cannot spontaneously generate appropriate situations that would elicit pride. Thus, there is convergence that a complete, verbal understanding of pride as well as shame, is not mastered until the approximate age of 8.

Cross-Cultural Differences in Pride and Shame

A review of the literature reveals that there has been far more cross-cultural attention devoted to shame than to pride. The studies described above were all conducted with samples of American children. In contrast to these norms, there is evidence that shame emerges in the behavioral repertoire and the vocabulary of Chinese children at much earlier ages than in the United States (Edelstein & Shaver, 2007; Shaver, Wu, & Schwartz, 1992). Shaver et al. found that shame was among the first words learned by Chinese children. By age 2, approximately 70% of Chinese children (according to parental report) knew the Chinese word for shame. In contrast, even by age 3, only 10% of American children knew the English word "shame." This is consistent with our own interview findings (Harter & Whitesell, 1989). Our youngest children, age 4, had a rudimentary understanding that shame was a "bad feeling" but they could not define it nor could they describe a meaningful cause. By ages 5 to 6, there was the verbal acknowledgment that their parents could be ashamed of them but it was not until about ages 7 to 8 that they acknowledged that they could be ashamed of themselves. Even then, the social origins of shame were evident in responses to our question of whether one could be ashamed of oneself if one were all alone. As one astute 7-year-old explained, "If I did something bad, I *might* be able to feel ashamed if I was all by myself, but it would sure help if my parents found out!"

Research reported by Wong and Tsai (2007) has revealed that Chinese parents are much more likely to use shaming disciplinary tactics than are American parents (see also Lagattuta & Thompson, 2007). Moreover, Chinese parents readily disclose their children's transgressions in front of strangers to induce shame and to socialize their children to behave appropriately. For these reasons, Chinese children come to experience shame and to learn the word "shame" at an earlier age than do children in the United States and England.

Several researchers (see Edelstein & Shaver, 2007) have pointed to the abundance of lexical terms for shame in the Chinese culture, suggesting that it is "hypercognized," given that shame is discussed more frequently and in greater detail than in the United States. J. Li, Wang, and Fischer (2004) document these contentions. In asking native Chinese to identify terms for shame, they discovered 113 different words reflecting various cultural facets of shame. Their hierarchical cluster analysis revealed two superordinate categories that distinguished between the self-focused *experience* of shame and *reactions* to shame where the focus was on the real or anticipated response of the other. Within the first category, three further distinctions were identified: (1) the fear of losing face, (2) the negative feeling state after one had lost face, and (3) guilt. Within the second category of reactions where others were aware of one's transgression, there were an additional three distinctions in the shame terminology: (4) disgrace, (5) the condemnation of shamelessness, and (6) feelings of embarrassment. It should be noted that other researchers have also reported that the distinctions between shame and guilt are much less pronounced in collectivistic cultures such as China than in the United States (see Fessler, 2007). In contrast, shame is more closely associated with sadness in American culture (Shaver et al., 1992).

Fessler (2007) has conducted cross-cultural research on the use of shame terminology in a collectivistic Southeast Asian fishing village (Bengkulu, Indonesia) comparing it to an individualistic cultural sample in southern California. In Bengkulu, shame is a common and salient feature of their discourse. When Bengkulu participants were asked to rate the frequency with which 52 emotion terms were employed in everyday conversation, the term "malu," readily translated as shame, was ranked second. In the

California sample, where participants were also presented with 52 emotion terms (common in the English language), shame was ranked 49th. Fessler has concluded that the lexical landscape of shame for Californians is relatively impoverished, by comparison.

That said, this conclusion does not mean that Californians were psychologically rudderless when it comes to the experience of self-conscious emotions. Rather, the emotion of guilt seems to overshadow shame in the experience of Westerners. Fessler (2007) found that guilt is associated with remorse, where the focus is on regret over psychologically hurtful actions toward others, typically leading to efforts at reparation. It is noteworthy that guilt is largely absent from Bengkulu culture. Rather, shame serves as a powerful social mechanism for regulating behavior, encouraging humility, respect, and subordination to others who are considered more important in the social order.

Fessler (2007) then points to a very interesting historical observation, namely, that the use of shame, as a means of regulating social behavior, has declined in the United States over the last century. We no longer resort to traditional forms of institutional shaming such as the dunce cap or the stockade, to punish wrongdoers. He notes that some have suggested that a return to public shaming as a sanction could result in greater social cohesion and more cooperation. That is, people would presumably be less likely to engage in actions that are driven by self-interest and more likely to perform acts that will benefit the group. As examples from our current judicial system, he cites judges who have ordered thieves to wear T-shirts advertising their convictions or drunk drivers who must display bumper stickers that expose their DUIs.

Having convincingly argued the merits of such tactics for redressing legal and social ills, Fessler (2007) then turns the argumentative tables by pointing to the potential downside of public shaming. He first reviews the benefits of shaming as a highly effective sanction; for example, it can produce greater social cohesion and harmony, a lower crime rate, and greater conformity to social goals. However, these are not without their costs. He returns to examples from the Bengkulu culture where he argues that shaming, as a means of social control, interferes with their motivation to achieve excellence. Rather, citizens of Bengkulu are focused on avoiding failure and its associated public punishment. For example, he describes how this pervades their educational and intellectual domains. Children at the end of the school year are more concerned about avoiding the disgrace of failing to advance to the next grade than they are to learn whether they are excelling at their studies.

Fessler (2007) further observes that shame holds greater social significance in Japan than in the United States, as a method of social control. As an example, he describes how in Japan, recycling programs are made more effective by requiring the use of transparent garbage bags that allow observers to discern whether one has appropriately sorted out the recyclables! Such societal tactics may well result in conformity to desired social goals. Other such techniques may well reduce the crime rate and promote more social cohesion. However, Fessler argues that this is a high price to pay, in order to guarantee security and prosocial behavior. It comes at the cost of diminishing innovation and creativity that are evidently not fostered in the Japanese educational system but rather are stifled. He sees this outcome reflected in Japan's manufacturing and economic efforts. These largely consist of copying or improving upon ideas and technology developed in other countries, an endeavor that they do quite well, but at some cost. In contrast, "U.S. culture is more likely to foster free-spirited innovation and experimentation, features that are vital to the economic and political success of the country" (p. 189). Thus, he concludes that there are intrinsic costs to the reliance on shame as the primary mechanism of social regulation.

There is far less cross-cultural research on the self-conscious emotion of pride. Stipek (1998) has reported that Chinese students were more likely to express pride for the accomplishment of a family member or relative, whereas American students were more likely to attach pride to their personal accomplishments. To the extent that Chinese do experience pride over their own achievements, it is in the service of actions that will benefit others.

Tracy and Robins (2007b) have also addressed the issue of pride cross-culturally. They have demonstrated that the pride expression appears to be universal. Even in preliterate societies, there is a recognition of the basic display rules (expanded posture, head tilted back slightly, arms often akimbo, with a slight smile). However, they also note that in many cultures, it is unacceptable to openly display pride; to do so may jeopardize one's social acceptance in the group. They cite a study by Eid and Diener (2001) that compared two individualistic cultures, the United States and Australia, to two collectivistic cultures, China and Taiwan. In both collectivist cultures, pride was considered undesirable, which Tracy and Robins interpret as a sign that the more negative manifestations of pride, in the form of hubris, may prevail. Those in collectivistic cultures eschew the arrogance and self-serving conceit that hubris implies. In contrast, in the two individualistic cultures pride was highly valued (see Chapter 8, where we return to a complete discussion of cross-cultural differences in the self).

Citing Stipek (1998), Tracy and Robins (2007b) concur that pride will be accepted and valued in collectivistic cultures to the extent that it is attached to accomplishments of the group, rather than to individual achievement. Thus, they conclude that pride must be activated by collective, rather than personal, self-representations and therefore must focus on the success of one's social network. As such, it is "collective pride," a term first coined by Piaget (1960). Collective pride is not absent in Western cultures, it is just not as salient, compared to personal pride in one's achievements. However, it can be observed, for example, in the pride that Americans take in the accomplishments of their sports teams, particularly when they reach the pinnacle of success (e.g., winning the World Series). Developmentally, Piaget placed the ability to experience collective pride at adolescence and noted that such glory is reflected upon the self. As the prototypical older adolescent in the cameo described in Chapter 3 comments, "When our team has a winning season and goes to the playoffs, everyone in the whole school is proud; what the team does reflects on all of us."

Just as collective pride is more common in collectivistic societies, so is collective shame (Lickel, Schmader, Curtis, Scarnier, & Ames, 2005; Tangney & Dearing, 2002; Tangney et al., 2007). Thus, the transgression by a family member or a member of one's in-group will bring shame upon the individual, as well. This serves as another means of socially controlling an individual's behavior. However, in some rare instances, collective shame can also appear in accounts by American adolescents. For example, one 17-year-old in our interview study lamented about how ashamed he felt as a member of the human race when he saw the movie *The Day of the Dolphins* (in which humans slaughtered their ocean protectors).

Features of the Negative Self-Conscious Emotions

Shame and Guilt

We begin with an analysis of the similarities and differences in shame and guilt, followed by attention to embarrassment and humiliation. Tangney and Dearing (2002) view shame and guilt as the two *moral* emotions (compared to embarrassment and humiliation), describing them as "emotional moral barometers" that provide salient feedback about our social and moral acceptability (see also Tangney, 2003). Ferguson, Brugman, White, and Eyre (2007) concur, describing how shame and guilt signal an individual's moral virtue or character. Of the two, Tangney considers guilt to be more moral than shame, given the prosocial behavior that it provokes (see also Lapsley, 2008). Shame is typically described as a more *public* self-conscious emotion (although as our developmental sequence reveals, one can be ashamed of the self when there is no observer).

Similarities

Tangney and Dearing (2002) first describe the *similarities* between shame and guilt. In addition to being negatively valenced, moral, self-conscious emotions, both also involve *internal* attributions, although the specific nature of these attributions differs. Both are experienced in interpersonal contexts. The negative events that give rise to shame and guilt are highly similar in that they frequently involve moral failures or transgressions. M. Lewis (2002, 2007, 2008) elaborates on this point, noting that there is no particular elicitor that distinguishes the two emotions; that is, no specific stimuli uniquely contribute to each emotion. What distinguishes them are cognitive—attributional features, to be described shortly.

Different Causes

There is considerable agreement among self-conscious emotion theorists and researchers as to the primary features that differentiate shame from guilt (see M. Lewis, 2007, 2008; Tangney, 2003; Tangney & Dearing, 2002). These are summarized in Table 6.1. Shame is provoked by transgressions or moral wrongdoings that violate others' ideals for the self as well as one's own ideals (see also Teroni & Deonna, 2008). The self is viewed as the cause, engendering self-blame. Shameful acts threaten one's social status and social identity, particularly when they are publicly exposed. Shame may also arise when one does not meet one's competence ideals, associated with achievement failure.

Guilt, on the other hand, results from the violations of standards or moral rules for how one *ought* to behave toward others. Guilt concerns prohibitions (Teroni & Deonna, 2008) in which the violations directly hurt another person, psychologically. Thus, acts are very specific or circumscribed. For example, on one occasion, an individual may stand up a friend given a planned engagement to celebrate the friend's birthday, choosing instead to go shopping at the best sale of the year.

Implications for the Self

In further contrasting shame and guilt, there are clear differences in the implications for the self. In the experience of shame, the I-self denigrates the Me-self in its entirety, leading to overall self-abasement (Giner-Sorolla, Castano, Espinosa, & Brown, 2008). The negative evaluations pertain to the self *globally*, in that one views oneself as a bad *person*, where attributions are internal and *stable*; from this perspective, shame-producing acts are considered to be relatively *uncontrollable* (Tracy & Robins, 2006). That is, they reflect a self that is fundamentally flawed, defective, or inadequate, thereby implicating the entire self (see M. Lewis, 2007, 2008; Tangney & Dearing, 2002). One's core identity, therefore, is threatened. Shame reflects painfully harsh and denigrating judgments *by* ourselves, *about* ourselves. We find ourselves to be defective, inferior, flawed, tiny, insignificant, dirty, and unworthy (Morrison, 2007). As such, shame is associated with low *self-esteem* that may either result from shameful acts or serve as a precursor to shame proneness (Tangney & Dearing, 2002).

In contrast to negative evaluations of the *global* self, as in the experience

TABLE 6.1. Features of Negative Self-Conscious Emotions

Causes	Implications for self	Role of the other	Emotional correlates	Behaviors/actions taken	Adaptive functions
			Shame		
Transgressions; moral wrongdoings that violate one's own ideals or others' ideals for the self; self as cause, self-blame; fear of others' evaluation; may be public exposure; incompetence or achievement failures. Threats to one's social status and identity.	I-self denigrates the Me-self; *global,* internal, and stable negative evaluations of the self; self as a bad person; actions relatively uncontrollable; self is fundamentally flawed, defective, inadequate; core identity threatened; low self-esteem; self-abasement. By age 8 can be ashamed of the self without an observer.	Others as potential shamers; loss of esteem in the eyes of others who serve as "social mirrors"; others negatively evaluate the self.	Dejection-based emotions; disappointment in the self; depression; hopelessness; defensive and destructive anger; fear of failure.	Attempts to hide from evaluating others; desire to disappear, shrink; avoidance of others, distancing from others; self is passive, immobilized; rumination; suicidal thoughts, behavior.	Inhibits arrogance; promotes self-awareness, humility; may serve to motivate soul searching and the revision of one's priorities and values; introspection; motivates self-improvement; can provide knowledge, feedback about the Me-self.
			Guilt		
Violations of standards or moral rules for how one *ought* to behave toward others; violations directly hurt others; acts violating prohibitions are *specific.*	I-self as agent is responsible; specific behavior evaluated as wrong; actions viewed as controllable; behavioral lack of effort; pangs of conscience.	Other as person who was hurt by actions of the self; other as passive victim; other as focus of guilty thoughts.	Agitation-type emotions (e.g., anxiety, tension, uneasiness) about a threat to the relationship; remorse, regret; fear of disapproval	I-self is mobilized to engage in acts of confession; apologies; efforts at reparation; empathy that motivates altruistic and prosocial behavior.	Restores emotional, relational bonds; motivates one to choose the moral path; repairs and strengthens the relationship; redistributes emotional distress; more adaptive than shame.

(continued)

213

TABLE 6.1. (continued)

Causes	Implications for self	Role of the other	Emotional correlates	Behaviors/actions taken	Adaptive functions
Embarrassment					
Public violation of social norms and scripts; social faux pas; unintended mishaps or accidents; awkward, clumsy, hapless behavior; unwanted public attention.	Relatively low level of responsibility or self-blame; lower level of self-devaluation; or self-derogation; transient drop in self-esteem. Sensitive to public evaluation, assume others are just as interested in one's behavior as is the self.	Observing public audience is a necessity; negative evaluation by others; however, others may be empathic.	Mortification, chagrin; fear of negative evaluations of others and exposure; exaggerated worry and concern.	Blushing, gaze aversion; awkward posture, behaving in a conciliatory manner to gain back approval from others and re-inclusion; may resort to humor; attempts at appeasement.	Reinforces social norms; serves to preserve the social order; reassures others of good intentions; evokes empathy, sympathy; forestalls social rejection; helps manage an awkward social situation.
Humiliation					
Put-downs, teasing, bullying, ridicule, mocking, harassment, torture by others; *hostile intent*; active, overt derogation; social rejection; acts of others judged as undeserved or unfair; others perceive a violation in standards of conduct.	Significant loss of self-esteem; lowered in the eyes of others; loss of dignity; painfully bad feelings; self is devalued and threatened; more intense than embarrassment. Feelings of insignificance, inferiority. Congruence with admitted character weakness of the self.	Observing public audience is a necessity; the larger the audience, the greater the level of humiliation; audience may laugh or join in the mockery; others are viewed as more powerful than the self.	Embarrassment; anger toward others; fury; sadness; depression; anxiety and fear of future humiliation.	Revenge, retaliation; violence toward perpetrators, including murder in the extreme; random violence toward others; desire to hide, escape, minimize event; self-harm; suicide for some as the ultimate escape from others and the self.	Least adaptive of the negative self-emotions; not experienced as functional by the victims; others may use it as a means of social control to secure the compliance and conformity of the victim.

214

of shame, guilt is provoked by *specific* acts that are evaluated as morally wrong or reprehensible, a distinction first articulated by M. Lewis (2000). Although the guilty I-self claims responsibility for the psychological harm inflicted on another, there is not the total condemnation of the self, as in shame. Thus, although the attribution is internal, it is *unstable* (i.e., not a characteristic trait), and *controllable* (Tracy & Robins, 2006). As a result, one's pangs of conscience can be overcome by actions on the part of the self to redress the situation, as we shall see, shortly, in examining the behavioral correlates of guilt.

The Role of the Other

The features of shame and guilt can also be distinguished on the basis of the role of the other. In the case of shame, others are potential shamers who negatively evaluate the self, if the act is observed or divulged. Thus, there is a loss of esteem in the eyes of others, real or imagined, who serve as "social mirrors," providing reflected appraisals of the blameworthy, shameful actions. The others in the guilt scenario are the persons who have been psychologically hurt by the actions of the self. They become passive victims as well as the focus of the guilty thoughts and pangs of conscience.

Emotional Correlates

What, then, are the emotional correlates of each of these self-conscious emotions; what other affects are experienced in conjunction with shame and guilt? For shame, the actor is first likely to experience dejection-based emotions. These include disappointment in the self and depression, or profound sadness, tinged with hopelessness. In certain cases there may be displays of defensive and destructive anger (Dost & Yagmurlu, 2008). If the shame-inducing act involved incompetence, then fear of continued failure may surface (McGregor & Elliot, 2005).

In the case of guilt, the actor is much more likely to experience agitation-related emotions such as anxiety and tension, as he/she is concerned about having threatened the relationship by his/her hurtful actions. Thus, there are also emotions of remorse and regret (M. Lewis, 2007; Tangney, 2003).

These emotions, in turn, are thought to motivate the different behavioral responses that ensue for shame versus guilt. When shame is experienced, there is typically an initial reaction of avoidance, as the individual seeks to disappear and distance him/herself from others whose negative evaluations, if not scorn, lead to feelings of dejection. Thus, the self may initially be immobilized and relatively passive. If defensive anger is experienced, a shamed individual may also resort to aggression (Baumeister & Bushman, 2007). Shame proneness is consistently linked to anger arousal, resentment, hostility, and irritability, in contrast to guilt where the opposite pattern of correlations is obtained (Tangney, Wagner, Fletcher, & Gramzow, 1992).

Shame is much more likely than guilt to provoke depression (see De Rubeis & Hollenstein, 2009). Moreover, studies have recently reported that shame (in contrast to guilt) is more likely to produce *rumination* (Dennison & Stewart, 2006; Orth, Berking, & Burkhardt, 2006). Dennison and Stewart, as well as Cheung, Gilbert, and Irons (2004), provide evidence for a mediational model in which shame predicts rumination that, in turn, leads to depression. These dynamics appear to be unique to shame (as opposed to guilt). If shame induces depression in the extreme, the individual is at risk for suicidal thinking and behavior much more so than in the case of guilt (Hastings, Northman, & Tangney, 2000).

Behaviors

The *action tendencies* for guilt are also quite distinct from those associated with the experience of shame. The I-self, consumed with guilt, is highly mobilized to engage in acts of confession, apology, and efforts at reparation (M. Lewis, 2007; Tangney, 2003; Tangney & Dearing, 2002). Thus, the individual is motivated to restore the relationship through acts of contrition and repair. Findings (see Tangney & Dearing, 2002) also reveal that those who express a proneness to experience guilt are much more likely to be *empathic* and thus engage in altruistic and prosocial behavior, if they commit a guilt-inducing violation that psychologically harms another. Similarly, guilt proneness is associated with benevolence and conformity to traditional as well as universal social values (Silfver, Helkama, Lönnqvist, & Verkasalo, 2008). Moreover, guilt appears to have some power to restrain and prevent aggression (Baumeister & Bushman, 2007).

Adaptive Functions

Finally, in this comparative analysis, we turn to the adaptive functions of shame and guilt, some of which have been anticipated in the preceding discussion. In general, self-conscious emotions are alleged to support the individual in adhering to group norms (Goetz & Keltner, 2007). However, there is considerable agreement that shame is much less adaptive than guilt (see Dost & Yagmurlu, 2008; Silfver, 2007; Tangney & Dearing, 2002). Shame is linked to destructive actions, whereas the behaviors emanating from guilt are viewed as constructive.

That said, shame does have several features that motivate the individual to engage in adaptive action. For example, shame is thought to inhibit arrogance and promote humility in some individuals who are able to control shame-induced anger and destructiveness. Shame may also serve to motivate soul-searching and introspection, which may lead the individual to revise his/her priorities and engage in self-improvement. As such, shame can provide feedback and knowledge about the Me-self. Shame may also function to enhance conformity to cultural standards of behavior (Tracy & Robins, 2007b). In drawing attention to larger societal concerns and consequences, shame represents a mechanism of social control. Thus, shame has been shown to have a clear interpersonal function in that it bolsters a sense of commitment to shared social goals.

There is considerable consensus, however, that guilt plays a far more constructive role in promoting such social goals. Acts to repair social relationships in the face of transgressions serve to restore emotional and relational bonds (Keltner & Beer, 2005). Guilt can produce approach-motivated behavior if an opportunity for reparation presents itself (Amodio, Devine, & Harmon-Jones, 2007). In this regard, guilt serves various relationship-enhancing functions. It motivates individuals to treat social partners well and to avoid transgressions. It enables less powerful partners to achieve a greater sense of equity and it redistributes emotional stress (Baumeister et al., 2001). With regard to this last function, the distress experienced by a victim of a hurtful act is somewhat balanced by the distress experienced by the transgressor. Finally, guilt motivates one to select the more "moral path" (Tangney & Dearing, 2002).

Child-Rearing Antecedents

The literature points to patterns of child rearing that distinguish between the antecedents of shame versus guilt. As observed earlier in this chapter, caregivers must first convey the *standards* of behavior that they initially expect of their toddler through modeling and instruction. Expectations regarding age-appropriate achievement behaviors as well as conduct are among the most common. Parents must then overtly evaluate their child's ability to meet such standards. Through such practices, young children begin to develop a rudimentary sense of their competence, behavioral conduct, and eventual morality.

Certain parental practices differentially lead to guilt, the more adaptive of the two emotions, compared to shame. Guilt is more likely to be produced if the parents focus on the consequences of the harm inflicted on others. In so doing, parents must clarify standards and place emphasis on the child's obligations and the need for personal responsibility. Thus, nurturant parents who employ "induction techniques" providing their children with age-appropriate explanations that promote insight and understanding of their behavior and its consequences, will be more likely to foster functional guilt (M. L. Hoffman, 2008). Such parenting techniques, including those that provide clarification of standards, are more likely to foster the internalization of standards associated with a toddler's reparations for a wrongdoing.

Shame will more likely be fostered, and be particularly intense, if the mother or father emphasizes the child's failure to meet high parental standards. Shame will also be induced if parents communicate that the child's failures reflect the fact that he/she is fundamentally flawed or deficient. If the child is made to feel inherently and consistently bad, and is expected to never be good enough or lovable, shame will be the self-conscious emotion that will ultimately be instilled (Barrett, 1995; M. Lewis, 2000).

Discrepancies between the child's behavior and particular types of expectations differentially predict the strength of guilt and shame reactions. Guilt is more likely to ensue if parents emphasize the discrepancy between the child's behavior and how he/she *ought* to behave. Shame, on the other hand, is more likely if parents underscore how the child is falling short of *parental ideals*, namely, how they *want* the child to behave (Moretti & Higgins, 1990). Barrett (1995) has also hypothesized that the precursors of shame will have more of an effect if there is a strong emotional bond between parent and child, such that parental values and associated feedback about performance are taken very seriously by the child.

Tangney and Dearing (2002) describe other mechanisms through which the family may influence the emotional displays of their children. One involves the parents' own affective styles that may directly have an impact through modeling by parents and the imitation by their children. They cite, as an example, a child who repeatedly observes his/her mother reacting with shame when faced with negative interpersonal exchanges. To the extent that the mother displays a shame-related shrinking posture, with downcast eyes, or shame-related verbal self-statements (e.g., "God, I'm so stupid"), the child will be more prone to adopt an emotional shame stance. On a broader scale, Tangney and Dearing point to an entire *shame-based dysfunctional family system* in which there are maladaptive patterns of communication, shaming tactics, and extreme family conflict or enmeshment.

Shame has been found to be extremely prevalent among those who as children were chronically and severely abused (see Harter, 1998, for a complete discussion). The blame, condemnation, and ostracism that parents, family, and society express toward abuse victims are incorporated not only into attributions of self-blame but result in powerful feelings of shame for the child's assumed role in shameful acts. Shame, as well as guilt, is also fueled by the perception that it is one's inherent badness that provoked the abuse rather than that the abuse was the *cause* of one's negative self-views and emotions.

M. Lewis (1992, 2008) also links the elicitation of shame to child sexual abuse, providing an attributional analysis. If the abuse is attributed to an internal, global, and stable cause, namely, the child's inherent negative characteristics, shame will result. Moreover, these effects are long lasting, extending well into adulthood. Feiring, Taska, and Lewis (2002) have demonstrated these effects in a longitudinal study where, consistent with our earlier analysis, abuse was highly related to both shame and depression.

Gender Differences

Gender differences are consistently reported for both shame and guilt, with girls expressing higher levels of both self-conscious emotions. Alessandri and Lewis (1993) have reported that girls experience more shame than do boys, consistent with the gender differences reported in the adult literature (H. B. Lewis, 1987; Tangney, 1995). Their studies with preschoolers and their parents reveal that in performing achievement-related laboratory tasks, girls expressed more shame over failures than did boys, despite no gender differences in actual performance. Interestingly, the parents of girls were observed to provide more negative feedback than did parents of boys (see also Eccles & Blumenfeld, 1985; Ruble et al., 2006). These investigators have concluded that the negative parental feedback promoted more unfavorable self-evaluations in girls, as it focused attention on their failures, which in turn predisposed the girls to experience shame.

Alessandri and Lewis (1993) relate their findings to the attribution literature (see Dweck & Leggett, 1988) where it has been demonstrated that girls are more likely to assume personal responsibility for failure and to focus on global, internal attributions than are boys. Girls have also been observed to have lower expectations for success and decreased achievement strivings in the face of failure or evaluative pressure. Thus, the differential treatment of girls and boys, both at home and in the classroom, would appear to contribute to girls' experience of more negative self-conscious emotions.

More recent studies support this conclusion. Walter and Burnaford (2006) have reported that adolescent girls reported more shame and guilt than did boys (see also Ferguson & Eyre, 2000). Tangney and Dearing (2002) find that the consistency in their own gender studies across diverse populations and ages is striking, with females reporting significantly higher levels of shame and guilt, as well as depression, than do males. M. Lewis (2008) reports that gender differences are particularly pronounced among maltreated girls who manifest more shame when they fail a task than do nonmaltreated girls. Maltreated boys, in contrast, show a suppression of shame in failure situations. Rather, boys who are the victims of trauma are much more likely to display anger in the laboratory situation, behaving aggressively and destructively toward the test materials, as they also engage in angry verbalizations.

From a somewhat different perspective, Pollack (1998), in his book

Real Boys, discusses how in the socialization of boys in our culture, males are actively shamed into not crying and not expressing fear. The purpose of such child-rearing techniques is to harden boys to become men who will meet the traditional standards of masculinity. Thus, young males must adhere to what he terms the "boy code." Pollack also observes that boys are also made to feel guilty if they express any forms of weakness, vulnerability, fear, or despair. These socialization practices, however, would not appear to support the adaptive functions of shame and guilt. Rather, they are more likely to suppress the active expression of these emotions, driving them into the psychological underground.

Roberts and Goldenberg (2007) take the issue of gender differences in self-conscious emotions to a broader canvas where they paint a picture of the shame, embarrassment, and self-loathing that women in our society express in evaluating their bodies, given current cultural standards (see the extensive treatment of this topic in Chapter 5, this volume). The failure to meet the punishing standards of attractiveness, exemplified by models and movie stars, is especially evident when appearance is made salient, leading women to experience more negative self-conscious emotions than men.

Embarrassment

Causes

In the self-conscious emotion family, embarrassment is a cousin of humiliation, and to a lesser extent, shame. The primary causes involve the faux pas, public violations of social norms of civility, and/or awkward and unintended mishaps or accidents that are observed by others (see R. S. Miller, 2007; Tangney, 2003). Thus, one may trip and fall in a public place, spill food on oneself in a restaurant, forget an acquaintance's name, engage in a gaffe, sport an open fly, or let out an uncontrollable fart, each of which leads to an awkward social situation in which one is conspicuous. These embarrassing, hapless moments have less direct implications for morality. Compared to shame and guilt, they are not nearly as serious as moral transgressions and failures that reflect badly on global and enduring attributes of the self, as in the case of shame (Tangney, 2003). Nor do they directly violate social norms that result in hurting another, as in the case of guilt. However, they do cause distress for the individual who feels exposed and incurs the social disapproval of the observing audience.

Interestingly, embarrassment is not always caused by social mishaps. It can also be experienced in situations where one is complimented, for example, in being praised during an introduction to a public presentation (M. Lewis, 2000, 2008). Embarrassment, when someone extols your virtues, appears to be caused more by the mere exposure of the self (rather than by negative evaluations). Robbins and Parlavecchio (2006) have developed this theme in their model of embarrassment that focuses on the unwanted exposure of the self. Thus, unwanted attention will provoke embarrassment whether the actions of the self are desirable or unflattering.

Implications for the Self

Compared to guilt or shame, embarrassment involves a much lower level of responsibility or self-blame, in large part because the causes are typically viewed as accidental. Nor is there marked self-devaluation or self-derogation, as the actions were unintentional. Nevertheless, individuals are sensitive to the potentially negative social evaluation of others, particularly if one is prone to embarrassment. R. S. Miller (2007) makes a cogent argument for the "spotlight effect," describing how we assume that observing others are as concerned about our social predicaments as we are. Years earlier, Elkind (1967) labeled this phenomenon the "imaginary audience" that emerges in midadolescence, namely the perception that others are as preoccupied with our behavior as we are. The interpretation that others are negatively evaluating the self in life's most embarrassing moments can lead to a transient drop in self-esteem.

Role of the Other

With regard to the role of the other, an observing public audience is necessary to invoke the experience of embarrassment. However, unlike the emotion of humiliation, others who observe the embarrassing event are not necessarily negative in their evaluations. It is true that some observers may laugh spontaneously. However, in other cases, they may be sympathetic to one's plight and even offer assistance.

Emotional Correlates

The emotional correlates of embarrassment can range from chagrin to mortification. Fear of exposure is often common, as one anticipates the negative appraisals of one's mishap. However, R. S. Miller's (2007) observations suggest that such worry and concern is exaggerated. These associated emotions are far less devastating than in the cases of either shame or guilt. They are also less debilitating than affective reactions to humiliation.

Behaviors

The behaviors linked to embarrassment include blushing, the immediate, involuntary physiological reaction that appears to be universal in nature (R. S. Miller, 2007). Other behaviors may include gaze aversion, an awkward or shifting posture, touching of the face or body, and a sheepish grin (see also M. Lewis, 2000, 2007). Subsequently, the individual may engage in conciliatory behavior, in the hope that he/she will be restored to the good graces of others. An appropriate reaction to an embarrassing behavior can be a desirable response to a social misdemeanor if it is sensitively calibrated to its context (R. S. Miller, 2007).

This observation ushers in a consideration of the social functions of embarrassment. It may evoke sympathy that diminishes the discomfort of awkward social situations and may forestall or prevent overt social rejection (R. S. Miller, 2007). R. S. Miller ends her treatment of embarrassment by asking whether embarrassment is a blessing or a curse. Although there are certainly adaptive advantages, there is also a downside to embarrassment that R. S. Miller likens to Leary's (2004) contentions concerning the curse of the self. Self-consciousness can be surprisingly costly (Leary, 2004). The heightened awareness of others' reactions toward the self and the exaggerated estimation of their interest and preoccupation with the mishaps that have befallen the self can cause unnecessary and excessive worry and grief (see also Rochat, 2009).

Humiliation

The fourth negative affect in the family of self-conscious emotions, humiliation, is distinct, first by its neglect in the literature. The primary focus in the field has been on shame, guilt, and to a lesser extent, embarrassment, as the chapter has thus far described. For example, in Tangney' and Fischer's (1995) *Self-Conscious Emotions* and in the last two editions of the *Handbook of Emotions* (M. Lewis & Haviland-Jones, 2000; M. Lewis et al., 2008), there were no index entries for humiliation. In the most recent comprehensive volume on *The self-conscious emotions* (Tracy et al., 2007), the only index entries for humiliation are for the chapter that Jeff Elison and I wrote on this topic (Elison & Harter, 2007). That is, until recently, humiliation has not appeared in the mainstream literature on self-conscious emotions. Negrao, Bonanno, Noll, Putnam, and Trickett (2005) note that attention to humiliation has also been conspicuously absent in the childhood sexual abuse literature where shame and anger have been the primary focus.

There are philosophical treatments of humiliation as well a clinical literature both of which focus on therapeutic implications for those who have been victims of humiliation. There are also nonempirical analyses that span a variety of disciplines. However, there is virtually no *research*. Yet humiliation has recently been revealed to be a very critical self-conscious emotion, particularly given its implications for our youth. Our own research in the last several years has attempted to address this gap. A few other investigators, during the last decade, have also come to realize the significance of this neglected self-conscious emotion and have devoted empirical attention to its study.

My own interest in the topic of humiliation has emerged gradually, as I began to study the media accounts of the now 12 high-profile school-shooting cases. The first of these began in 1996, when Barry Loukaitis, age 14, from Moses Lake, Washington, fired on his middle school algebra class, killing three students and wounding one. As the number of cases grew to 12, it became increasingly clear that humiliation was a root cause and that the violence represented revenge. In every case, the shooters described how they had been ridiculed, taunted, teased, harassed, or bullied. The humiliation they experienced came at the hands of peers (who mocked their inadequate appearance and their lack of social skills or athletic behavior). A few had been spurned by someone in whom they were romantically interested. Still others were publicly humiliated in their classrooms by a teacher or school administrator. Each of these events led to an experience of profound humiliation (see Harter, Low, et al., 2003).

All of these school shooters were White, middle-class male youth, from small rural or suburban communities scattered across the country. They eventually sought revenge in the extreme, gunning down classmates indiscriminately. "I killed because people like me are mistreated every day," explained pudgy, bespectacled Luke Woodham, age 16, from Pearl, Mississippi, whose gunfire ended the lives of two students, injuring others. "My whole life I felt outcasted, alone," he lamented. In Peducah, Kentucky, 15-year-old Michael Carneal was tired of being teased and picked on by his schoolmates. He took a gun to school, shooting to death three students and wounding five others, as he fired upon a prayer circle just outside the entrance to his high school. Another shooter, Mitchell Johnson, age 13, complained that "Everyone that hates me, everyone I don't like, is going to die!" He and Andrew Golden, age 11, shot and killed one teacher and four students, wounding 10 others, after they set off a false fire alarm at their middle school. This drove people to vacate the school, providing the boys with sitting-duck targets as they fired from a nearby knoll. Like many male youth who grew up in a gun and hunting culture, they were excellent marksmen. In fact, newspaper reports likened them in skill to police swat teams.

The media accounts eerily continued and literally came a bit too close to home. Columbine, the high school in Littleton, Colorado, has become the metaphor for these school-shooting events. The school is 15 minutes from where I live in Colorado, and therefore the incident was very prominent in my thinking and in our news for months. In his Internet manifesto, Eric Harris, age 18, the older of the two shooters from Columbine High School, described how classmates, primarily the jocks, "ridiculed me, chose not to accept me, and treated me like I was not worth their time." A member of the Trenchcoat Mafia (the name given pejoratively to Harris, Klebold, and friends by the popular jocks) described how he and Klebold, the second shooter, were constantly "cornered, pushed day after day, we were ridiculed and bashed against lockers." It is noteworthy that those labeled by the jocks as members of the Trenchcoat Mafia were not a gang, they had no special symbols or rituals, and they were not, for the most part, very close friends. Rather, they were a small confederation of rejected losers in the eyes of others, who loosely formed a group because they could not garner the social acceptance or respect from the more popular students. Harris and Klebold, in the deadliest event of its kind for teenagers, shot and killed one teacher and 11 students, wounding countless others.

In all of these tragic cases, a history of humiliation culminated in violent revenge causing the death of peers and, at the hands of certain shooters, the death of a teacher and school administrators. Harris's manifesto, written just a few days before the shooting incident, described the constant humiliation by peers. As another member of the infamous Trenchcoat Mafia told reporters, "Tell people that we were harassed and sometimes it was impossible to take; eventually, someone was going to snap!" He noted that the torment often became vicious. He described walking to school with a knot in his stomach, dreading to face the continual bullying and humiliation. Central to the events that these boys described was the presence of an audience who witnessed the harassment, often laughing or joining in the mockery.

It should be noted that humiliation-fueled violence is not always restricted to harm toward others as it has been with the school shooters. It may also be directed toward the self. In two incidents, Columbine and a 2005 Red Lake shooting, the male adolescents successfully suicided. In another case, an attempted suicide was averted by police. Other school shooters expressed the wish to die at their own hands, but had not prepared, accordingly, or were stopped in their efforts.

These cases were particularly compelling because the dynamics in the lives of these young males so closely approximated the antecedents, correlates, and consequences of self-esteem that have been documented in our own model (see Chapter 3). In this model, previewed in Chapter 3 on adolescence, and applicable to those in the 8 to 18 age range, the determinants of low global self-esteem include lack of peer and parental support, as well as a sense of incompetence or inadequacy in domains that are judged to be important to the self or the peer group. As more and more details were revealed, it became clear that these boys clearly did not have the support of parents or peers; in fact, they were actively rejected. Nor were they competent in areas deemed important by the peer culture (e.g., looks, social appeal, and athletic ability). Moreover, several had signs of depression, some of clinical proportions for which they were taking prescription drugs. Suicidal ideation, typically driven by extreme depression, was evident in the wishes and behavior of several of the school shooters. We will return to our own research documenting a revised model in which peer rejection and humiliation, as well as anger and homicidal ideation, were added to the model.

McGee and DeBernardo (1999) have also presented a profile of the high-profile school shooters, describing many of these same features. They observe that demographically these White, middle-class males, an average age of 15, came from either rural communities or small cities. The psychological profile that they describe is consistent with our own description in that these boys were regarded as unattractive and socially inadequate loners. McGee and DeBerndo also describe a history of psychological stressors including social rejection and experiences of humiliation.

Leary, Kowalski, Smith, and Phillips (2003) have provided a similar case study of the school shooters. Consistent with our own analysis and that of McGee and DeBernado (1999), they describe the teasing, bullying, and ostracism that most of these males experienced. They describe how the relentless cruelty produced feelings of shame and humiliation. They conclude that social rejection alone was not the only factor that provoked their vengeful acts. As we have argued (Harter, Low, et al., 2003), histories that produce depression, low self-esteem, and hopelessness also contribute to violent retaliation. Leary et al. also note that a significant number of the school shooters had histories of suicidal ideation, and also observe, as our own findings document, that these male youth had an interest in bombs or firearms. Moreover, their analysis reveals that the school shooters also had a fascination with death and sadism.

The features of humiliation are summarized in Table 6.1. Despite the lack of rigorous research on the topic of humiliation, thoughtful analyses of its dynamics, bolstered by our own research and a few recent studies, have emerged (see Elison & Harter, 2007, for a more complete review). Discussion here will focus on how humiliation can be differentiated from shame, guilt, and embarrassment in each of the six categories identified in Table 6.1. As with the other self-conscious emotions, these categories target the causes of humiliation, implications for the self, the role of others, the emotional correlates, and behavioral actions and outcomes, as well as adaptive functions. Within the family of self-conscious emotions, humiliation shares certain similarities with embarrassment, although there are clear differences that will be highlighted.

Causes

With regard to the causes or determinants of humiliation, clearly bullying, taunting, harassing, mocking, and torture, in the extreme, by others have all been identified as powerful prototypical antecedents (see review in Elison & Harter, 2007). Gilbert (1997) describes humiliation as "an experience of external attack" (p. 133). One feature that differentiates humiliation from embarrassment is the *hostile intent* of others who deliberately engage in acts designed to humiliate the victim (see also Hartling & Luchetta, 1999; Jackson, 2000; Klein, 1991; Statman, 2000).

Several theorists have argued that humiliation is more *other-focused*, whereas shame is more *self-focused* (Gilbert, 1997; Klein, 1991; S. B. Miller, 1988; Sarphatie, 1993). According to Sarphatie, shame is always self-inflicted, whereas humiliation is inflicted by others. Klein concurs, arguing that humiliation is a self-conscious emotion that is experienced when one is ridiculed, scorned, or belittled by others, whereas shame is experienced when one fails to live up to the moral ideals of the self or others. Thus, humiliation is an emotional reaction to put-downs, harassment, and bulling by hostile others because of the victim's implicit *violation of social norms*. In contrast, shame is a more self-focused reaction that results from actions of the self that willfully violate social expectations. Humiliation, therefore, requires the negative attribution of blame to *another*, whereas shame requires that blame be placed on the *self*.

That said, just what are the implicit social norms, violated by the *victims* of humiliation? I would argue that in the context of the school shootings, a norm violation is in the eye of the beholder, namely, those who commit acts of harassment and bullying. For example, at Columbine, the victims were condemned for the unconventional way they dressed (e.g., Gothlike black and trench coats), being unsociable, and violating the social standards that the jocks demanded and rewarded, namely, participation in sports.

This observation can be linked to another feature of humiliation identified by several theorists, namely, that the derogation by others is judged to be unfair or undeserved (see Gilbert, 1997; Hartling & Luchetta, 1999; Statman, 2000). For example, the victims of humiliation who became school shooters were not overtly confronting those who held the social reins. That is, they did not openly flaunt their own values. Rather, in their implicit violation of social norms, they passively adhered to their own life-style, which happened to offend those peers in positions of social power. As a result, it is understandable why the victims would feel unfairly judged and that the harassment was undeserved.

Humiliation and embarrassment share certain features; for example, both require an observing audience that may be judgmental. However, embarrassment is far less intense and involves a much lower level of self-blame, in large part because the actions that provoke embarrassment are typically viewed as unfortunate and unintended accidents. The social norms of civility that are violated are much less serious and the acts and experience are fleeting. Compared to shame and guilt, there is less self-devaluation in the case of embarrassment and humiliation if they are experienced as unjustified and undeserved (Elison & Harter, 2007; Jackson, 2000; Pulham, 2009). Pulham's dissertation findings have revealed that the negative evaluations of an audience may be more easily discounted when the self is viewed as not responsible for an act, compared to shame where the blame falls directly on the self.

Often the same act may provoke either embarrassment or humiliation depending upon the attributions as well as the reaction of the observing audience. For example, some years ago a very flat-chested friend of mine told me of a painful summer experience during her adolescence in which she was wearing a two-piece swimsuit with a heavily padded top. At a crowded public pool, she proceeded to jump off of the high-diving board with a rather impressive dive that caught people's attention. However, upon hitting the water, she went in *one* direction but her padded top flew off upon impact and went bobbing along the water's surface in the opposite direction!

Two potential self-conscious emotions could have ensued. If she viewed this as a rare and unfortunate accident that also evoked the sympathy of the onlookers, she might have escaped with the mere experience of embarrassment. In contrast, if she berated herself for wearing such a top in the service of vanity, particularly given her decision to jump off of the high dive, and if the audience reacted with uncontrollable laughter, relentlessly ridiculing her as she desperately tried to recover the top half of her bathing suit at the other end of the pool, then she would be much more likely to experience intense, public humiliation.

Implications for the Self

This anecdote ushers in the second category in our analysis of self-conscious emotions, namely, the implications for the self. If the self is seriously devalued in the eyes of others, if one loses one's dignity and experiences a major loss of self-esteem, then intense humiliation, a very painful emotion, will result. The emotional intensity is much greater in the case of humiliation, compared to embarrassment.

Another determinant of the likelihood and intensity of humiliation depends on whether the act that provokes it is viewed as congruent with one's relevant self-concept, particularly one's perceived weaknesses. For example, if one views the self as a klutz, then spilling food on one's clothing and the floor in a popular restaurant, and then tripping in an attempt to recover the food on the floor, will simply reinforce one's trait attributions of clumsiness. In turn, this will produce a more intense feeling of humiliation and the fearful anticipation of future such experiences. This self-congruence hypothesis has been documented in recent research by both Pulham (2009) as well as Elison and Harter (2007).

Role of the Other

The role of the other, the third category in this comparison of self-conscious emotions, has already been touched on in that an audience is a prerequisite for the experience of humiliation (Harter, Low, et al., 2003; Harter, Kiang, et al., 2003). Our findings have revealed that the larger the audience, the more intense the feelings of humiliation. Moreover, humiliation is intensified if the observing others laugh or join in the mockery. When others are demeaning, cruel, and lack empathy, low self-esteem will be implicated. In a dissertation by McCarley (2009), we found evidence for the hypothesis that low self-esteem as a global self-evaluation sets the stage for the experience of humiliation. Thus, the lower the *trait* self-esteem that one brought to the situation, the more intense was the humiliation. Tangney and Dearing (2002) have also suggested that low global self-esteem may make one prone to negative self-conscious emotions. In addition, a transient drop in *state* or transitory self-esteem will also be experienced as a result of the humiliating event.

Emotional Correlates

There are also clear emotional correlates of humiliation. The humiliated individual will most likely experience initial embarrassment. As Elison and Harter (2007) point out, if a person feels humiliated, it is likely that he/she will also experience embarrassment. If one merely feels embarrassed, he/she will not necessarily experience humiliation. However, the emotional correlates that accompany humiliation extend far beyond fleeting embarrassment. The victim feels anger toward the perpetrator, if not rage. The constellation of associated emotions also includes sadness and depression, as well as anxiety and fear over future such humiliation and attacks against the self.

Behaviors

The intense emotional reactions provide causal links to the behaviors that can be provoked. Humiliation, and its correlates, particularly anger and fury, are highly likely to fuel acts of revenge, as in the case of the school shooters, who were driven to violence given a chronic history of victimization (Harter, Low, et al., 2003). Participants in Jackson's (2000) study of the narratives of young adults reported anger toward others and a desire for revenge, after being humiliated. R. H. Smith, Webster, Parrott, and Eyre (2002) have reported that humiliation, more so than shame, was strongly correlated with hostility.

    As Garbarino (1999), author of *Lost Boys: Why Our Sons Turn Violent and How We Can Save Them*, also points out, social rejection by peers and neglect by parents leads to anger and depression, culminating in acts of violence toward peers and, in certain cases, toward parents. With regard to the latter, Kip Kinkel, the 15-year-old school shooter from Springfield, Oregon, felt neglected by his parents as well as rejected by classmates. He shot and killed both of his parents, before proceeding to school, where he fired into a crowd of students, killing two and wounding 22 others.

Garbarino (1999), in his analysis of such violence that was based on interviews with incarcerated youth, is one of the few to mention the humiliation experienced by boys who have committed violent acts. However, he implies that humiliation is always linked directly to shame, as if the two affects were synonymous. As my own analysis has revealed, clear differences between these two self-conscious emotions are postulated, based on the literature.

In our own revision of the original model of the causes, correlates and consequences of self-esteem, we added or modified certain variables, to examine the dynamics that emerged from the analysis of the lives of the school shooters (Harter, Low, et al., 2003). Peer approval was modified to include peer rejection that also reflected humiliation. In addition to depression, as a consequence, we added anger-induced physical aggression. In addition to suicidal ideation as an outcome of these processes, we added homicidal ideation. The most relevant features of our revised model, empirically tested with adolescents, included the depression composite (depressed affect, low self-esteem, and hopelessness), which was predicted by social rejection/humiliation that, in turn, predicted both suicidal and homicidal ideation. Anger-induced physical aggression directly predicted homicidal ideation. Thus, humiliation and its affective correlates, particularly anger-induced aggressive feelings, directly impact feelings of revenge in the form of homicidal intentions.

In another open-ended interview study (Harter, Kiang, et al., 2003), we asked college students about their behavioral reactions to humiliation. Acts of revenge or retaliation were common. While the majority of college participants indicated that they would direct their revenge toward the perpetrator, some responded that they would act violently toward anyone. This was a common feature in the school shootings where the targets appeared to be random, as the shooters recklessly fired into crowds of students.

Less common responses to humiliation among the college student sample were (1) attempts to escape from the humiliating perpetrators, and (2) psychological efforts to minimize the insult (Harter, Kiang, et al., 2003). In a follow-up study, a dissertation by McCarley (2009), a path model revealed that those with low self-esteem, which predicted humiliation, were more likely to report that their strategy would be withdrawal or escape from the humiliators and the situation. A weaker path revealed that low self-esteem predicted vengeful retaliation. A stronger predictor of retaliation was anger associated with humiliation. To a lesser extent, anger was predictive of minimization, as a coping strategy to deal with the humiliating experience.

Humiliation and Violence within the School Setting

We end this chapter with a return to the issue of humiliation and violence within the school setting. Our own formulation differs from many who study bullying and victimization, linking it directly to revenge and violence. Our own approach has been to postulate and demonstrate that humiliation is a critical emotional mediator. Bullying provokes humiliation in the victim that, over time, can erupt into violence as a form of retaliation. As noted earlier, anger and fury associated with humiliation can lead to indiscriminant violence where innocent peers, and in some cases teachers, become random targets.

In our own research (Harter, Low, et al., 2003), we have also explored young adolescents' reactions to hypothetical events that simulated the types of harassment experienced by the school shooters, albeit in somewhat milder forms. We constructed vignettes that portrayed incidents in which the target character is ridiculed, put down, or harassed, by peers, in two cases, in a third by someone in whom they were romantically interested, and in a fourth, by a teacher. A sample *peer* vignette reads as follows: "Jason is coming to school and is walking toward the school building. A small group of kids comes toward him and start to tease him about what he is wearing and how he looks. As he tries to get away, they shove him and make loud insulting comments that all of the other kids can hear. Some of the other kids join in the harassment and others laugh. (This wasn't the first time something like this had happened to Jason.) Imagine you are Jason/Jennifer." (There were separate versions for each gender.)

Two features of all four of the vignettes are noteworthy. First, there is a peer audience that either laughs at the victim or participates in the harassment. Secondly, each vignette ends with a statement to the effect that this is not the first time something like this has happened to the target child, thus implying a history of insult and ridicule. These features characterized the harassment experienced by the actual school shooters and have been found, in our own research, to be critical (Harter, Kiang, et al., 2003).

At the end of each vignette, the participant was asked to imagine that he/she were the victim. What followed were questions, all rated on a 4-point scale, about (1) *emotional reactions* (how humiliated you would feel in front of others, how angry at the perpetrator, how depressed), (2) *cognitive* reactions (how unfair was the act, how difficult would it be to get the incident out of your mind), and (3) *behavioral reactions* (along a continuum from doing nothing, at one extreme, to planning a way to get back at the perpetrators by seriously harming them or thoughts of harming anyone, it wouldn't matter who they were, at the other extreme). This second form of harm was included given the fact that the school shooters engaged in firing into a crowd of students, randomly.

We first determined that the mean level of rated humiliation was 3.1

on the 4-point scale clearly indicating that the vignettes we created did elicit feelings of humiliation. There was enough variability in the humiliation ratings to reveal that humiliation was highly correlated with anger toward others ($r = .41$), depression ($r = .56$), unfairness ($r = .40$), and difficulty of getting the event out of one's mind ($r = .51$). Thus, the findings revealed a constellation of correlates that are consistent with the claims in the literature.

A major goal of this research was to develop a profile of those who, in *response* to a humiliating event, indicated that they would act violently (plan a way to get back at the perpetrators by seriously harming them and/or harming anyone, it wouldn't matter whom) versus those who would not respond violently. Among this middle school sample, the violent ideators (compared to the nonviolent ideators) reported significantly greater anger toward the perpetrators, more blame toward the perpetrators, and greater difficulty in getting a humiliating event out of their mind. Violent ideators also reported more depressed affect, lower self-esteem, and greater hopelessness, variables in our model of the causes and correlates of self-esteem. In examining the *antecedents* of self-esteem from our general model, we found that the violent ideators reported highly significant differences reflecting lower peer likability and more negative evaluations of their attractiveness, as well as lower social support from both peers and parents. A separate measure of peer rejection also revealed marked differences between the two groups.

More proximal correlates revealed that the violent ideators reported greater preoccupation with violent media (movies, TV, music, video games) and more interest in, and access to, weapons and bombs. Many of the actual school shooters were attracted to violent media and all, obviously, had access to weapons. Many were fascinated with guns and some with bomb making. Literature, reviewed in Harter, Low, et al. (2003), reveals that exposure to violent media desensitizes youth to killing, leading to the greater likelihood of committing violent acts themselves. The military has long employed violent video games as training devices to desensitize combat soldiers in order to provoke them to kill the enemy.

Finally, in this study, we sought to determine whether school personnel could identify those at risk for violence. As reported in Chapter 3 on adolescent development, a comparison of teacher ratings and student ratings of the potential for violence indicated that teachers were unaware of a significant number of adolescents harboring violent thoughts. This is not to indict teachers, as their job definition does not include such detection. The point is that there are self-report strategies that can help to identify such individuals who are at risk, not only for harmful acts toward others but also toward themselves. The identification of such youth may well help to prevent incidents of both homicide as well as suicide (see Harter, Low, et al., 2003).

Within the last decade, others have turned their attention to the role of humiliation and violence within the school setting. Phillips (2007) describes the dynamics of bullying and "punking" in middle school and high school environments. Punking is the practice of verbally and physically assaulting victims. It includes public shaming and humiliation, typically by males where other males are the victims. Both bullying and punking are purposeful strategies to affirm masculine norms of toughness, strength, dominance, and control (see also Pollack, 1998).

Olweus (2008) describes bullying as one of the biggest social problems affecting children in our schools today, observing that periodically we read of yet another suicide by a victim of persistent bullying and related humiliation. He advocates greater awareness of the problem as well as intervention and prevention programs to reduce the incidence of such victimization. Olweus cogently argues that it should be a fundamental right for a child to feel safe within the school setting and to be spared the oppression and repeated, intentional humiliation provoked by bullying.

Mattaini (2008) also addresses this concern, observing that rates of harassment, bullying, threats, coercions, humiliation, and intentional exclusion among children and adolescents are much higher than most adults realize. Even school personnel are not aware of the extent of this problem. Mattaini observes that one-third of high school students do not feel safe at school. Moreover, many find the school environment so socially toxic, emotionally threatening, and violent that they would prefer not to attend school at all.

The problem extends beyond high school into the college campus environment where bullying in the form of hazing has become institutionalized (Denmark, Klara, & Baron, 2008). Hazing involves initiation activities that intentionally include physical challenges or pain, required actions that also produce embarrassment and humiliation. Throughout the current treatments of this topic is the recurring theme of *hostile intent,* identified as a primary cause of humiliation.

K. Williams and Nida (2009) have recently addressed the interesting question of which is worse, bullying or ostracism? They observe that bullying not only involves physical pain and suffering but takes an emotional toll in the form of embarrassment and humiliation that can have lingering effects for years. Despite the aversiveness of being bullied, the victims may derive some satisfaction from realizing that they must be important enough to be the object of such harassment. In contrast, the essence of ostracism is the feeling that one is an invisible victim whom others ignore or overtly reject.

Perhaps even more despicable is humiliation at the hands of adults within the school setting. Some of the vignettes we crafted in our research were modeled on two real-life events that occurred in the middle school that became our natural laboratory. In one case, a teacher intercepted a note that was being passed from one student to another. The teacher read the contents out loud to the entire class. The audience effect was pronounced as laughter ensued, enhancing the humiliation of the note writer. In another classroom the teacher loudly chastised an eighth-grade boy for picking his nose, which provoked laughter among his classmates. The humiliated student started crying, violating the "masculine boy code" (Pollack, 1998). He bolted from the room, running to the principal's office, in tears, where he called his father, begging to be taken home. From a teacher's perspective, humiliation is an effective practice to produce conformity to classroom norms of conduct, and thus it represents a tool in the service of social control. However, from the perspective of the humiliated student, it constitutes a painful emotional experience that can lead to self-derogation, loss of dignity, and associated emotions such as depression and social anxiety.

Gervis and Dunn (2004) have documented the use of humiliation practices by athletic coaches in the United Kingdom. Their focus was the emotional abuse routinely heaped on elite child athletes. In this retrospective study, the athletes recalled numerous examples of such coaching practices, including belittling, humiliating, rejecting, ignoring, and threatening behaviors. The study participants reported feeling humiliated, stupid, worthless, depressed, fearful, and angry, as a result of their coaches' tactics. These athletes' reactions were not only in response to their coaches' behavior at the time but had long-lasting effects.

Perhaps retaliation was not an option for these child athletes, given that an adult authority figure was the humiliator. As a result, reactions were more likely the loss of self-worth and depression as well as minimizing the situation. Thus, the saga of humiliation ends on an unfortunate note that was underscored earlier in comparing the functions of the four negative self-conscious emotions. Humiliation is the least adaptive of these affects and the most emotionally painful, from the perspective of the victim.

Chapter 7

Self-Processes and Motivation in the Classroom

The role of self-perceptions in the classroom is important, not only for psychologists but for educators, where the relationship between scholastic self-concept and classroom motivation is a major theme. Intrinsic versus extrinsic motivation has been a major focus. Findings (see Harter, 1981, 1996) reveal that those with more positive perceptions of their academic competence are much more likely to display intrinsic motivation, whereas those with more negative evaluations of their classroom competence report a more extrinsic motivational orientation. However, what are the dynamics of this relationship and how do we conceptualize the directionality of effects?

Moreover, how does the academic environment itself shape children's and adolescents' perceptions of their scholastic competencies as well as impact the type of motivation they display? How do systematic *changes* in educational practices within the classroom, as children move along the path from elementary school to middle and junior high school, influence changes in self-evaluative processes and motivational orientations? Here, the work of Eccles and colleagues (see Eccles & Roeser, 2009) is of paramount importance. In addition, how do the processes observed in normally achieving students apply to special groups such as learning disabled and gifted children?

In our own work, we initially pitted intrinsic motivation against extrinsic motivation. Subsequently, we operationalized each independently, allowing us to determine how they might conspire to influence performance outcomes. By treating each separately, we were able to construct a typology of students that represents different *combinations* of motivational styles. We further broadened our conceptualization to include *internalized motivation*, a cornerstone of self-determination theory (Ryan & Deci, 2009). According to this theory, students first introject the academic values instilled and modeled by significant others, and eventually come to own these standards that highlight the importance of scholastic diligence and success.

What are the implications of these efforts for possible interventions in the classroom? For example, what motivational orientations should be fostered, in order to promote learning? Should teachers concentrate on basic scholastic skills or should they focus on enhancing scholastic self-concept and self-esteem, an issue about which there is controversy? Moreover, how important is it that students' perceptions of their scholastic competence be *realistic*?

Other than test anxiety, student *emotions* have been given short shrift. We suggest that anxiety mediates the relationship between perceived scholastic competence and motivational orientation. We have also addressed the distinction between *self-conscious emotions* (e.g., pride and shame) and *externally directed emotions* (e.g., anger, frustration, happiness, relief), exploring their relationship to perceived scholastic competence and motivational orientation.

Several contemporary educational issues are also examined: (1) students' ability to voice their opinions in the classroom, (2) gender bias in the classroom, (3) same-gender versus coeducational environments, and (4) the impact of sports participation on self-processes among adolescent female athletes. Finally, implications for educational reform are addressed.

The Link between Perceived Scholastic Competence and Classroom Motivation

Considerable research now indicates that students' perceptions of their scholastic competence bear a strong relationship to their motivational orientation (intrinsic vs. extrinsic) in the classroom (see Eccles & Roeser, 2009; Eccles, Wigfield, & Schiefele, 1998; Eccles et al., 1984; Grum, Lebaric, & Kolenc, 2004; Harter, 1981, 1992, 1996; Lepper, Corpus, & Iyengar, 2005; Marsh & Hau, 2003; Ryan & Deci, 2009). Our own work is first described, followed by a more comprehensive review of the literature.

In our own seminal studies, we have operationally defined perceived scholastic competence as how smart one feels relative to others, how well assignments are understood, how easy it is to figure out assignments, and how quickly one can perform academic tasks (Harter, 1985). In assessing a child's motivational orientation (Harter, 1981) we initially pitted an intrinsic orientation against an extrinsic orientation, in a forced-choice format. We identified the following three dimensions: (1) preference for challenge *versus* preference for easy work assigned, (2) desire to work to satisfy one's curiosity *versus* working to please the teacher and to obtain good grades, and (3) independent mastery attempts *versus* dependent on the teacher.

Initially (Harter, 1981) we merely examined the correlations between perceived scholastic competence and each of these dimensions, finding that perceived scholastic competence was strongly related to *challenge* ($r = .57$), *curiosity* ($r = .33$), and *mastery* ($r = .54$). In subsequent studies (see Harter & Connell, 1984) we combined the three motivational subscales into one motivational composite, which bore a strong relationship to perceived scholastic competence in both elementary ($r = .52$) and junior high ($r = .58$) school samples. Thus, among normative samples, students who feel scholastically competent report more intrinsic motivation compared to the less competent students who opt for a more extrinsic orientation.

We have also demonstrated the robustness of this relationship among learning-disabled children as well as gifted students. In a sample of elementary school mainstreamed learning-disabled students, Renick and Harter (1989) demonstrated that perceived scholastic competence was highly correlated with the motivational composite ($r = .53$). In a dissertation with sixth-grade gifted students (Zumpf, 1986), we first divided pupils into those above and below the group's motivational mean, discovering that even within this intellectually select group, the perceived scholastic competence score of those above the mean (on a 4-point scale) was 3.6 compared to 3.0 for those below the mean, a substantial difference. Thus, across a range of grades (third through ninth) within our normative samples, and among two special education populations, the learning disabled and gifted, there is ample evidence that perceptions of scholastic competence are directly related to self-reported motivational orientation in the classroom.

In an early effort to address the directionality of this relationship (Harter, Whitesell, & Kowalski, 1992), we postulated that competence-related affect (e.g., feeling good or badly about one's work, worrying about whether one could complete assignments, being fearful of getting bad grades) would serve as a mediator. Path-analytic techniques revealed a chain in which perceived scholastic competence influenced competence-related affect, which in turn impacted motivational orientation. Thus, the more scholastically competent children reported more positive emotional reactions, which in turn led them to report a greater intrinsic motivational orientation. In contrast, those who felt that they were less able academically reported more negative emotional reactions, as well as a more extrinsic motivational orientation.

Behavioral Evidence

The findings just described all relied on self-report measures, employing correlational procedures. Therefore, in a master's thesis by Guzman (1983), we employed a *behavioral* index of one dimension of motivational orientation, namely, preference for challenge. We were specifically interested in whether *state test anxiety* mediated the relationship between perceived scholastic competence and behavioral preference for challenge. Test anxiety was defined by emotional reactions (jittery, tense, nervous, shaking) in addition to *worries* about not being able to perform as fast as others, getting the wrong answers or a poor grade, and concerns that others will think you are stupid.

Test anxiety is one of the few emotions that has been extensively researched (Pekrun, 2009). Pekrun has demonstrated that anxiety is the most frequently mentioned emotion in student narratives about what feelings they experience in the academic setting. Pekrun, Goetz, Perry, Kramer, and Hochstadt (2004) have reported that test anxiety is positively related to student expectations of failure and negatively related to their self-evaluations of academic ability. Moreover, failure-related anxiety has been found to reduce intrinsic interest and motivation (Pekrun, 2009). Finally, test anxiety increases over the elementary school years and into middle and junior high school; it remains at relatively high levels thereafter.

We tested a model of the relationships among perceived scholastic competence, test anxiety, and preference for challenge in a simulated classroom environment. Groups of 8 to 10 middle school students sat in a small classroom (with desks in a circle), where research assistants were described as young university teachers who would grade them, clocking (via a visible stopwatch) how long it took every student to complete each problem. Participants were instructed to raise their hand (in front of all of the other students) when they had completed a given problem. Thus, the situation contained elements of both surveillance and social comparison that have been found to undermine intrinsic motivation (Lepper & Gilovich, 1981).

Anagram tasks work well in these simulated classroom conditions because they can be described as an index of their verbal ability, a skill important to their English performance in school. Five levels of difficulty were included (three-, four-, five-, six-, and seven-letter anagrams). During a practice phase, students attempted anagrams at each difficulty level, to get a feel for their own ability level on this task. In a second-choice phase, they were presented with eight pages of three- to seven-letter anagrams and told that on each page they could pick whichever difficulty level they preferred. They were also given letter grades for their performance: they needed to get all eight correct to obtain an A, six correct for a B, four correct for a C, two correct for a D, and none correct would constitute a fail. After the grading system was explained, they were given the anxiety measure followed by the anagram task.

The findings revealed that level of perceived scholastic competence (which had been assessed earlier in their regular school classrooms) was highly predictive of their reported level of anxiety or worry, as well as their difficulty level choices. The more scholastically competent the child felt, the lower the anxiety/worry score, and the more difficult were the anagrams selected. The less competent the child felt, the more anxiety/worry he/she reported to be feeling in the situation, and the easier were the anagrams selected. These findings suggested that the anxiety/worry component may have mediated the relationship between perceived scholastic competence and their difficulty level choices. In order to examine this possibility, we partialled out the effects of the anxiety/worry component, finding that the relationship between perceived competence and difficulty level choice was no longer significant. These results strongly suggest that perceived competence influences level of anxiety/worry, which in turn, determines the difficulty level that a child is willing to attempt in a behavioral problem-solving situation.

Thus, this study expands our interpretation of the link between perceived scholastic competence and motivational orientation, suggesting the mediating role of emotion. Meece, Wigfield, and Eccles (1990) have reported that the effects of achievement (and by inference, perceived scholastic competence) on anxiety are more likely than the effects of anxiety on achievement, consistent with our interpretation. In addition to the importance of emotion to classroom learning, behavioral choices in our preference-for-challenge paradigm have implications for educators. The student who actively avoids challenge will miss learning opportunities that can hone and enhance needed academic skills.

Developmental Decline in Intrinsic Motivation across the School Years

We have also demonstrated dramatic declines in intrinsic motivation over grades 3 through 9 (Harter, 1981) as children gradually shift to a more extrinsic motivational orientation, reflecting increasingly less interest in cognitive challenge, fewer independent mastery strivings, and diminished curiosity as a motivation for learning. This shift reflects a corresponding preference for easy work, a greater extrinsic desire to please the teacher and obtain good grades, and greater dependence on the teacher for solutions to class assignments.

When we first reported these findings (Harter, 1981), we offered the speculation that children were adapting to the demands of a school culture that increasingly reinforces an extrinsic motivational orientation. As the educational focus gradually shifts to the products of one's learning, evaluated through grading practices, children show an accompanying disinterest in the learning process itself, as revealed by their waning intrinsic motivation. Shortly, we will review more comprehensive analyses of the decline of intrinsic motivation, which is supplanted by an extrinsic motivational orientation (e.g., Eccles et al., 1984).

Another dramatic developmental trajectory further suggests that children are systematically mastering the standards by which schools operate (Harter, 1981). We identified two other constructs: (1) independent judgment, and (2) internal criteria for success/failure. Independent judgment assesses students' understanding of what is expected of them in the classroom, having gradually internalized the standards and ground rules established by teachers. Internal criteria for success and failure reflects the degree to which students have internalized the performance standards of educators, allowing them to evaluate themselves, accordingly. We have colloquially referred to these subscales as "knowledge of the rules of the game called school."

The findings reveal a dramatic grade-related *increase* in scores on these two subscales. Thus, as students move through the school system, they increasingly acquire information about how the educational system operates. They come to understand the practices to which teachers adhere and they internalize the standards by which their own classroom performance is evaluated. We would submit that this *increase* in knowledge of the rules of the game called school is intimately related to the *decrease* in students' intrinsic motivation. The more students appreciate the shifting standards of performance, the more many children opt for an extrinsic orientation that ultimately undermines intrinsic interest in learning.

Eccles's Analysis of Motivational Declines between Elementary and Junior High School

The 1970s and early 1980s ushered in a spate of experimental studies demonstrating that extrinsic rewards for learning severely undermined children's intrinsic mastery motivation (see Deci, 1975; Lepper & Greene, 1975). Lepper and Henderlong (2000) have reviewed 25 years of research documenting the detrimental effects of extrinsic reinforcement on children's natural intrinsic interest in mastery and learning. Lepper and Gilovich (1981) have further demonstrated that surveillance, as well as social comparison, contributes to decreases in intrinsic motivation. In the mid-1980s, the stage shifted to a direct examination of these processes within the classroom. Eccles and colleagues (1984) have offered a thoughtful indictment of our educational system for practices that undermine our students' intrinsic interest in mastery and learning.

Eccles et al. (1984) initially provided an extensive summary of findings documenting classroom declines in motivation and put forth the first comprehensive analysis of why these trends have existed and persisted within our educational system. They argued that the educational establishment is responsible for the decline in intrinsic motivation as well as for why attitudes toward school learning and achievement become increasingly negative as children progress through the school system. They observed that the classroom environment, itself, as reflected in teacher values and practices, changes as students move into middle or junior high schools in ways that directly impact students' self-perceptions and motivation.

Here is a summary of their trenchant critique. As students make these educational transitions, the classroom environment becomes more impersonal (teachers focus on their own particular school subject to the detriment of personal relationships with students). The structure of the school becomes more *formal* in its demands. There is increasing emphasis on a student's *ability*, whereas in elementary school there was more focus on *effort* as the path to learning. Evaluation is predicated on a student's performance on tests, designed by the teacher as well as by standardized test developers. Thus, the focus shifts from the *process* of learning to an evaluation of *products* or *outcomes* that define achievement. Moreover, these outcomes become more *public*, as exemplified by the public posting of grades, the major metric of performance. The learning environment becomes more *competitive*. Competition is exacerbated by the increasing emphasis on *social comparison*, as students are encouraged to assess their ability relative to others. Grading on a curve is designed to separate students from one another, forcing students to locate themselves on a hierarchy of performance where all but those at the top of the academic totem pole fall short.

Eccles et al. (1984) review findings in the late 1970s and early 1980s that speak to the negative consequences of these changes. One set of consequences involves the impact on the *self* that, in turn, may impact motivational orientation. A review of the extant literature of the time reveals that when the evaluative beacon focuses on the ability of the self in comparison to others, rather than on learning itself, interest and motivation are attenuated. Eccles et al. report that students express negative attitudes about drills, testing, grading on a curve, competition, and the emphasis on right versus wrong. Negative perceptions of these palpable changes in classroom practices lead to the decline in students' perceptions of ability, as they make the transition to middle and junior high schools (see also Jacobs et al., 2002). Moreover, as noted earlier, anxiety over one's scholastic performance increases across grade level, particularly during these transitions. Thus, a constellation of grade-related changes in the teaching and learning environment negatively impact both perceptions of scholastic competence and classroom motivation.

Generalization of Grade-Related Changes to Learning-Disabled Students

The decline of intrinsic motivation is not limited to regular classroom students but extends to learning-disabled children. We have compared normally achieving children to mainstreamed learning-disabled children who spent the majority of their school day within the regular classroom setting. They were staffed into a learning disabilities resource room for special remedial help in areas where they had particular deficiencies (Renick & Harter, 1989).

Figure 7.1 presents a comparison of the trends for normally achieving and learning-disabled students across grades 3 through 7. The findings highlight dramatic *similarities* between the two groups as well as *differences*. First, the developmental trends are virtually identical. With increasing grade level, the learning-disabled students also reported a systematic *decrease* in intrinsic motivation. Furthermore, both groups demonstrated a systematic *increase* in the internalization of the standards of judgment and criteria for success put forth by teachers. Thus, the learning-disabled students displayed the same developmental trajectories across grade level that were demonstrated by normally achieving students.

The *difference* between the normally achieving and learning-disabled students can be observed in the *mean level* of these scores, which for the learning-disabled students are systematically more extrinsic at every grade level, for both factors. This greater extrinsic orientation among the learning-disabled students can be interpreted as quite realistic, given their intellectual limitations. With regard to the *motivational* components, greater avoidance of challenge, efforts to please the teacher, and dependence on the teacher to master material would appear to be adaptive responses. Similarly, for what we have labeled the *informational* components, greater reliance on the teacher's judgment and a greater need for extrinsic feedback are realistic strategies that may ensure some modicum of success.

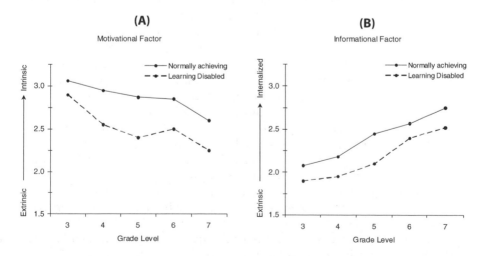

FIGURE 7.1. Intrinsic versus extrinsic components by grade and type of student.

These findings caution us against making value judgments about the unequivocal desirability of an intrinsic motivational orientation. For children with certain cognitive deficits, a more adaptive strategy for minimizing failure and maximizing successful performance may understandably entail a more extrinsic orientation. Thus, we need to consider students' motivational orientation in relation to their particular strengths and weaknesses, rather than tout intrinsic motivation as the optimal orientation for all.

Individual Differences in Grade-Related Motivational Shifts toward an Extrinsic Orientation

The implication, thus far, is that systematic changes within the educational environment attenuate the intrinsic motivation of all students, particularly during transitions to middle and junior high school. Such is not always the case, however. A minority of students actually show *increases* in intrinsic motivation. A third group of students report no major changes in their level of motivation, along the intrinsic–extrinsic motivation continuum (Harter et al., 1992; Riddle, 1986).

Our own analysis has focused on how the grade-related changes in educational practices identified by Eccles and her colleagues (1984) first impact perceptions of academic competence that, in turn, will result in changes or stability in motivational orientation. As argued in more detail elsewhere (Harter, 1996), such transitions bring with them a new *social reference* group. Typically students from several elementary feeder schools make the shift to a single middle or junior high school. Thus, the majority of the student body constitutes individuals whom one has not previously encountered in the classroom setting. The pedagogical changes identified by Eccles et al. (e.g., social comparison and an emphasis on ability) exacerbate the need for students to reevaluate their competence relative to those in the new social reference group. Some may feel *less* scholastically competent, some *more* competent, and still others may experience no change in their level of competence. These changes, therefore, will force students to reevaluate their positions in the scholastic pecking order. We will provide evidence, shortly, that changes in perceived scholastic competence drive corresponding changes in motivational orientation.

Eccles et al. (1984) make a related point, arguing that the effects of educational transitions and related changes in practices will, in part, depend upon a student's *ability* level. They are likely to increase anxiety among those students who do not perceive themselves to be scholastically capable. They cite findings suggesting that environmental settings that focus attention on ability, rather than the academic task at hand, have debilitating effects on the motivation of all but the most scholastically competent and confident individuals.

We have examined these hypotheses in our own work (Harter et al., 1992; Riddle, 1986). We employed a 7-month longitudinal design, testing students in the spring of their sixth-grade elementary year and then in the late fall of their seventh-grade junior high school year, following the transition. The junior high school drew from four different elementary schools, confronting the seventh graders with a substantially large new social reference group, three-fourths of whom were unknown to them. Measures of perceived scholastic competence and motivational orientation were administered at each time point. For the second administration, we selected late fall in order to ensure that as junior high school students, they had already received sufficient teacher feedback on assignments and classroom tests, as well as one report card. We were particularly interested in the hypothesis that changes in students' perceptions of competence would be predictive of changes in their motivational orientation. Thus, we first identified three subgroups of students, those whose perceptions of scholastic competence across the two time periods (1) increased, (2) decreased, or (3) remained the same.

The perceived scholastic scores of these three groups at the two grade levels are presented in Figure 7.2. The changes of those whose perceptions either increased or decreased were marked. We speculated that the enhanced salience of ability feedback in combination with greater emphasis on social comparison in junior high school, within the context of a new social reference group, caused students to reevaluate their scholastic competence. As a result, a sizable number of students reported altered conceptions of their academic ability.

In order to test the hypothesis that changes in motivational orientation

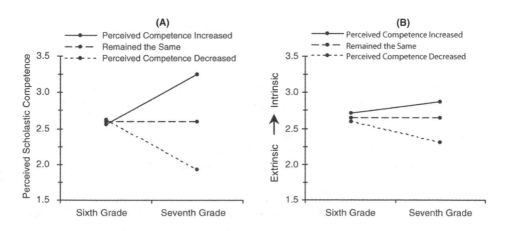

FIGURE 7.2. Perceived competence and motivational orientation by change groups over time.

paralleled these shifts in perceived scholastic ability, we examined the motivational composite (preference for challenge, curiosity, and independent mastery) for the three perceived competence change groups. Students whose perceptions of competence increased also manifested corresponding increases in intrinsic motivation. Students whose perceptions of their scholastic competence decreased showed a corresponding shift toward extrinsic motivation. Those with no changes in perceived scholastic competence showed no shifts in motivational orientation. Thus, the pattern provides support for the hypothesis that changes in perceived scholastic competence across the transition to junior high school predict corresponding changes in motivational orientation.

Our methodology, however, does not directly establish the directionality of effects. Might it be that changes in educational practices first impact motivational orientation that, in turn, lead to alterations in students' academic performance that are mirrored in their perceptions of their competence? Further research, employing more specific methodologies and more sophisticated statistical procedures are needed to tease apart the directionality of effects.

Marsh and colleagues (Guay, Marsh, & Boivin, 2003; Marsh & Hau, 2003; Marsh, Trautwein, Lüdtke, Köller, & Baument, 2005) have embarked on a related endeavor to address the directionality of academic self-concept and actual academic achievement. Employing statistically sensitive techniques and longitudinal designs, they have found considerable support for a *reciprocal effects model*, revealing that academic self-concept is both a cause and an effect of achievement. Thus, self-concept has an effect on achievement but achievement also causally influences self-concept. This model has been documented in a meta-analysis of studies that includes cross-cultural comparisons (Marsh & Craven, 2006).

Students' Perceptions of Changes in Classroom Educational Practices

The previous interpretation of our findings relies on *inferences* about changes in the educational classroom environment as students progress from one grade to the next. We had no direct evidence that the educational practices in these schools increasingly focused on the salience of ability, emphasized social comparison and competition, and stressed the importance of grades and the product of one's performance. Thus, we conducted a follow-up study in which we asked students directly to evaluate their educational environment with regard to changes in these practices. Middle school students in grades 6, 7, and 8 were asked to compare current school practices with those in the preceding year.

The findings (Harter et al., 1992) revealed that the vast majority of students indicated that educational practices in their classrooms had changed in the direction of a greater emphasis on those dimensions that foster a more negative evaluation of scholastic competence and a more extrinsic motivational orientation. That is, they reported increases in the more external emphasis on competence evaluation, academic performance, and social comparison that, in turn, would make their own ability more salient and attenuate intrinsic interest in learning. Thus, we were able to demonstrate that a number of the changes that have been postulated would appear to exist within our local school settings, at least in the perceptions of middle school students.

Eccles's More Recent Analysis of the Mismatch between Educational Practices and Adolescents' Developmental Needs

Eccles and colleagues (see Eccles & Midgley, 1989; Eccles & Roeser, 2009; Eccles et al., 1998) have provided a compelling developmental analysis of numerous *mismatches* between the psychological needs of young adolescents and the educational practices that students must endure, the perspective of person–environment fit.

1. Just as young adolescents are appropriately yearning for *autonomy* in making decisions, teachers become more controlling, for fear of raging hormones and adolescent uncontrollability. Thus, students are given less choice in decision making within the classroom learning environment, stifling their need to practice more mature, psychological skills.

2. Just at the stage of development when young adolescents are searching for adult surrogates, as they struggle to become somewhat independent of parents, the job definition for teachers shifts. The new agenda is to focus on teaching their particular school subject, rather than offering students emotional and psychological support. In our experience, such teachers are outspoken in indicating that they did not enter their profession to address what they consider to be "touchy-feely" goals. Some openly acknowledge that they are uncomfortable treading on this territory because they lack the training and the desire to intervene in the psychological and emotional lives of their students.

3. At a period of their life when adolescents are becoming increasingly more self-conscious, cognizant of the ever-present evaluation by others (real or imagined), the educational system increases its emphasis on social comparison through many teacher practices (e.g., posting of grades and evaluative verbal feedback in front of other students). Marsh and Hau (2003) confirm that students actively compare their academic achievements to those of their peers, in forming their own academic self-concept. Studies

of self-conscious emotions (see Chapter 6) reveal that humiliation is a natural and painful emotional reaction to negative feedback in the presence of an audience. Furthermore, embarrassment is not merely a reaction to the public display of social mishaps but can be triggered by praise for successes that are publicly acknowledged. Self-conscious adolescents would appear to be particularly vulnerable.

Social comparison is rampant at many levels. Within the regular classroom setting, it is increasingly evident as students make the transition to middle and junior high school. The context broadens with ability grouping within one's classroom. Eccles and Roeser (2009) review findings revealing that lower-track students report being labeled "dumb" by teachers and peers, causing them to feel less committed to school and less successful, academically. The comparative canvas broadens even further as certain adolescents are segregated into special education classrooms, leading to the potential stigmatization of students so assigned.

The comparative lens also focuses on the aptitude of entire schools. For example, in Colorado there is the statewide administration of the Colorado Scholastic Aptitude Performance (CSAP) tests; scores for Denver-area schools are published in the newspaper. These comparisons are not lost on students. When we recently conducted a study in one of the lowest-achieving schools in Denver, the students spontaneously volunteered that they were the "Denver dummy school." Comparisons escalate when districts are compared to other districts, and when inner-city schools are compared to suburban schools. Thus, social comparison spirals upward within the educational system, ultimately leading to collective pride or shame, experienced by one's entire school or district.

4. At a time when adolescents' increasing cognitive-developmental skills might foster increasing preference for challenge, many of the assignments, for example, rote-learning exercises, do not fulfill these new cognitive-developmental needs. When our own daughter took a ninth-grade chemistry class, she came home one Friday distressed and bored over a weekend assignment where she had to memorize the periodic table. This is not an intrinsically interesting task for most adolescents, nor is the practical utility obvious. She was truly turned off to "science" as defined by the school system. Since it was a sunny spring day, I suggested that we conduct a *real* experiment in the garden. So we planted onion sets in two different rows, one where the sets (that resemble Hershey kisses for the nongardener) were planted upright and in a second row, they were planted upside down. She eagerly but impatiently waited out the 21 days when we had our answer. Both rows of healthy scallions were identical! Our daughter was incredulous. "You mean that under the ground the ones we planted upside down knew how to turn themselves right-side up?" She had answered her own scientific question in the natural laboratory of our garden. To this day, she

remembers nothing about the periodic table (and obviously, she did not pursue a career in chemistry!) She became a successful elementary school teacher in imparting such lessons to her pupils and her inquisitive young son. This experience hit home, revealing how the many nonchallenging and noninteresting classroom assignments can dampen students' enthusiasm for (in this case) science, as it has traditionally been taught (see Harter, 2011).

Eccles and Roeser (2009) identify two additional mismatches. As children progress through puberty, they need more sleep and their natural sleep cycle dictates the desire to go to bed later in the evening and wake up later in the morning. They note that many secondary school systems now typically demand early rise times for adolescents. As a result, many teenagers experience daytime sleepiness that undermines their ability to arrive on time, alert, and prepared to learn. (Over the years, when we have been given the first period to administer our measures, we have witnessed many early morning heads on desks and constant yawning.)

Finally, Eccles and Roeser (2009) describe a mismatch that is relevant for female students. Here, they introduce the concept of "girl-friendly" classrooms. They address pedagogical strategies for teaching math and science to girls. Females, they point out, respond more positively to math and science instruction if it is taught in a cooperative and/or individualized manner, rather than in a competitive atmosphere. Their review of the literature further reveals that if these subjects are taught from an applied and more person-centered perspective, as opposed to an abstract theoretical point of view, it will be more effective. Finally, they note that an experiential approach, coupled with the lack of subtle sexism that often occurs in teaching math and science to girls, will enhance their interest and motivation.

Social Comparison among Learning-Disabled and Gifted Students

It is of interest to ask whether the social comparison processes that have been identified for normally achieving students are observed in special populations. We (Renick & Harter, 1989) addressed this issue among learning-disabled students documenting, as have others, that these students clearly do make use of social comparison information in judging their own scholastic competence. The findings in the literature are equivocal with regard to the impact on perceived scholastic competence (see Erlbaum, 2002; Zeleke, 2004). We have demonstrated that the effect upon these evaluative judgments depends upon the type of classroom setting, mainstreamed into the regular classroom versus segregated in full-time special education classrooms, in interaction with the developmental level of the student (children vs. adolescents).

At the elementary school level, we found that learning-disabled students reported more positive scholastic competence if they attended special education classes full time; in contrast, the self-perceptions of those who were mainstreamed were more negative. We interpreted these findings in terms of social comparison processes. We inferred that those elementary school students in the special education setting were comparing themselves to other learning-disabled students who favored more positive self-evaluations. The mainstreamed learning disabled students were forced to compare themselves to a majority of normally achieving students, leading to the realization that their performance was less adequate, causing more negative evaluations of their scholastic competence. These findings are consistent with Pekrun's (2009) observation that students' self-evaluations of ability tend to be higher in low-ability, compared to high-ability, classrooms.

Marsh and Hau (2003) report similar findings among students in the second through sixth grades, where learning-disabled students in special education classes reported significantly more positive self-concepts in reading and math, compared to those who remained in regular classroom contexts. Our interpretation of such differences assumes that elementary school learning-disabled students in the self-contained classroom were comparing themselves to others in that setting.

We have, however, observed just the opposite pattern at the *middle* school level. Those learning-disabled children in self-contained special education classrooms reported more negative scholastic self-concepts than those who were mainstreamed into the regular classroom. What might be possible for the reversal of effects? We reasoned that these young adolescents had become cognitively aware of the psychological implications of their placement. That is, those in the special education environment were making their comparisons at the *classroom* level, and felt stigmatized, as a result. If they were comparing their entire classroom to the mainstreamed environment, then they would come up short. Middle school students placed in the regular classroom profited from identifying with the higher-functioning students in that setting, leading to more positive evaluations of their scholastic competence. This interpretation requires an appreciation for those cognitive-developmental advances in early adolescence that permit students to make more sophisticated judgments about the implications of their placement.

Our examination of social comparison processes among *gifted* children came at the invitation of a suburban school district that had initiated a program to segregate their fifth- and sixth-grade gifted and talented students in self-contained classrooms where the curriculum was tailored to their advanced intellectual level. It was the educators' hope that such a program would lead to more positive student evaluations of their scholastic self-concept and would also enhance their level of intrinsic motivation, offsetting the normative decline that our previous findings had demonstrated. In a dissertation by Zumpf (1986), we administered our measures of perceived scholastic competence and motivational orientation at the very beginning of the program and then at the end of the school year, 8 months later.

Contrary to the hopes of the school administrators, we did not find increases in either scholastic self-concept or intrinsic motivation over the course of this program. If anything, we found a slight decline in perceived scholastic self-concept. Marsh and Hau (2003) have also reported declines over time in academic self-concept for those in gifted and talented programs, compared to a normative comparison group. In the regular classroom setting, gifted children stood out in terms of their intellectual ability. As McCoach and Siegle (2003) have documented, gifted children report higher academic self-perceptions and higher grade-point averages (GPAs) than the general school sample, when integrated into regulated classrooms. We interpreted our own findings as suggesting that segregated gifted placement stimulated social comparison with other, equally talented students with whom they were competing, driving their self-evaluations in a more negative direction.

It should be emphasized that the decline in perceptions of scholastic competence for the entire gifted classroom was not dramatic. Rather, the pattern was more complex. We first divided students into three groups, those whose perceived scholastic competence increased, decreased, or remained the same over the course of the academic year program. Since the gifted students were drawn from several schools in the district, they faced a new social reference group of similarly gifted individuals to whom they now compared themselves. The salience of intellectual *ability* was marked, given that this was the selection criterion placing them in the program.

When we examined changes in motivational orientation we found that those gifted students whose perceptions of their scholastic competence increased reported corresponding increases in intrinsic motivation. Conversely, those whose perceptions of competence decreased showed a parallel shift toward a more extrinsic orientation. Those reporting no change in perceived competence also reported no significant changes in their motivational orientation. Thus, even within this intellectually select group, we documented the same processes observed with normally achieving students. Changes in their academic environment provoked a reevaluation of their academic ability that, in turn, led to changes in their motivational orientation.

In this study, we had the opportunity to conduct individual interviews with students at the end of the year-long program. We were particularly interested in those gifted students who reported *increases* in their scholastic competence (approximately 20%, compared to 30% reporting no change and 50% who acknowledged a decline in perceived ability). The focus of our interview was the role of social comparison. Those comparing themselves to other gifted children reported decreases in scholastic competence. Among those who reported *increases* in perceived competence, many articulated the fact that they did *not* compare themselves to the other gifted children in the program. Rather, they compared their achievements to their *own past performance* in the regular classroom setting, describing how much more they were learning in the gifted program and how much more scholastically able they felt, as a result. Sample comments included "I don't really care how the other students are doing, all I care about is how *I* am doing, compared to last year, before the program"; "It doesn't make sense to compare myself to the other students, that isn't relevant to my own improvement"; "How hard I work and whether the schoolwork is interesting and challenging is what really matters, not what other kids do or think"; and "If I am interested in my own schoolwork, not other kids', I will put in the effort and then I will feel smarter than before."

These findings highlight the distinction between two different comparison processes, a "self-referential" or "internal" frame of reference versus a "social comparative or external frame of reference" (D'Amico, Carmeci, & Cardaci, 2006; Marsh, Trautwein, Lüdtke, & Köller, 2008). The external frame of reference involves a comparison with others, a practice fostered by many teachers. In contrast, the self-referential frame of reference involves a comparison between one's own abilities in different competence domains ("I'm better at math than English") or "temporal" comparisons ("I'm smarter this year than last year"). Oyserman, Bybee, Terry, and Hart-Johnson (2004) suggest that the latter type of comparison allows students to play a role in self-regulating their own future behavior (e.g., "I may not be doing well in school this year, but to make sure I do better next year, I have signed up for summer tutoring").

Our interview findings have implications for teacher training and educational reform. Instead of forcing children to compare themselves to other students, a much better strategy would be to encourage children to compare their progress to their own past performance, noting realistic gains and improvements due to their own mastery efforts (see Eccles & Roeser, 2009). Such a strategy should lead students to appreciate increasing levels of achievement driven by their own behavior, independent of the performance of other students.

We can relate these observations to the work of Dweck (see Dweck & Master, 2009), who has identified two types of intelligence beliefs held by students. Those possessing what Dweck calls an *incremental theory* of intelligence believe that ability is malleable and that the more *effort* they put into learning, the more intellectually competent they will become. In contrast, those who contend that intelligence is fixed, whom Dweck labels as *entity* theorists, are less likely to exert effort and therefore will typically not report gains in their intellectual ability. Entity theorists also worry more about their ability, which interferes with their performance, leading to less effort and to declines in their perceived competence given little intrinsic motivation to perform (see also Dweck & Grant, 2008).

Other investigators have found support for this framework. For example, Robbins and Pals (2002) have reported that undergraduates, identified as *entity* theorists, adopted performance goals rather than the learning goals of *incremental* theorists. Furthermore, entity theorists displayed a helpless response pattern, whereas incremental theorists displayed a mastery orientation. Finally, entity theorists reported declines in self-esteem during their college years in contrast to incremental theorists whose self-esteem increased. Applying Dweck's (Dweck & Master, 2009) framework, it would appear that those gifted children in our study, whose perceived academic competence increased in the program, were incremental theorists who made temporal comparisons that highlighted their own personal mastery efforts, rather than comparing themselves to others.

Intrinsic *versus* Extrinsic Motivation or Intrinsic *and* Extrinsic Motivation?

Our motivational composite, pitting intrinsic motivation against extrinsic motivation, does have conceptual and empirical utility, as well as appeal (see Lepper et al., 2005). Moreover, it is clearly predicted by perceived scholastic competence among normally achieving students as well as learning-disabled and gifted children. That said, in middle and junior high school specific school subjects such as math, science, social studies, and English become increasingly differentiated leading us to ask whether students report the same or different motivational orientations across these subjects (Harter & Jackson, 1992). We further questioned whether intrinsic and extrinsic motivations should be viewed as opposite poles along a single dimension or whether they might coexist as independent determinants of classroom learning.

We examined these issues by making two methodological changes to our typical question format. On the original intrinsic versus extrinsic motivation, we had questions such as the following:

Some kids like hard work because it is a challenge.	BUT	Other kids prefer easy work they are sure they can do.

Very True for Me	Sort of True for Me		Sort of True for Me	Very True for Me
____	____		____	____

Students first choose whether they are more like the students described on the left side of the statement (those who like hard work) or more like the students described on the right side of the statement (who prefer easy work). They then go to the statement that is most like them and make a second decision: Is that statement "very true for me" or just "sort of true for me"? Thus, they make only one response choice (among the four) per question; they check either the left side or the right side but not both sides. Items are counterbalanced such that sometimes the intrinsic choice is on the left and sometimes it is on the right. An item like the one above would be scored 4, 3, 2, 1, where intrinsic motivation is given the higher scores and extrinsic motivation is given the lower scores. An item where the extrinsic motivational description was on the left would be scored 1, 2, 3, 4.

There were two modifications to this question format: (1) Students made separate judgments of their motivational orientation across four school subjects (math, science, social studies, and English; and (2) students were given the option of checking that *both* orientations are true for them, a choice placed in the middle of the item (see example below).

Some kids like hard work in MATH because it is a challenge.			Other kids prefer easy work in MATH that they are sure they can do.	
Really True for Me	Sort of True for Me	BOTH SIDES ARE TRUE	Sort of True for Me	Really True for Me
_____	_____	_____	_____	_____

The rationale for this second adaptation was that, in reality, many students are motivated by both intrinsic factors *and* extrinsic incentives and rewards (Harter & Jackson, 1992). They may be inherently interested in a particular school subject, displaying curiosity. However, they also see the need to get good grades, they wish to please the teacher, and when help *is* needed, they ask for it appropriately. In our own academic histories, most of us would probably acknowledge that despite intrinsic curiosity and preference for challenge, we realized that to be truly successful in school, a microcosm of our larger society, we also had to adhere to certain extrinsic demands that would, in part, be an important pathway to achievement.

Some years later, others (see Covington, 2009; Lepper et al., 2005) came to a similar conclusion. Covington argues that a positive, additive relationship between extrinsic and intrinsic rewards is more often the rule than the exception. He contends that extrinsic rewards, for example, money or praise, can serve intrinsic goals as long as they support valued goals. Covington clarifies his argument, observing that extrinsic rewards can either advance a love of learning, if they serve positive, task-orientated goals, or interfere with intrinsic motives for learning if they are pursued for the purpose of self-aggrandizement. Successful students most likely value the intrinsic appeal of learning as well as the fulfillment of academic requirements that are necessary to achieve eventual educational and occupational goals.

Lepper et al. (2005) present a similar argument, adapting our original instrument that pitted an intrinsic against an extrinsic orientation (Harter, 1981). Their solution was to translate the extrinsic and intrinsic content into separate Likert scales, thereby allowing students to endorse both orientations, should they so desire. They have concluded that intrinsic and extrinsic motivation can and do coexist in the classroom; the intent is to determine how much of each motivation a child displays. This was precisely what our (Harter & Jackson, 1992) study addressed.

Our findings (Harter & Jackson, 1992) revealed four patterns that described student motivations:

1. The first pattern identified those students who reported very strong differences in motivational orientation across four subjects; math, science, English, and social studies. Many students reported higher intrinsic motivation for English and social studies but extrinsic motivation for science and math. The opposite, less common configuration was observed for those who displayed an extrinsic orientation for English and social studies in contrast to an intrinsic motivation for science and math.
2. A second pattern defined those students who endorsed the *middle* choice, indicating that they were both intrinsically and extrinsically motivated across most, if not all, school subjects.
3. A third pattern captured students who reported that they were intrinsically motivated in all school subjects.
4. A fourth pattern, the opposite, defined those students who indicated that they were primarily extrinsically motivated across all school subjects.

In summary, the first pattern reveals that certain students exhibit a more situation-specific stance, indicating that they are more intrinsically motivated in some school subjects and more extrinsically motivated in others. The second most common pattern, reflects the fact that many students are not unilaterally either intrinsically or extrinsically motivated across school subjects but that *both* orientations operate across school subjects. The third and fourth patterns speak more to traitlike behavior for certain subgroups of students. These students report that they are either totally intrinsically motivated across all school subjects, the third pattern, or totally extrinsically motivated across all school subjects, the fourth pattern.

From a larger theoretical perspective, our research raises the issue of whether intrinsic versus extrinsic motivation is best conceptualized as a *trait* or is more situation specific, where situation, in this case, refers to academic school subjects. Whether certain behaviors are best characterized as generalized traits or more situation specific has been a long-standing debate in the field. Certain theorists (e.g., Mischel, 1973; Mischel & Morf, 2003) have made a compelling case for situation specificity. Others have made thoughtful arguments for the utility of more generalized traits (e.g., Epstein, 1981; Kendrick & Funder, 1988).

We have not identified with either camp. We have proposed that the construct of motivational orientation itself should not be conceptualized as either a trait or as situation specific (Harter & Jackson, 1992). That is, there may be a group of individuals who display intrinsic motivation in some situations, whereas their behavior is more extrinsically motivated in others. However, neither did we espouse the strong form of the antitrait position, namely, that behavior in all individuals is best characterized as situation specific. Rather, we have argued that there exist certain subgroups of children who *behave* in traitlike fashion; that is, their behavior is consistently intrinsic or extrinsic across situations. Thus, the motivational orientation construct per se is *not* a trait, because many individuals do show situation specificity.

The Relationship of Motivational Orientation to Perceived Scholastic Competence for Specific School Subjects

As reported, previous findings have documented a strong relationship between intrinsic motivation and perceptions of scholastic competence. In the Harter and Jackson (1992) study cited above, we also found a similar relationship at the school subject level. Perceived scholastic competence in a given school subject strongly predicted motivational orientation for that domain of study. The unevenness observed in some student report cards may well be a function of this relationship. Poorer grades are going to be obtained for those school subjects where students feel both incompetent and extrinsically motivated, whereas better grades will be more likely awarded in those school subjects where a student feels competent and intrinsically motivated.

Intrinsic Motivation Compared to Internalized Motivation

In the preceding discussion, our primary motivational constructs have targeted intrinsic and extrinsic motivation. However, thoughtful observations of child behavior will reveal that these are not the only motivational forces at work, particularly for behaviors that initially require adult guidance, supervision, and support. What ultimately motivates children to clean their rooms, take out the garbage, feed the dog, share a favorite toy with a not-so-likable cousin, study for a test in the school subject one likes the least, and refrain from retaliating, given a sibling's provocation? When these become seemingly self-motivated behaviors, it is highly unlikely that they are being driven by intrinsic interest, curiosity, inherent pleasure, or enjoyment in the process per se.

A more plausible interpretation is that these behaviors represent the *internalization* of rewards, values, standards, and attitudes that were initially external (i.e., modeled and demanded by adult socializing agents). That is, behaviors initially under the control of extrinsically established contingencies come to be performed because the child has learned that these behaviors are important and therefore he/she internalizes these values. Thus, the child becomes capable, eventually, of engaging in self-reward for performing these behaviors and is no longer completely dependent upon external rewards from the significant others in his/her life. There is ample historical precedent for such an internalization process, in Freudian concepts of the superego and the ego ideal (Freud, 1952), and in the early theorizing of social learning theorists (e.g., Aronfreed, 1976).

Others (see Ryan, Connell, & Deci, 1985) began to develop a more comprehensive theoretical model of these and related constructs, postulating that extrinsically motivated behaviors could become subject to an internalization process that would allow them to become autonomous. On their surface, behaviors propelled by internalized motivation seem to share many of the features that define intrinsic motivation, in that individuals experience both as freely chosen and volitional, as well as personally engaging. However, Ryan and Deci (2009) make an important distinction in clarifying that intrinsic motivation is driven by inherent *interest*, whereas behaviors propelled by *internalized* motivation are predicated on the fact that they come to be *valued* as personally important and relevant to what eventually become self-selected goals. In developing their self-determination theory, Ryan and Deci have provided an analysis of an emerging sequence that includes intermediate stages toward the endpoint of *internalization*. Between an extrinsic and internalized orientation are stages of "introjected" behavioral regulation where there is still an awareness of the extrinsic roots of the standards and values that partially govern performance. The individual, at these intermediate stages, has not yet totally "owned" an internalized motivation that drives his/her behavior. Thus, engagement in school learning is not yet totally self-determined until the final endpoint of this process.

In our own earlier empirical efforts (see C. Chandler, 1981; Connell, 1981; Harter, 1992), we examined the distinction between intrinsic and internalized motivation, incorporating both into a measure that also tapped extrinsic motivation. This self-report instrument differed from our original questionnaire in that it did not employ a forced-choice format. Rather, we opted to assess each of these three motivational sources independently. Lepper et al. (2005) adopted a similar, partial strategy some years later, arguing that intrinsic motivation needed to be distinguished from extrinsic motivation, assessing each independently. They also urged that a separate measure of internalized motive could be potentially useful and informative, which our own study had demonstrated, some years earlier. Our procedure, therefore, allowed the student to indicate that more than one source of motivation could be simultaneously operative.

The questionnaire we developed consisted of three subscales: intrinsic, internalized, and extrinsic motivation. Items were worded as statements to which the child could respond on a 4-point scale: Very True, Pretty True, Only Sort of True, and Not Very True. Each item began with the stem "I do my schoolwork because" and several related reasons were included. On the intrinsic subscales, reasons included "Because what we learn is really interesting," "Because it is challenging," "Because I'm really curious," and "Because I enjoy trying to understand things I do not already know." Thus, it tapped those features reflected in the intrinsic pole of our earlier scale, namely, preference for challenge, curiosity, independent mastery, and enjoyment of the learning process, itself.

The *internalized* motivation subscale included the following reasons for why I do my schoolwork: "Because I've learned for myself that it's important for me to do it well," "Because I just know, without having to be told, that I should do my schoolwork," "because it's important to get a good education," and "If I do well now, it will mean better things for my future education and my ability to get a good job." Thus, some of the reasons focus on future goals and aspirations.

The *extrinsic* motivation subscale focused on performance, in order to either obtain rewards and approval or avoid external sanctions and disapproval. Both parents and teachers were included as sources of external motivation. Reasons that emphasize more immediate consequences included "Because my teacher will be pleased with me if I do," "Because I will get something extra or special privileges from the teacher for getting the work done," "Because the teacher will give me a bad grade if I don't," "Because my parents will be mad or annoyed with me if I don't do well," and "Because my parents will be happy with me if I do well.

A major goal in constructing this instrument was to identify a *typology* representing different combinations of these three motivational dimensions. We began by identifying students whose scores presented combinations of high (top-third) or low (bottom-third) values across the three dimensions. Given three dimensions, there were eight possible combinations of high and low scores. Of these eight, four patterns stood out with sufficient frequency to suggest that these were the primary constellations that defined our sample of middle school students. These four types, labeled A, B, C, D, are described in the table below.

Type	Intrinsic	Internalized	Extrinsic
A	High	High	Low
B	High	High	High
C	Low	Low	High
D	Low	Low	Low

The *Type A* student claims to be both intrinsically interested in learning as well as motivated for internalized reasons, having come to value school performance as important. This type of student does not endorse extrinsic motivation, presumably because he/she no longer needs extrinsic rewards and sanctions to motivate engagement in schoolwork.

The *Type B* student endorses all three sources of motivation. Unlike the Type A student, this group appears to still need the extrinsic rewards and sanctions, to maximize performance. One may speculate that for such children, the internalization process was not supported, and therefore motivation cannot be sustained in the absence of external contingencies. These students may typify an intermediate, *introjected* stage, identified by Ryan and Deci (2009).

The *Type C* student displays a pattern that is the opposite of the Type A student in that neither intrinsic nor internalized motivation play a primary role. Rather, the only source of motivation appears to be external rewards and privileges, in combination with the avoidance of sanctions or disapproval from teachers and parents.

The *Type D* student plummets to a motivational nadir in that none of the sources we included appear to be motivating. Although it is possible that unidentified sources are operative, such students report little, if any, motivation for classroom learning. These are the most challenging and frustrating students, for teachers.

Correlates of These Styles: Perceptions of Competence, Affect, and Teacher Acceptance

Having established the most prevalent motivational patterns, we next addressed how these patterns were related to children's perceptions of their scholastic competence, their affective reactions to their school performance, and perceived teacher acceptance. The pattern of findings, presented in Figure 7.3, is quite consistent across the measures of competence, affect, and teacher acceptance.

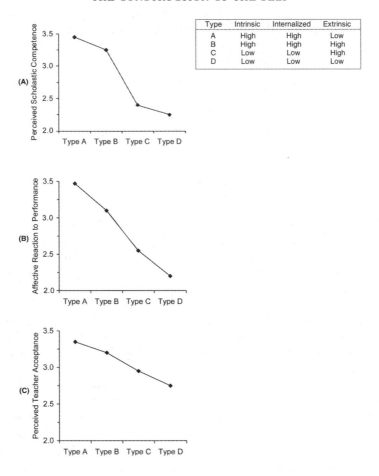

Type	Intrinsic	Internalized	Extrinsic
A	High	High	Low
B	High	High	High
C	Low	Low	High
D	Low	Low	Low

FIGURE 7.3. Competence, affect, and teacher acceptance by type of student.

The Type A student, high on both intrinsic and internalized motivation but low on extrinsic motivation, reports high scholastic competence as well as the most positive affect, and experiences the highest level of teacher acceptance. Students high on all three motivational sources (Type B) follow closely behind, although their scores are lower on all three correlates.

The Type C student, predominantly motivated by external rewards and sanctions, shows quite a different pattern, particularly with regard to negative perceived competence and affect. For perceived competence, there are differences of almost an entire scale score point, compared to the Type B profile. These students feel relatively badly about their performance and would appear to opt for an extrinsic motivational orientation. These individuals show virtually no self-motivation of either form, intrinsic or internalized. While they do report relatively high levels of extrinsic motivation, such an orientation sustains only marginal academic performance, and thus does not garner a great deal of teacher support.

The most extreme, negative perceptions are held by Type D students, defined as low on all three sources of motivation. These students feel the least competent, experience the most negative affect, and report the lowest teacher acceptance of all four motivational profiles. It is highly likely that the actual performance of such unmotivated students is relatively poor, given that no incentives or sanctions—intrinsic, extrinsic, or internalized—appear to be motivating. That such students should receive or perceive the lowest level of teacher support is also understandable, given the difficulty teachers must have in responding positively to students who are so disinterested in learning.

Discrete Emotions and Their Relationship to Perceived Competence and Motivation

As others have thoughtfully argued, emotions are functionally critical for student motivation and performance (see Pekrun, 2009; Weiner, 2007). Pekrun observes that there is a paucity of research on classroom emotions, other than anxiety. In reviewing what little other research has been conducted, Pekrun makes the distinction between a *two-dimensional* approach, parsimonious in differentiating between positive and negative affective reactions, and the *discrete emotions* approach where a broad range of specific affects are identified.

We have already presented our own work revealing that both general affective reactions to one's academic performance, as well as test anxiety, mediate motivation and behavioral preference for challenge. In more recent studies we have examined discrete emotions, identifying the affects that children experience in response to their scholastic successes and failures. We concur with Pekrun (2009) and Wiener (2007) that emotions are intimately related to cognitive attributions and to motivational constructs.

With regard to discrete emotions, in a dissertation by Kowalski (1985) we presented children with lists of both "good feelings" and "bad feelings," asking them to choose the most salient positive and negative emotions in response to academic success and failure, respectively. We have distinguished between *self-conscious affects* (e.g., proud or ashamed of oneself) and *externally directed emotions* (e.g., happy and angry). Weiner (2007) has made a similar distinction in his extensive work, identifying self-conscious affects such as shame and guilt that are provoked by failure attributed to *internal* and controllable causes such as lack of effort and those emotions in which attributions for success and failure are directed to *external* causes under the control of others (or chance).

Among the positive feelings that we examined, pride was the single self-conscious emotion that was included. Five other positive affects—namely, happy, excited, surprised, relieved, and grateful—were possible choices. Among our list of negative emotions, three self-conscious emotions were included: ashamed, mad at the self, and guilty. The remaining negative emotions were frustrated, sad, mad, and worried (as a proxy for anxiety, which may not be in the vocabulary of some middle school children).

Self-Conscious Emotions, Externally Directed Emotions, and Links to Perceived Competence

The relationship between combinations of emotions children reported for their scholastic successes and failures and their perceived scholastic competence was of initial interest. Three combinations were addressed: (1) self-conscious emotions for both success and failure (e.g., proud over successes and ashamed or guilty over failures); (2) a self-conscious emotion for one outcome and an externally directed emotion for the other (e.g., proud about successes and frustrated over failures, or happy about successes and mad at self over failures); and (3) externally directed emotions in response to both successes and failures (e.g., happy over successes and sad about failures, or relieved over successes and frustrated about failures).

Kowalski's (1985) results indicated that children reporting *self-conscious emotions* for *both* success and failure reported the highest level of perceived competence (3.10 on a 4-point scale). Those students who experienced one self-affect and one externally directed emotion reported lower perceived competence scores (2.90). Those who acknowledged no self-conscious emotions but only externally directed emotions reported the lowest perceived competence (2.70). It makes intuitive sense that pride in response to personal, academic success should be associated with positive perceived competence. In fact, a recent study by L. Williams and Desteno (2008) demonstrated that pride serves as an incentive to persevere on an effortful, challenging task.

However, why should the more highly competent student also experience a *negative* self-affect in response to failure? Interestingly, one of our historical scholars of the self, Cooley (1902), offered some insights. For Cooley, the most desirable combination of emotions is found in the competent individual who not only feels pride in his/her accomplishments but who can take responsibility for personal failures and can constructively criticize the self, and experience negative self-affects in the process.

Self-Conscious and Externally Directed Emotions: Links to Motivational Orientation

Contemporary theorists (see Pekrun, 2009) emphasize that emotions, particularly negative affects, consume cognitive resources that can undermine motivation and related achievement. For example, anger can be detrimental to scholastic motivation and shame can interfere with students' effort and related academic performance. Positive affects, in contrast, can enhance academic motivation and can foster divergent thinking and flexible problem solving. Pekrun reviews the relatively few findings in the literature demonstrating that emotions profoundly impact students' engagement and academic motivation.

Our own research (see Harter, 1992) has examined the relationship that the two types of affective reactions bear to our three motivational orientations. We first identified only two subgroups of students for the purpose of contrast: those who reported self-conscious emotions in response to both academic successes and failures, and those who indicated that they experienced externally directed emotions in reaction to both successes and failures. Among the first group are students who might have reported feeling proud over successes and mad at themselves over failures. Among the second group, a typical pattern might involve relief over successes and worry, or anger at others, over failures.

The pattern of results is presented in Figure 7.4. Among those experiencing self-conscious emotions in response to their successes and failures, *internalized* motivation represents the strongest source, followed by intrinsic motivation. Extrinsic motivation is less critical for these individuals, particularly negative forms such as disapproval and sanctions. Thus,

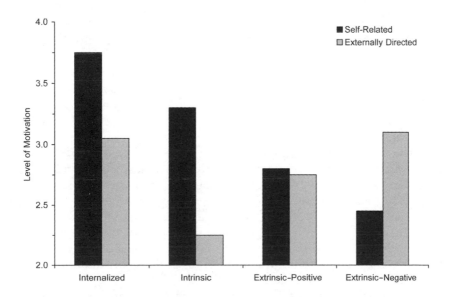

FIGURE 7.4. Level and type of motivation by self-related versus externally directed emotions.

students who experience self-conscious emotions in response to success and failure are those who report high levels of self-motivation, particularly an internalized orientation. Among those students who react with more externally related emotions, the level of intrinsic and internalized forms of motivation is markedly lower than for those reporting self-affects. In addition, extrinsic motivation, primarily the negative forms such as reactions to disapproval and sanctions, is much higher than among those who report self-conscious emotions. Thus, it is not only the valence of emotional reactions (positive vs. negative) that is critical in mediating motivational orientation but the specific or discrete emotions, as well.

It is clear, therefore, that we need to attend to the discrete emotions experienced by child and adolescent students, in addition to the more general affective reactions to classroom performance. Our pattern of findings is consistent with recent treatments of the links between cognition, emotion, and motivation (see Pekrun, 2009). Our findings reveal that one type of cognition, perceived scholastic competence, is intimately related to general as well as discrete emotional reactions, and to motivational constructs, defined as intrinsic, extrinsic, and internalized orientations. However, our results do not address the issue of *directionality*. The "which comes first" question among these variables has not been empirically addressed. In future studies of these relationships, the possibility of feedback loops (see Pekrun, 2009) merits consideration, because the effects may well *not* be captured by linear, sequential models.

The Accuracy of Scholastic Competence Self-Evaluations

Throughout this chapter, perceived scholastic competence has been central as a predictor of motivational orientation and as a correlate of self-affects and externally directed emotions in the classroom. Yet a nagging question lingers. How critical is it that these perceptions be accurate; how important are *realistic* self-appraisals?

The educational transitions that have been discussed present new developmental tasks to be mastered, which may cause doubt and anxieties about one's abilities. They can challenge existing self-representations, leading not only to alterations but potential inaccuracies in the evaluations of one's perceived competence. The literature demonstrates that there are individual differences in the degree to which self-evaluations are veridical with more objective indices (see Harter, 2006a; Leahy & Shirk, 1985; Phillips & Zimmerman, 1990). Might inaccuracies be predictors of outcomes critical to the interest of educators?

We became interested in the issue of whether individual differences in the accuracy of scholastic competence judgments among middle school students would predict one particular dimension of intrinsic motivation, behavioral preference for challenge. We determined accuracy by comparing teachers' ratings of each student's academic performance to the student's own perceptions of his/her scholastic competence, reasoning that teachers would be relatively accurate judges of their students' actual scholastic performance. We next created three groups, dividing students into "overraters," those whose perceived competence scores significantly exceeded the rating of the teacher; "underraters," whose scores were significantly lower than the teacher's ratings; and "accurate raters," whose scores were congruent with the teacher's.

We employed a slight variation of the anagram task procedure described earlier in this chapter. We brought small groups of middle school students into a mock classroom. All groups had approximately the same number of overraters, underraters, and accurate raters (as determined by an earlier administration of our questionnaires in the students' school classrooms). They were given workbooks containing anagrams of different difficulty levels, and were first instructed to attempt anagrams of each difficulty level (so that we could establish baseline ability level for each student).

In the second *choice* phase, students were told that the anagrams they would do would be more like a test. They could choose whatever level of difficulty they preferred, and they would be graded for how well they did (A, B, C, D, or fail). To create the atmosphere of social comparison and monitoring by teacher surrogates, students had to raise their hand after they had completed each anagram and were then timed. In creating this type of classroom environment, we anticipated that children's perceptions of their academic ability would be particularly salient.

Given this preference-for-challenge paradigm, we were interested in the difficulty level that each accuracy group selected in the second "test" phase, relative to each student's ability level established during the first "game" phase. The findings revealed that both underraters and overraters selected much easier anagrams than their ability scores (from the first game phase) revealed, unlike the accurate raters who selected anagrams commensurate with their demonstrated skill level.

We could interpret the underraters' selection of the easier anagrams, presumably because they inaccurately underestimated their academic ability, just as they did in their actual classroom. However, why should the *overraters* with unrealistically high estimates of scholastic competence select easier anagrams? These overraters had selected anagrams that were congruent with their moderately low actual ability rather than with their inflated sense of competence. This suggests that, at some level (conscious or unconscious), overraters were aware that they were not nearly as competent as their self-reported evaluations implied. It would appear that to protect what may be a fragile and distorted sense of scholastic ability, they were driven to select the easiest anagrams in order to avoid failure and its implications for the self.

These findings are important for several reasons. First, consider the over-raters. If they are selecting easier tasks in a simulated classroom setting, then they are likely to choose less difficult tasks in other areas of their life. To the extent that they are actively avoiding challenge wherever possible, this may well limit opportunities for new learning and problem solving, jeopardizing their acquisition of higher-order skills in many domains. From the perspective of educational interventions, promoting more realistic self-evaluations among overraters should be a first step. This leads to the seemingly counter-intuitive strategy of initially lowering their perceptions of competence. However, if these students become more accurate in their assessment of their abilities, abandoning their defensively unrealistic views of their competence, then skill training appropriate for their actual ability level may lead to academic improvement. To the extent that their skills are enhanced, then higher levels of perceived competence may ensue and realistic evaluations could be reinforced. For underraters, there would be a similar goal, namely, to instill realistic self-evaluations. However, the strategy would be very different. These students need confirmation of their positive academic abilities; interventions would demonstrate to them that they are more competent than they believe. Pointing out their actual performance on assignments, tests, and so on may be an initial avenue. However, there are undoubtedly other causes of their unrealistic assessments of their abilities that may be beyond the intervention efforts of classroom teachers. For example, harsh parental feedback that their children are not living up to perfectionistic standards can represent one possible cause. Psychological counseling interventions such as family therapy may well be needed to determine the ultimate causes for the underestimation of one's scholastic abilities.

Our findings have broader implications. One controversial issue is whether the goal of an educational or psychological intervention should be the *enhancement* of self-perceptions, for example, in the domain of scholastic competence, or whether efforts should promote *realistic* evaluations, where the focus is on accuracy. There are those who tout enhancement as the primary goal, such that students will feel good about themselves. However, others point to the dangers of promoting unrealistically high domain-specific evaluations and urge that interventions promote more realistic self-perceptions (see Damon, 1995). Our own research on the negative effects of both overrating and underrating one's scholastic competence clearly suggests the importance of promoting realistic self-appraisals that ultimately will serve the goals of learning and achievement. These issues will be a focus in the final chapter as will the role of self-esteem in the classroom.

Contemporary Issues in the Classroom

A number of contemporary issues dot the landscape of self-perceptions and performance of students in the classroom. The first relates to female adolescents' ability to voice their opinions in the classroom, an issue first introduced by Gilligan (see Gilligan et al., 1989) who has contended that females lose their voice beginning in midadolescence. At about the same time, the American Association of University Women (AAUW; 1992) placed the blame on the psychological shoulders of educators who were accused of classroom practices that were detrimental to girls, producing negative effects on their self-esteem. Sadker and Sadker (1994) also made claims that schools were shortchanging girls, relegating them to the "silent ghetto" of the classroom. They pointed to numerous practices that represented *gender bias* against girls, in favor of boys. It was suggested by some that same-gender classrooms would protect girls and allow them to flourish.

Since these claims, the gender tide has turned. A number of authors (see Pollack, 1998) have suggested that today it is the boys who are having difficulty in school, for a number of reasons including the lack of understanding of boys by teachers. Pollack recommends single-gender educational environments for boys, to redress this concern. Thus, the field has shifted to greater concern over boys and those factors that attenuate their performance. Each of these themes are briefly reviewed, introducing our own recent research. First, the issue of gender and level of voice is addressed. Attention next turns to gender bias in the classroom. Then, the topic of same gender versus coeducation is addressed. Finally, the role of sports participation for female students is considered, with an eye toward whether it is positively associated with academic performance and self-esteem.

Level of Voice

Gilligan has devoted much of her career to the study of women and girls, given that so little attention has been paid to females in past theory and research. The field of psychology seemed, for many years, to be based on studies of men, by men, and for men. In her studies of voice (Gilligan, 1993; Gilligan et al., 1989), Gilligan and colleagues argue that prior to adolescence, girls know their mind and can clearly express it. She presents four primary motives for why girls lose their ability to express their opinions as they move into midadolescence, in what is still primarily a patriarchal culture. These motives include the following: (1) girls realize that they are on the path to womanhood and begin to adopt the societal "good woman stereotype," which is to be nurturant, caring, dependent, and *quiet*; (2) girls' realization that women's voices are not appreciated or reinforced in this society, be it in the corporate world of work, with its "glass ceiling," in politics, or in other influential realms; (3) imitation of their own mothers who have suppressed their voice; and (4) fear of the loss of relationships or rejection if they were to speak their mind honestly. In support of her conclusions, Gilligan has spent considerable time listening to adolescents in focus groups. She has also employed sentence completion methodologies, as well as interview techniques.

We approached this issue within our framework in which lack of voice was considered to be a manifestation of *false-self* behavior, given the suppression of one's thoughts and feelings. In contrast, the ability to express thoughts, opinions, and feelings was conceptualized as a reflection of *true-self* behavior. Adolescent responses to open-ended questions confirmed this assumption. We have investigated the issue of voice employing a self-report methodology that built upon these open-ended responses, crafting questionnaires (Harter, Waters, & Whitesell, 1997; Harter, Waters, Whitesell, & Kastelic, 1998). It was important in our approach to include males as well as females. One can hardly make generalizations that imply gender differences if one does not include both genders. Thus, males and females have answered questions to assess level of voice across five different relational contexts: teachers, parents, male classmates, female classmates, and close friends.

Employing a cross-sectional methodology, across grades 6 though 11, we initially discovered that there were few significant differences in level of voice between females and males, nor was there any interaction with grade level. That is, there was no dip in level of voice for girls in midadolescence. In fact, girls showed small but systematically higher levels of voice than did boys, a difference that was highly significant with close friends. More recent findings (Bassen & Lamb, 2006) have also contested the claims regarding girls' loss of voice during adolescence, reporting that girls' assertiveness did not decline between seventh and tenth grades.

Of particular interest in our own research were the vast individual differences *within* each gender, the more important finding. What could account for such demonstrable individual differences? We examined two possible contributors. The first was social support for voice, across each source of support. The second was gender orientation (feminine, masculine, androgynous). The effects for social support were dramatic for both females and males at all grade levels. Across each of the five contexts (parents, teachers, male classmates, female classmates, and close friends), those with low levels of support reported low levels of voice, those with moderate level of support reported moderate levels of voice, and those with high support for voice reported the highest level of voice.

Self-reported gender orientation as a predictor was clearer for females and interacted with relational context or source of support. Androgynous females reported higher levels of voice than did feminine girls in what we have labeled the "more public domains," that is, in school. Thus, voice with teachers, male classmates, and female classmates defined the public domain. In the more private domains, with close friends and parents, there were no differences between the androgynous and feminine girls. These findings led us to the conclusion that Gilligan's analysis may well apply to feminine girls, who stifle their voices in public contexts but who can more freely express their opinions and feelings in private relationships (Gilligan, 1993;

Gilligan et al. 1989). It is of interest that in our Denver sample 65% of the female adolescents reported an androgynous orientation, 34% reported a feminine orientation, and only 1% reported a masculine orientation.

We do not contest the initial observations of Gilligan and colleagues (1989) nor the AAUW (1992) report that appeared over two decades ago. However, we would suggest that there have been changes in female adolescents' views of themselves and their ability to express their opinions. One can point to many influences that have yet to be examined empirically. Some credit the women's movement as one factor. Many may cite gains for women in education (where graduate degrees for women now exceed those for men in many fields), in their professional status within the workplace, in their earning power, and in politics. Some adolescent females have families that want their daughters to express themselves. Some females, with the support of their peers, agree to express their true selves. Some request the same type of treatment in the classroom. (Our daughter never lost her voice; I wonder why!) Our newer work (Harter & Buddin, 2011) directly documents the effects of parental modeling and support for voice on the level of voice among high school adolescents (see Cooper, Groterant, & Condon, 1983).

However, our framework in which the ability to voice one's opinions is equated with *true-self* behavior and the failure to express oneself to others is considered to be *false-self* behavior has certain limitations. I was first alerted to this possibility when a very bright Chinese American graduate student wrote extremely insightful papers throughout our graduate seminar. However, she never opted to share her thoughtful observations during our discussions. When I privately pointed this out to her, urging her to participate, she bravely countered my suggestion, replying, "So you want me to be a false self?" By that she meant that *not* speaking up was her *true self*, which I understood to reflect how her self-effacing tendencies were genuine and appropriate, given her Chinese American heritage.

I was intrigued by the possibility that certain adolescents, for a variety of reasons, might share the perspective that *not* voicing one's opinions could well represent *true-self* behavior. Thus, I addressed this issue in open-ended survey questions asking adolescents how *not* expressing yourself could reflect *true-self* behavior. A content analysis of their responses fell into three categories: (1) Adolescents cited temperamental or personality characteristics, such as being shy, nervous, not wanting to brag, or not wanting to stand out; (2) another reason focused on keeping private thoughts to oneself or protecting one's deepest personal secrets; (3) a third reason involved not wanting to share one's thoughts or opinions with someone whom one didn't trust. Thus, there were very defensible justifications for suppressing one's voice that were considered to reflect one's true self.

This led me to question whether the fourth quadrant in this 2 × 2 conceptual matrix might also exist. That is, could the *presence of voice*, the outspoken expression of one's thoughts and opinions, constitute *false-self* behavior? Three possible manifestations came to mind: (1) There are normative adolescent exaggerations about the qualities of the self—braggadocio (e.g., "I'm awesome!")—which typically produces eye-rolls among observers; (2) there are tactical self-promotion strategies that typically reflect self-distortion and unrealistic self-appraisals, with displays of narcissism in the extreme; (3) another version represents excessive, inaccurate claims of knowledge, typically opinions that have little validity but which are foisted on vulnerable others; this is the "phony leader with the bullhorn" approach where one may, in the short run, attract gullible followers.

Thus, I have recently expanded the original conceptualization to include two other possibilities, first that *failure* to overtly express oneself can reflect, for some, *true-self* behavior. Secondly, voicing if not broadcasting one's thoughts and opinions can represent certain forms of *false-self* behavior, to the extent that it reflects distortions or unrealistic perceptions of the self. The ideal goal, it would seem, is to express oneself in a respectful manner such that what one has to say can actually be *heard* and genuinely *understood* by others. Only this form of expression will truly facilitate communication and foster healthy relationships.

Gender Bias in the Classroom

As noted above, a number of scholars, notably the Sadkers (Sadker & Sadker, 1994), have identified numerous examples emerging from their own observations, demonstrating gender bias against girls. It should be noted that while they reported these findings in their book, an examination of their grant proposals and TV appearances dates the actual work as quite some years earlier, in the 1980s. This is not a criticism but a consideration of whether practices and students' attitudes may have changed since their earlier efforts, at least a quarter of a century ago.

In a study designed to determine whether young adolescents detect gender bias in the classroom, Harter, Rienks, and McCarley (2006) examined the very dimensions to which the Sadkers (Sadker & Sadker, 1994) have called our attention. Among middle school students, we found that 75% of students (80% of females and 68% of males) felt that teachers were unbiased, treating boys and girls equally. Thus, in contrast to the claims of the Sadkers and the AAUW (1992) report, students in this representative middle-class, Denver public school environment did not perceive gender bias. Perhaps the school climate has changed in light of the sensitivity to this issue on the societal stage, including seminars and training programs for teachers.

Among the minority of those students who did perceive bias, most reported bias against boys, not girls. Students of both genders reported that boys receive more negative attention from the teacher leading to disciplinary actions. This pattern is in keeping with Pollack's (1998) claims that it is boys who are being shortchanged in the classroom. His thesis is that teachers, primarily female in today's schools, do not understand the emotional needs of boys but rather see boys as troublemakers who primarily require discipline.

We also hypothesized that the smaller group of students who *did* see bias against their own gender would report more negative classroom outcomes. This prediction was borne out in their lower self-concept as a student, less intrinsic motivation, and lower levels of voice in the classroom, as well as less teacher support for voice. Thus, on the basis of a representative Denver sample, there is little evidence that middle school children today, as a group, experience teacher bias. For the small subgroup that does see bias against their gender, we need to ask the unanswered question of whether bias is the *cause* of negative outcomes, or whether those with lower self-concepts, more extrinsic motivation, and lack of voice are more likely to report bias, as an effect.

Same- versus Integrated-Gender Classrooms

Fortunately, given our interest in this topic, a local Denver public high school (drawing from upper-middle class, primarily Caucasian families) decided to introduce same-gender classrooms for incoming ninth graders, retaining mixed-gender classrooms, as well. The impetus for this educational experiment was a concern that their high school boys were falling behind, academically, and were less successful on the standardized state-mandated CSAP tests, compared to their girls.

We engaged in a collaborative study (Rienks & Harter, 2006). A positive design feature was the random assignment of ninth-grade students to single-gender and mixed-gender classes. Results were complicated given a very complex design; however, the following findings were of interest. The majority of ninth graders of both genders preferred coed classes, although a small minority expressed their preference for same-gender classrooms. Reasons for favoring coed classes ranged from familiarity, "It is what I have always been comfortable with," to appreciation for gender differences, "It makes discussion a lot more interesting," and "I like a mix because each gender has something different to offer," and to more social aspects, "It's more fun to be with boys and girls." Those who preferred *single-gender* classes often said they would feel more comfortable. "I don't have to worry about what I say or what I look like" and "I am not very good at English and I like my class this year (all boys); it has helped me a lot." Several boys in an all-male special education class for math indicated that they preferred this situation to regular coed classes because they didn't want to feel stupid in front of the girls.

When preferences are examined by school subjects, more girls than boys preferred single-gender classes for math (13% vs. 9%), science (14% vs. 9%), gym (42% vs. 13%), and health (43% vs. 18%). Differences for gym and health classes were primarily due to girls feeling less athletically competent than boys and embarrassed in coed classrooms. Boys and girls have similar preference rates for single-gender classes in English (15%) and history (8%). However, overall, coed classes are general preferred to single-gender classes.

That said, students who did prefer single-gender classes reported that they got better grades in single-gender classrooms, that they could be more serious about their work, and that it was easier to be themselves. They indicated that it was harder to pay attention in coed classes. Interestingly, boys, but not girls, reported that they were better behaved in coed classes. In all-male classes, they became more rowdy.

In both environments, gender main effects in math and English grades revealed that girls outperformed boys. Overall, girls also reported more positive outcomes such as self-concept as a student, intrinsic motivation, and task orientation. This pattern is consistent with recent claims that boys are falling behind girls in the academic arena (Pollack, 1998). With regard to *level of voice*, there were no overall gender difference in level of voice, contrary to Gilligan's (1993) assertions, but consistent with our own earlier findings. However, students in single-gender classes reported higher levels of voice than those in coed classes, acknowledging that they feel more comfortable speaking up and sharing their opinions within single-gender environments.

The Effects of Sports Participation on Self-Processes within the School Setting

The premise that sports involvement is beneficial can be traced to the ancient Greeks, who believed that a healthy body produced a healthy mind. The justification for athletic programs in schools and communities rests on the assumption that sports participation not only has physical but also social and psychological benefits, some of which transfer to academic motivation in the classroom (Hines & Grove, 1989). More recently, Chen and Ennis (2009) have suggested that sports should be integrated into the total educational curriculum so that physical education is not merely an "add on" but an anchor to the motivation of students in all of school learning.

A dissertation by Freyer (1996) addressed this issue among high school female basketball players. Historically, sports opportunities within the educational system have been much more prevalent for males than for females. In 1972, the Title IX Education Act created new opportunities for females to participate in sports by prohibiting gender discrimination in funding for any organization that received federal assistance (see Brake, 2010). The women's movement also provided an impetus for females to enter into the sports arena, by challenging those traditional gender role stereotypes that prevented women from aspiring to athletic competition. Thus, there has been a dramatic increase in the number of female children, adolescents, and young adults engaged in athletic activities. More recently, the issue of sports participation for females has become even more timely and controversial, given the backlash against Title IX in which opponents have made claims of reverse discrimination. They argued that certain male sports programs (e.g., wrestling) have been dismantled or eliminated in order to achieve the goal of proportionality, equalizing opportunities and funding for women's programs (see Brake, 2010). These issues provoked us to examine whether sports participation currently produces psychological, social, or educational benefits for female athletes who play competitive varsity basketball (Harter & Freyer, 2012).

We cast a broad net, identifying 11 possible benefits, grouped into three categories:

1. *Sports/physical* domains targeted development of athletic skills, healthy competitiveness, increased physical fitness, and enhanced physical appearance.
2. *Social benefits* addressed enhanced social status, finding a social niche, and enhanced parental support.
3. *Personal attributes* included a greater sense of responsibility, improved academic performance, self-confidence, and enhanced self-esteem.

We raised three research questions:

1. *Motives.* What motivates high school females to participate in sports, initially? To what extent do female high school athletes feel that sports participation will lead to enhancement in each of the 11 domains we identified?
2. *Effects of participation.* Do such athletes feel that participating in sports actually leads to gains in these 11 arenas? That is, do they perceive a *link* between sports involvement and benefits in each domain?
3. *Outcomes.* Do those who perceive links for each domain report better outcomes compared to those who do not see a link? For example, do they feel more fit, report higher self-esteem, feel more motivated, scholastically, and so forth?

What did the findings reveal? An analysis of the *motives* for participation indicated that reasons involving the more proximal sports and physical skills (e.g., to gain athletic skills, to become fit) were the most important, followed by personal attributes (e.g., self-esteem, academic success) and social benefits (e.g., enhanced social status).

Of particular interest was the perception of the *links* between participation and all 11 outcomes. Across all 11 domains, these female athletes felt that sports involvement leads to improvement in all domains, even though some domains may not have been a major reason for their initial participation in the sport (e.g., improved academic performance).

In addressing the *relationship between perceived links and outcomes*, athletes who perceived links reported significantly higher outcome scores in all three general categories than did those who did not perceive such links. Those acknowledging the links reported better outcomes compared to nonlink participants, for sports/physical domains, social benefits, and personal attributes. Thus, the entire constellation of findings indicates that sports participation is far more important to these girls than merely a means to develop athletic skills. It has much broader consequences that include the enhancement of their self-esteem, confidence, academic motivation, responsibility, and social approval. We concur, therefore, with Chen and Ennis (2009), who urge that educators integrate athletic activity into the total educational curriculum.

Eccles and Roeser (2009) also review studies that tout the benefits of sports participation. Involvement in athletics lowers the likelihood of school dropout and also leads to higher rates of college attendance. Furthermore, it enhances educational and occupational attainment during early adulthood, especially among low-achieving male athletes. Other studies reviewed reveal that participation in school-based extracurricular activities is linked to high school GPA, strong school engagement, and higher educational aspirations. Extracurricular participation can also lead to enhanced self-esteem and the adoption of positive educational values, as well as increase the student's social capital, as our own study has clearly demonstrated.

Despite the benefits of sports participation, current educational practices do not conform to these conclusions. Physical education programs and recess are increasingly on the curricular hit list in many schools across the nation. What are the causes of such trends? Financial constraints represent one reason. However, more important causes reside in the current value system of our educational institutions. Academic achievement on standardized tests now heads the list as an important goal that holds teachers as well as entire schools and districts accountable. Funding is now often tied to students' public academic performance. This preoccupation precludes a serious investment in athletic activities that could well improve fitness and provide the many other psychological benefits demonstrated by our own research and studies by others (see Chen & Ennis, 2009; Eccles & Roeser, 2009).

This unfortunate trend comes at a time when childhood obesity is at an all-time high in our nation. Contributing to this epidemic are less than healthy school lunches containing too much fat, too many carbohydrates, and high caloric content, as well as sugar-laden carbonated drinks and snacks available in school vending machines. Fast-food consumption outside of school is common and meals at home are often no more nutritious. As a sports enthusiast and former high school and college athlete, I was appalled at several of the sponsors for the 2010 Winter Olympics. These included Coca-Cola, McDonald's, and Kentucky Fried Chicken! There are obvious conclusions to be drawn about our priorities.

Implications for Educational Interventions and Reform

Considerable evidence now reveals that students who are intrinsically motivated and inherently interested or engaged in the learning process will more effectively master classroom assignments and achieve at higher levels (see Eccles & Roeser, 2009; Harter, 1996; Lepper et al., 2005; Ryan & Deci, 2009; Skinner, Kindermann, Connell, & Wellborn, 2009). Low-achieving students who report negative perceptions of their scholastic competence are more likely to display an extrinsic orientation, attending to external rewards and sanctions. The analysis by Eccles and colleagues (see Eccles & Roeser, 2009) points to many features of our educational system that represent a mismatch between the psychological needs of students and the practices that teachers employ, particularly as students make the transition to middle or junior high school. These practices (e.g., social comparison, competition for grades, focus on ability) all conspire to produce negative perceptions of scholastic competence and attenuate intrinsic mastery motivation in the classroom.

From these observations, a number of changes seem warranted in order to prevent students from falling further into this educational abyss. To begin with, the flagrant use of external rewards and sanctions must be tempered. Assignments that are intrinsically interesting and reflect age-appropriate levels of challenge must dominate the curriculum. The excessive emphasis on individual differences in *ability*, coupled with a focus on the *product* of one's achievements, should be supplanted with a recognition of the importance of *effort* that students put into the *process* of learning. Students should be encouraged to realize that ability is malleable (see Dweck & Master, 2009), and that effort cannot only be personally rewarding but will cause them to become smarter. Cooperative learning projects, as opposed to the current competitive atmosphere, can reinforce such goals, particularly for female students, as can the reduction of the sexism to which girls are sometimes subject.

Perhaps the most insidious practice of teachers in the classroom is the rampant use of public social comparison. These practices escalate at a period of development during which adolescents are highly *self-conscious*. As an alternative, fostering students' comparisons with their *own past performance* will prove less personally devastating and considerably more motivating, as they observe demonstrable progress due to the fruits of their own autonomous labor (see also Ryan & Deci, 2009). For many, autonomy is essential to success in the classroom.

Given the seeming reasonableness of these suggestions, why has there been no ground-swell movement among educators to implement these practices? Resistance stems, in part, from the current educational agenda. The call to action is driven by high-stakes achievement testing, accountability demands, a narrowing of the curriculum, and external pressures for students to conform and perform (see McCombs, 2007; Ryan & Deci, 2009). McCombs points out that many beginning teachers may well espouse the values underlying the suggestions offered. However, they are discouraged by current school policies that focus on economic efficiency, high-stakes testing, and accountability demands.

Ryan and Deci (2009) have argued that if entire schools are held hostage to rewards and sanctions contingent on test outcomes, it will have deleterious effects on classroom practice, student motivation, and ultimate learning. They argue that the application of such rewards and sanctions is an inherently *controlling* intervention. In a study on the effects of high-stakes testing, they demonstrated that these evaluations led to teaching to the test, the narrowing of curriculum choices, more drill and redundancy, and fewer hands-on learning opportunities. For students, these practices led to lower intrinsic motivation, poor transfer of "rewarded" test outcomes, and increased dropout rates of at-risk students (see also Locker & Cropley, 2004).

Combinations of Motivational Orientations

During the 1970s, extrinsic motivation was initially viewed as the villain, as experimental studies revealed that the application of tangible rewards undermined intrinsic interest (see Deci & Ryan, 1985; Lepper & Henderlong, 2000). Subsequently, this drama shifted to the stage of classroom learning where it was demonstrated that external sanctions and rewards interfered with students' intrinsic mastery motivation (see Deci & Ryan, 1985; Eccles & Roeser, 2009; Eccles et al., 1984). School policies and practices were indicted as the cause of demonstrable developmental decline in intrinsic motivation. More recently, scholars have come to the realization that intrinsic and extrinsic motivation need not be antagonistic foes. In certain forms, these two orientations can conspire to enhance learning and achievement.

Our own work (Harter & Jackson, 1992) has demonstrated that for many students, the combination of extrinsic and intrinsic goals enhances performance. The addition of *internalized* motivation contributes to the most positive outcomes (e.g., perceived scholastic competence, positive affect toward school learning, and teacher acceptance). Internalized motivation can be fostered by parents and teachers who instill the values of effort and achievement in the classroom, values that such children come to "own" as self-directed goals. Thus, educators can capitalize on this union of motives, employing practices that bolster students' appreciation for the importance of effort and achievement, in the service of current and future aspirations.

Covington (2009) views this issue through a somewhat different lens, arguing that tangible reinforcement and praise can enhance intrinsic motivation *if* they serve positive, task-oriented goals. For example, success-oriented students are most likely to value the intrinsic appeal of learning for the sake of learning, while fulfilling requirements to obtain the good grades necessary to achieve eventual occupational goals that are desired and personally meaningful. Lepper et al. (2005) have also argued that a combination of these motivations can, under certain circumstances, enhance levels of achievement. They observe that it is certainly plausible that children might come to enjoy learning and challenge and may be more likely to master material if they are also receiving high marks and positive feedback. Thus, the most effective practices will combine intrinsic, extrinsic, and internalized motivations.

In a dissertation by Lane (1998) we obtained findings revealing student benefits, if teachers adopt both intrinsic and extrinsic goals. Lane identified two different teaching orientations that were labeled *student centered* and *content centered*. Student-centered practices emphasized student autonomy and independence, mastery-oriented goals such as preference for challenge, the partnership between teacher and student, validation of the student, support for the expression of student opinions, and an emphasis of the relevance of the material to be learned. These themes were consistent with an intrinsic orientation to learning. Content-centered practices focused on the teacher as the expert authority, the importance of teacher opinions, the teacher as a role model, an emphasis on the content of the material, and the use of teaching algorithms. These practices were consistent with an extrinsic orientation toward achievement.

We identified a typology of four different teaching styles. Relatively few teachers exemplified just one orientation. A small percentage (19.4%) were categorized as primarily student oriented, emphasizing intrinsic learning goals. That same percentage (19.4%) of teachers primarily espoused extrinsic achievement goals. A fourth of the teachers (25.8%) *strongly* endorsed both intrinsic student-oriented and the more extrinsic content-centered orientation, and the largest subgroup (35.5%) gave their *moderate* endorsement to the combination of the two learning goals. Thus, a total of 61.3% of the teachers embraced both teaching orientations.

Our findings revealed a direct relationship between the teacher typology and student outcomes. The students of those teachers who endorsed both student-centered intrinsic goals *and* content-centered extrinsic goals reported higher levels of both intrinsic and extrinsic motivation, had higher GPAs, better achievement test scores, and higher self-esteem (compared to the teachers who were either primarily student centered or primarily content centered).

The pattern of findings, therefore, leads to the conclusion that *teachers* whose styles emphasize both intrinsic *and* extrinsic motivational orientations, in the service of learning *and* achievement, produced the most positive outcomes for their students. The implications for teacher education are clear. Teachers should be selected or trained to stimulate both kinds of motivational orientations, provided that their extrinsic style does not focus on sanctions and external rewards that can undermine intrinsic motivation. Rather, the judicious use of praise or rewards should complement students' interest in the process of learning, the joy of personal mastery, and the inherent rewards of effort.

The operative word, here, is "judicious." Considerable controversy swirls around the use of praise and rewards in the classroom designed to enhance self-esteem (see Chapter 9, where the arguments are presented). There has been a resurgence of "feel-good" approaches designed to enhance students' feelings of worth, independent of whether student efforts are realistic or praise worthy. Some (e.g., Damon, 1995) view these priorities as misguided, in that they lead to inflated perceptions of competence and self-esteem. Damon contends that the importance of self-esteem as a psychological commodity has been greatly exaggerated. Furthermore, the effusive praise that parents or teachers heap on children to make them feel good is often met with suspicion by children. Moreover, it interferes with the goal of building specific skills in the service of genuine achievement. Cote (2009) has also decried the "cult of self-esteem" that has gripped schools in this country. This controversy is evaluated in depth in Chapter 9.

The Broader Stage of Proposals and Programs for Major Educational Reform

The piecemeal suggestions offered above represent specific suggestions for interventions in the classroom to improve student motivation and associated realistic perceptions of competence. Others have painted a much broader picture to illustrate how our entire educational system requires reform. A review of this burgeoning literature extends well beyond the scope of this chapter. That said, I will point to two cogent analyses of various new future directions that have been offered by psychologists and educators who have effectively straddled the conceptual divide between basic research and educational application. Two primary players on this stage are Eccles (see

Eccles & Roeser, 2009) and McCombs (2007), each of whom reviews critical literature in support of their arguments.

Eccles and colleagues have focused on secondary school reform, building upon their analysis of the mismatch between the psychological needs of young adolescents and the educational practices that do not speak to these needs, as discussed earlier. Their analysis and research have been taken seriously by the Carnegie Corporation on Adolescent Development that in 1989 issued a publication entitled *Turning Points* (see Eccles & Roeser, 2009), calling for educational reform directed toward young adolescents.

Some of the key recommendations that are most relevant to the theme of this chapter include the following:

1. Create small learning communities that will allow personal relationships to emerge between teachers and students. Such an environment, in turn, should provide opportunities for students to experience an appropriate level of autonomy within a close social network. It should foster student engagement and identification with the school institution.
2. Teach a core academic curriculum that includes opportunities for service (e.g., helping within the community and tutoring of younger students, which benefits both). Such interventions can promote the connection of students to the community, allowing young adolescents to offer their skills and develop real-world experience.
3. Ensure success for all through the elimination of *tracking*, the promotion of cooperative learning, provisions for flexible scheduling, and adequate resources to meet the learning needs of every student.

The impetus behind the recommendation to do away with tracking presumably stems from the detrimental effects described earlier, namely, lowered perceptions of scholastic competence, an undermined sense of self-efficacy, and reduction in genuine intrinsic interest in learning. However, educators that I know, including our daughter who teaches third grade in a public school, are divided on this issue. Our daughter has developed a compromise where students are assigned to ability groups within the classroom that are highly flexible in their membership. That is, if a student improves in a given subject, he/she is moved back into the regular curriculum. Her program for students who need remedial help emphasizes their progress relative to their own past performance, which fosters personal effort and instills pride in their accomplishments. (She must be doing something right because in only her third year of teaching, she won acclaim as the best elementary teacher in the entire county.) Elementary school would appear to be the place to initiate such reforms. If students make observable gains in their skill level, prior to middle or junior high school, then they may not

need to be tracked or suffer the psychological consequences of being stigmatized when they become young adolescents.

Eccles (see Eccles & Roeser, 2009) laments the fact that at the secondary school level the efforts spearheaded by the Carnegie (1989) recommendations have been disappointing. Many districts attempted to switch
from a junior high school format to the creation of middle schools. However, these changes have been rather superficial attempts. Eccles observes
that these new middle schools looked a great deal like the old junior high
schools except that now they contained grades 6–8 rather than grades 7–9.
That is, the infrastructure changed but the recommended philosophically
based educational practices were not instituted.

Subsequent programs reviewed by Eccles and Roeser (2009) seem to
have met with more success (see also Junoven, Le, Kaganoff, Augustine, &
Constant, 2004). These scholars have argued that K–8 structures might be
more successful at implementing the types of classroom characteristics most
supportive of continued academic engagement and positive youth development. Three programs stand out, in the estimation of these scholars, efforts
that seek to better meet the psychological needs of adolescents. One is the
Coca-Cola Valued Youth Program, described in Eccles and Roeser (2009).
It builds upon teenagers' desire to make a difference in the community and
includes a tutoring component where at-risk teenagers mentor elementary
school students who have also been identified as at risk. In tutoring younger
children, academically challenged youth are provided with an opportunity
to help others do well in school, which in turn bolsters their own feelings
of pride and success.

Another intervention, the Teen Outreach Program (J. P. Allen, Kuperminc, Philliber, & Herre, 1994) provides a national volunteer service program designed to help adolescents both understand and evaluate their
future life options. In a context featuring strong social ties to adult mentors, the program fosters the development of relevant skills, as well as a
sense of autonomy.

A third intervention program touted by Eccles and Roeser (2009)
has been developed by Oyserman and colleagues (see Oyserman, Gant,
& Ager, 1995) and seeks to explore with students the "possible selves"
that can emerge as a result of school engagement. The focus is on African
American students' realistic future occupations and the pathways they need
to take, including increased current commitment to educational success, in
order to attain these eventual goals. One premise is that traditional programs in many schools have retained past practices and curricula that do
not support the optimal level of learning or preparation for adult development for many young people, including adolescents of color (e.g., African
Americans, Latinos, and Native Americans). Others, deeply immersed in
these issues (see Cooper, 2011), concur and offer their own suggestions for
school interventions in the lives of ethnic, minority youth.

McCombs (2007), another research psychologist who has turned her interests and devotion to the academic stage, has focused on what she terms "learner-centered practices" that she argues are essential for school reform. The learners, in her view, are not only the students but also the teachers. McCombs takes, as her educational launch pad, the guidelines reflected in the American Psychological Association's *Learner-Centered Psychological Principles* that she and colleagues have crafted. These principles were designed to provide a context for positive learner development, motivation, and achievement (see also McCombs & Miller, 2008).

Of particular relevance to this chapter are those principles that target motivational and affective processes. The learner's motivation is best fostered by natural curiosity and intrinsic interest, stimulated by tasks of optimal novelty and challenge. Providing for the learners' choices, opinions, and appropriate decision making is also essential. If these goals are attained, students will be much more likely to exert effort in the service of effective learning and achievement that will be gratifying. These recommendations are consistent with the claims of others (e.g., Eccles & Roeser, 2009; Ryan & Deci, 2009) who argue that in order to ensure student motivation, educators must provide support for autonomy, competence, and relatedness.

What do these principles imply for teacher practices in the classroom? McCombs and colleagues (see McCombs, 2007) have identified four critical practices: (1) creating positive teacher–student relationships, (2) honoring student voice, (3) supporting higher-order thinking skills, and (4) adapting to individual differences. Therefore, teachers must view each student as unique and genuinely capable of learning. In addition, teachers must be willing to share power and control with students in a collaborative learning partnership. As Eccles et al. (1984) argued over 25 years ago, many middle and high school teachers fear that they will lose control over potentially unruly young teenagers whom they assume are primarily driven by raging hormones. As a result, they clamp down autocratically on their students offering few, if any, opportunities for autonomy, expression of opinions, choice, and a sense of control.

McCombs (2007) further observes that most teachers are not totally learning centered: they also realistically engage in practices that target objective achievement goals. In today's educational world, teachers must effectively balance learning-centered practices with the demands of accountability, often predicated on student achievement and test performance. These observations are consistent with the dissertation findings by Lane (1998), who found that the majority of high school teachers in her study displayed a combination of student-centered intrinsic practices and content-centered techniques that focused on extrinsic goals such as test performance and GPA. Students so taught reported the highest level of both intrinsic and extrinsic motivation, as well as the most positive objective outcomes.

McCombs (2007) has concluded that there has been an imbalance in traditional teaching methods. For too long, teaching practices have not sufficiently included the student-centered components of this combination that, as demonstrated in her and others' research, clearly contribute to enhanced student motivation, effort, learning, and positive self-perceptions.

Many of these issues are revisited in the concluding chapter that touches on the controversy surrounding contemporary educators' efforts to promote the positive self-evaluations of students, often to the detriment of skill development. Just how far should teachers go in their use of praise, enhancement of students' feelings of worth, and the creation of positive teacher–student relationships? Where does one draw the line, so as to avoid practices that lead to unrealistically inflated self-perceptions that ultimately interfere with desired learning and mastery goals?

Chapter 8

Cross-Cultural and Multicultural Considerations

For the past few decades cultures have been characterized as either *indi- vidualistic* or *collectivistic*. The seminal works of Hofstede (1980), Markus and Kitayama (1991), and Triandis (1989) identified the basic val- ues and dimension that define these two orientations. These orientations, in turn, have been hypothesized to provoke psychological and behavioral *consequences* such as self-construals, cognitive modes of thinking, and emotional tendencies. This chapter focuses on (1) the values and dimen- sions defining each cultural orientation, and (2) associated self-construals and their psychological correlates.

This chapter reviews the literature on the links between cultural descriptors and their consequences in Western versus Eastern cultures. How child-rearing and schooling practices impact the socialization of both cultural values and psychological consequences will then be examined. In much of this burgeoning literature, a given country is treated as a proxy for cultural orientation. For example, the United States is the prototype for a Western culture, whereas China, Japan, and Korea have typified an Eastern cultural orientation. Criticisms of this perspective will be reviewed.

The past decade has witnessed numerous other critiques of this dichot- omous classification of cultures. Two themes predominate. First, the *con- ceptual* foundations of such a distinction have been challenged, given the observation that all cultures involve both individualistic and collectivist manifestations. Moreover, many scholars now assert that the psychological makeup of those within each type of culture includes both independent *and* interdependent self-construals. The second challenge is *methodological*, for example, critics point to the inappropriateness of administering self-report instruments developed in Western cultures (primarily the United States) in Eastern cultures where they are deemed psychometrically flawed and culturally insensitive.

Finally, the chapter next turns to issues of race, bicultural identifications, and acculturation. A central racial question asks why in the United States do African Americans consistently report higher levels of self-esteem than European Americans as well as other minority ethnic groups such as Asian Americans and Hispanic Americans? Models of acculturation have undergone transformations in recent years. The predominant frames of reference focus on successful adaptation within the United States. Bicultural models now command center stage, highlighting the intersection of accepting the values of one's culture of origin and incorporation of the predominant values of the adoptive culture. One may accept the tenets of both cultures, a bicultural stance. Alternatively, one can totally assimilate to the new culture (rejecting the traditional values of one's culture of origin), or one may continue to embrace the values and traditions of one's culture of origin, eschewing the mainstream culture. The consequences of each of these choices will be explored.

Individualistic versus Collectivistic Cultural Dimensions and Values

A considerable body of literature has been devoted to the distinction between individualistic and collectivistic cultures. Building upon the efforts of Hofstede (1980) and Triandis (1989), Markus and Kitayama (1991) offered a seminal analysis of how individualistic versus collectivistic cultures dictated correspondingly different self-construals, namely, different dimensions of self-evaluation. Many cross-cultural scholars have elaborated on these distinctions (see Cross & Gore, 2003; Cross & Markus, 1999; Fiske & Fiske, 2007; Heine, 2001; Kitayama, Duffy, & Uchida, 2007; H. Li, Zhang, Bhatt, & Yum, 2006; Markus & Hamedani, 2007; Morling & Kitayama, 2008; Oyserman, Coon, & Kemmelmeier, 2002; Triandis, 2009). I will first focus attention on the values and dimensions that characterize these two cultural orientations (see Table 8.1) before describing the associated self-construals and their psychological correlates (see Table 8.2). As Oyserman et al. (2002) have cogently argued, too often the presumed defining cultural dimensions (individualist vs. collectivistic) are confounded with their associated self-construals (independent versus interdependent) in terms of both conceptualization as well as research methodology. Thus, it is critical to distinguish between these two themes. Because the focus of this volume is the *self*, more emphasis will be placed on self-construals and their psychological correlates.

Table 8.1 summarizes the values and defining dimensions for each cultural orientation. The United States represents the prototypic

TABLE 8.1. Values and Defining Dimensions for Each Cultural Orientation

Individualism	Collectivism
Value of inherent, personal *uniqueness*. Separateness of individuals, distinct from one another.	Value of duty to in-group (vs. out-group) unity, *harmony* within the in-group.
Emphasis on pursuit of personal goals. Freedom of individual *choice*, control over outcomes.	Conformity to, priority of, group goals (subordinate to personal goals).
Individual achievements, task accomplishments, valued.	Standing, status in the group more important than personal accomplishment.
Success attributed to personal ability, failure to external factors (or bad luck).	Success attributed to help from others, to effort, failure to lack of effort.
Relationships, group membership, needed to attain, advance, self-determined personal goals.	Sacrifice for the common good to maintain favorable interpersonal relationships within the in-group.
Emphasis on equity and competition.	Emphasis on equality and cooperation.
Relationships impermanent; may leave relationships when costs outweigh the personal benefits.	Obligations to group goals, social roles, leads to more permanence of the in-group.
Open and direct communication, expression of emotions.	Refrain from direct expression of emotions, opinions, to preserve harmony.
Value self-affirmation; use of "I" and "Me" predominant in the language. Pronouns obligatory.	Value group affirmation; language does not require the use of "I" and "Me." Can drop these pronouns.

individualistic culture, whereas China, Japan, and Korea are typically described as collectivistic. Oyserman et al. (2002) have observed that too many studies simply use *country* as a proxy for *culture*, failing to directly examine the particular features presumed to differentiate the two cultural orientations.

As Table 8.1 indicates, a primary manifestation of an individualistic orientation inheres in the individual's personal *uniqueness*. To be psychologically *separate* from other individuals, to be *distinct*, to stand out, is critical. The cultural mandate is the *autonomous* pursuit of personal goals. In so doing, the individual must display *freedom of choice*, as well as personal control over outcomes. In contrast, collectivistic cultures place major value on *duty to the in-group* where the focus is on within-group *harmony*. The distinction between the in-group and out-groups is more pronounced among collectivistic cultures. In addition, *conformity* to group goals is given top priority, and such collective goals take precedence over personal goals. Markus and Kitayama (1991) make use of cultural maxims to illustrate this point. They note that Americans learn that "It is the squeaky wheel that gets the grease." In countries such as China and Japan, a proverb cautions that "The nail that sticks up shall be hammered down."

Several cross-cultural scholars point to popular culture for examples of this distinction. Cross and Gore (2003) note that advertising reflects one avenue through which social norms and cultural values are expressed. In the United States, the emphasis is on uniqueness and personal choice. As an example, they cite one ad that purports "The internet isn't for everybody. But then you are not everybody" (H. Kim & Markus, 1999). Markus and Kitayama (2003) have observed that American advertising makes salient the perspective of the actor. "Whether the product is perfume, soap, cars, computers, or software, the message is clear and insistent—be free, declare your independence, think differently, ditch the Joneses, find your own road, be a driver, not a passenger, be an original, you can do it" (p. 24).

Consistent with this theme, in 2009 I encountered a plaque in a boutique that mandated: "Dare to be different, be the YOU-nique person God created you to be." A 2010 TV ad for an American-made printer touts: "My (business) plan is to outsmart, to outshine, to see things from a different perspective, and to get the competitive edge." These both highlight key features that define individualism. In stark contrast is a plaque advertised in a Buddhist catalogue that portrays a common purpose: "We are here to awaken from the illusion of our separateness."

Cross and Gore (2003) describe one American automobile advertising campaign that backfired. The product was the Dodge Caravan and the ad touted the importance of being "different." The campaign was so successful that this model became the best-selling make in that class of vehicle at the time. Ironically, buyers found themselves among the many other buyers on the "collective" highway, all of whom presumed that their purchase would confirm their uniqueness!

Contrasting advertising themes are observed in certain Asian countries. Kim and Markus (1999) give an example of a Korean ad claiming that "Seven out of 10 people are using this product." Such an ad trades on the value of conformity to group norms and social trends. Ads like this are typical in this culture. Markus and Kitayama (2003) summarize their message: "Be like us, follow this trend, try to do it in the traditional way, be a good role member (a good teacher, student, employee), here is the way to be" (p. 24).

Within individualistic cultures, individual achievements are highly valued. Personal *task* accomplishments are particularly salient. In collectivistic cultures, by contrast, one's standing in the group is more important than personal achievements. Moreover, attributions for success among those in individualistic cultures differ from those in collectivistic cultures. Individualism fosters attributions about personal ability where the self is primarily responsible for his/her success. The causes of failures, if they are revealed, are more likely the result of bad luck or external factors, for example, a backstabbing competitor, an unappreciative boss, a downturn in the market beyond one's control, and so forth. Contrasting attributions for success and failure can be observed in cultures where collectivism prevails. Success is typically attributed to help from others, consistent with an emphasis on interpersonal relationships with members of the in-group. Alternatively, the focus is on *effort* (rather than personal ability). Failures are viewed as personal, reflecting the lack of effort.

In another interesting example of cultural differences in media messages, Markus, Uchida, Omoregie, Townsend, and Kitayama (2006) analyzed cultural differences in the reporting of the 2000 and 2002 Olympics. American reporting of successful performances highlighted the athletes' independent, autonomous contribution and their personal, dispositional skills and talents. Explanations for Japanese athletes' success were couched in terms of their interpersonal network of support from family and their coaches. Japanese cameras typically captured the athlete in the company of coaches and team members, in contrast to the image of the individual American athlete.

The focus on in-group unity and harmony as well as the importance of interpersonal commitments among collectivistic cultures has led certain scholars to erroneously conclude that such commitments are not critical values in individualistic cultures. Relationships *are* important to the individualist. However, they serve a different function. Group membership, as well as support from others, serves to advance the individual's self-determined goals, within a context of equity and competition. The contemporary watchword is "networking." A request for help, if successful, signifies the individual's social skills and interpersonal efficacy. From this perspective, relationships can be relatively impermanent. Thus, Americans may willingly leave a relationship when the costs outweigh the personal benefits. One is not duty bound to the group. Before the current recession in this country, the job mobility of upper-middle-class Americans was at an all-time high. People readily moved from one company to another, from one university to another, from one sports team to another, and even from one profession to another, if it seemed to their personal advantage. Economic factors have attenuated this trend to some extent, but it is still viewed as an upwardly mobile route to success.

In contrast, those in collectivistic cultures are expected to sacrifice for the common good in order to maintain favorable, harmonious interpersonal relationships within their in-group. The obligation is to one's social role within the collective and it serves to establish more group permanence. Thus, within the group one is more duty bound, where equality and cooperation are the predominant values. Within the business world, negotiation strategies that avoid confrontation and litigation are the norm (Cross & Gore, 2003).

Features of their language also divide individualistic and collectivist cultures. With English, as well as most Western European languages, grammatically constructed sentences are obliged to include both a subject and an object, often in the form of pronouns at the beginning of a sentence. This is not a requirement in the languages of many collectivistic cultures, a phenomenon known as "pronoun drop," for example, "went home" (see Cross & Gore, 2003; Kashima, & Kashima, 1998; Kitayama et al., 2007). Kitayama and colleagues observe that this is not merely a matter of linguistic convention. They observe that English speakers need to make salient to listeners that it is "I" speaking and it is "me" to whom you had best attend. Thus, the use of "I" and "me" serves to support the cultural value of self-affirmation. Collectivistic cultures value *group affirmation*, which does not demand the excessive use of "I" and "me." Pronouns such as "we" and "us" are more common (Gardner, Gabriel, & Lee, 1999; Kitayama & Park, 2007).

In the same vein, Cross and Gore (2003) contrast the English speaker, who must be in the foreground as the central focus of an utterance, with the Japanese speaker who is merely an implicit element of the situation. They give, as an example, the English sentence "I cut my hair," which in Japanese would be translated "cut hair." The English statement would be offered even when an American had visited his/her hairstylist. Cross and Gore highlight their point by asking who, in fact, did the actual cutting! They cogently observe that English emphasizes the agency of the person who chooses to have his/her hair cut and not the role of the hairstylist who cut the hair. They preface their argument with the observation that in Japanese, there is simply no one translation for each of the English pronouns "I", "me," or the possessive "mine." There are many available terms from which one can select depending upon the situation, interpersonal considerations, and other contextual factors.

Communication styles vary in other respects between individualistic and collectivistic cultures. The expression of one's thoughts and feelings is more direct, to the point of being confrontational in some situations, for the individualist who is encouraged to openly assert his/her uniqueness and personal perspective. In contrast, collectivists refrain from the direct and open expression of personal thoughts, opinions, and emotions because to give them expression might offend in-group members and disrupt valued harmony. Moreover, the direct expression of feelings such as anger among Westerners is viewed by Easterners as arrogant and immature. This also applies to the expression of positive feelings, because a focus on one's accomplishments is frowned upon and is tantamount to hubris (Cross & Gore, 2003).

Religious Underpinnings of Individualistic and Collectivistic Orientations

In China, *Confucianism* has been the traditional, ideological cornerstone for centuries, and, to a lesser extent, other Asian cultures have embraced its tenets. The supreme virtue is captured by the term "ren," which is translated as "sensitive concern for others." Associated values include connection to others, similarity to others, and harmonious relationships (see Cross & Gore, 2003). These serve as the foundation for understanding expected behavior within a social and moral order.

Y. Wang and Ollendick (2001) expand on the virtues valued within the Confucian ideology. They concur that the self is defined in terms of relationships and as such is socially situated, defined and shaped by relational contexts. The spiritual development of the self or self-cultivation (termed "Xiu-ji") is emphasized and can be attained if guided by specific virtues that include "Jen" (humaneness), "Yi" (righteousness), "Li" (ritual propriety), "Chung" (loyalty), "Shu" (reciprocity), and "Hsiao" (filial piety). Y. Wang and Ollendick describe how the majority of these virtues serve to maintain the harmony of hierarchical relationships (see also J. Li & Yue, 2004, who review empirical evidence supporting these values and related behaviors in contemporary Chinese culture). For those within the group, adherence also provides a sense of security.

Within this context, individual autonomy is devalued (Wang & Ross, 2007). In fact, there is a specific term, "Ke-ji," meaning to conquer or overcome one's individuality. An appreciation for this stance is instilled in childhood where individuality is actively discouraged and suppressed as a form of selfishness. On the surface, this might appear to contradict the social role prescriptions dictated by Confucianism. However, the self *is* encouraged to engage in individual agency in the realm of morality, where one exercises judgment about right and wrong, as well as in the domain of academic achievement. As will be discussed in a future section, agency and even autonomy clearly exist in collectivistic cultures, although their function and manifestations would appear to differ from their role in individualistic cultures.

Wang and Ross (2007) point to an interesting feature of the Confucian intellectual tradition that colors contemporary Asian thought. There is a reverence for the past, a trust in the wisdom of the ancients that is not contested. Wang and Ross contrast this uncritical acceptance with the Western tradition of independent thinking that challenges the intellectual claims of scholars and religious figures of the past. Religious tenets and scientific theories are questioned and such scrutiny may result in their being modified or even overturned, in contrast to the Chinese focus on the precise memorization of ancient texts that are the standards of wisdom.

Against this strong Eastern traditional background, one can ask what historical, religious, intellectual, and philosophical movements might have influenced the emergence of an individualistic cultural perspective. Kitayama et al. (2007) argue that many of the modern Western ideals of thought can be traced to ancient Greek civilization. Socrates' exhortation "Know thyself" represents the harbinger of a stance wherein one chooses personal goals, highlights one's distinctiveness from others, and promotes an authentic self.

The religious upheaval in Western Europe during the 16th century gave rise to Calvinism and Protestantism that challenged Catholicism and introduced an emerging model of the independent self (Kitayama et al., 2007). During the 18th-century Age of Enlightenment, philosophers (e.g., Rousseau, Locke, and Voltaire) also fueled the flame, highlighting the individual thinker. Ambitious Western European immigrants transplanted such ideas to American soil where they found their way into the political, ideological, and religious foundations of a fledgling country. As such, they served as a foundation for the "rugged individualism" that came to chacaterize Americans.

Empirical Support for the Distinction between Individualistic and Collectivistic Cultures

To what extent are these distinctions supported by empirical cross-cultural research? One of the most comprehensive treatments can be found in a meta-analysis by Oyserman et al. (2002), who sought to empirically evaluate the theoretical assumptions underlying the distinction between individualism and collectivism. The findings revealed that Americans emerged as higher in individualism and lower in collectivism than most other countries. However, the patterns were similar to those of Western European countries (e.g., Germany) and English-speaking countries (e.g., Australia).

Oyserman et al. (2002) note that the meta-analysis did *not* support the assumption that European Americans represent the gold standard of individualism. African Americans emerged as the most individualistic. Both groups scored higher on this dimension than did Asian Americans. In contrast, Latino Americans were just as individualistic as European Americans. With regard to collectivism within the United States, Asian Americans and Latino Americans displayed higher levels than both European Americans and African Americans. These investigators raise the interesting question of whether or not ethnic minorities within the United States resemble those from the countries (outside of the United States) that represent their cultural heritage. The data, however, are too few in number to make meaningful comparisons. We return to this issue, when the topics of acculturation and biculturalism are discussed.

The evidence for cross-national differences in individualism versus collectivism relies heavily on comparisons between North Americans and Asians from four East Asian countries: the People's Republic of China, Hong Kong, Taiwan, Japan, and Korea (Oyserman et al., 2002). Differences between the greater individualism of Americans and the greater collectivism of Asians are greatest when the Asian comparison is with those from the People's Republic of China, Hong Kong, and Taiwan. These distinctions are less pronounced when Japanese and Koreans comprise the Asian contrast group. Oyserman and colleagues conjecture that collectivism is historically more typical within Chinese culture, whereas Japanese and Korean cultures have other traditional roots that are more distinct from the Chinese. They urge that more attention be paid to differences between Asian countries and cultures, rather than overemphasizing similarities among all East Asian cultures. The meta-analytic findings, therefore, revealed smaller differences between Americans and both Japanese and Koreans for individualism as well as collectivism in contrast to comparisons with the Chinese.

In keeping with these findings, Hong, Ip, Chiu, Morris, and Menon (2001) predicted that the Chinese would be more likely than Americans to focus on collective duties when their cultural identity was evoked. In contrast, Americans were predicted to focus on individual rights. In addition, a comparison of the spontaneous self-concepts of Hong Kong Chinese and Americans supported these predictions, which anticipates our next topic.

Associated Self-Construals and Psychological Consequences

Markus and Kitayama (1991) posited that the two cultural orientations, individualism and collectiveness, impacted corresponding self-construals, namely independent versus interdependent concepts of self. Other psychological consequences such as self-esteem and the extent to which the self is enacted as a consistent, stable entity versus variable or changeable have been related to these construals. However, as Oyserman and colleagues (see Oyserman & Sorensen, 2009; Oyserman et al., 2002) as well as Singelis (1994) have urged, one must first clearly distinguish between the values that define each cultural orientation (Table 8.1) and the self-construals as well as the psychological consequences to which they are presumed to give rise (Table 8.2). Individualism versus collectivism defines distinctions in cultural *values*, whereas self-construals represent the extent to which these values are incorporated into an independent versus interdependent *self*. Discussion now turns to this latter distinction, summarized in Table 8.2.

For Markus and Kitayama (1991), the *independent* conceptualization of the self is one of *separateness* from others, of *autonomy* (see also Singelis, 1994). The self is defined as *distinct*, pursuing its own personal goals. The self strives to be *unique,* to *stand out* from the crowd, hopefully by being superior. One also places such self-attributes on display. In communicating with others, one is open and direct with regard to thoughts, opinions, and emotions.

TABLE 8.2. Associated Self-Construals and Psychological Consequences

Independent	Interdependent
Self is defined as separate, distinct, *independent* from others, promoting one's own personal goals.	Self is defined as *connected* to others, pursuing in-group goals.
Self is *unique*, *stands out* from others, should be different, superior to others.	Self strives to occupy one's proper role, to *fit in*, so as to achieve social harmony within the in-group.
Self is *direct* in communicating with others, including expression of emotions.	Self refrains from direct communication, is reluctant to express emotions that disrupts group harmony.
Self-esteem is important, defined by meeting standards of uniqueness, distinctiveness. Self-esteem is high.	Self-esteem not salient as a goal. Self-esteem is moderate and lower than those with an independent orientation.
Many *self-enhancement* strategies to ensure high self-esteem that may not be realistic.	*Self-effacing* tendencies, modesty, that are associated lower self-esteem. Self-criticism.
Individual accomplishments, personal success, are sources of self-esteem.	Harmonious relationships are sources of self-esteem, meeting in-group goals.
Thinking is linear, reflecting analytic logic, clarity, minimizing ambiguity.	Thinking is dialectical, tolerating contradiction and and ambiguity.
Autobiographical memory focuses on distinctive, personal accomplishments.	Autobiographical memory emphasizes connectedness, interpersonal relationships.
Self is unitary, *consistent*, stable across situations. Contradictory multiple selves cause conflict.	Self is flexible, variable, changes to accommodate the situation. Contradictory attributes not in conflict.

In contrast, *interdependent* self-construals are typified by representations of self in relation to significant others. In-group goals are pursued. The self strives to occupy proscribed and proper roles, to *fit in*, so as to achieve social harmony within the group. Connectedness to others is paramount. The interdependent self refrains from direct communication, because the open and uncensored expression of thoughts, opinions, and emotions may disrupt group harmony.

For those with an independent construal, s*elf-esteem* is a highly sought-after commodity. In the United States, the primary criteria for evaluating one's sense of worth include how successfully one demonstrates the cultural values of independence, autonomy, and uniqueness. Cultural assessments of self-esteem reveal that it is high, in comparison to countries characterized by a more interdependent self (see Cross & Gore, 2003). In such countries (e.g., Japan) self-esteem is not a salient personal goal and therefore not highly sought after. R. Brown (2008) has reported that American college students view high self-esteem as not only desirable but a necessity, whereas Japanese students admit that it is potentially desirable but not a personal requirement. Levels of self-esteem among Asians are moderate and significantly lower than for individuals in the West. However, given that most of these instruments were developed in the United States, their appropriateness and cultural sensitivity can be questioned, a topic to which we return.

Self-Enhancement Strategies versus Self-Effacing Tendencies

In the service of promoting high self-esteem, numerous *self-enhancement strategies* have been documented in the United States and, to a lesser extent, in other Western countries. These strategies can be contrasted to *self-effacing* tendencies among Eastern countries that involve *modesty* and *self-criticism* toward the goal of *self-improvement*. Heine (2003) defines self-enhancement as the tendency to dwell on, elaborate, and exaggerate *positive* aspects of the self, relative to personal weaknesses. In contrast, self-improvement involves the tendency to dwell on, elaborate, and exaggerate *negative* aspects of the self, relative to personal strengths, in an effort to correct perceived shortcomings.

North Americans are notorious for not only viewing themselves positively but making *unrealistic* evaluations of their positive attributes (Cross & Gore, 2003; Heine, 2007; Heine, Lehman, Markus, & Kitayama, 1999). This self-enhancing style takes other forms. For example, Americans take credit for their successes, but attribute failures to external or situational factors. If forced to face negative evaluations of the self, the individual can access positive information that counters the negative feedback (Steele, 1988). Another tactic is to make "downward comparisons," highlighting the less adequate performance of others, thereby looking more competent, in comparison. A meta-analysis by Mezulis, Abramson, Hyde, and Hankin (2004) reveals strong tendencies for Americans to demonstrate a self-serving attributional bias, namely, making more internal, stable, and global attributions for positive, compared to negative, personal outcomes. Asian samples, in contrast, did not display such strong biases. The authors conclude that there is no *universal* attributional positivity bias.

Heine et al. (1999) previously observed that the need for positive self-regard is also not universal. Many elements of Japanese culture, for example, are incongruent with self-enhancing motivations. The predominant tendency is *self-criticism* that serves as a motive for *self-improvement*. The Japanese tend to view everyday situations as opportunities to be self-critical and also welcome such scrutiny from others (see also Heine, 2003). Findings from Kanagawa, Cross, and Markus (2001) have corroborated the more negative self-evaluations of the Japanese in the service of self-criticism that is viewed as socially desirable. Moreover, discrepancies between the ideal and the real self are greater among the Japanese than Americans (Heine,

2003). Among Americans, where such discrepancies exist, they threaten one's self-esteem and provoke depressive reactions. In Japan, such discrepancies signal the need to improve the self, motivating one to strive to meet the cultural ideal (Heine et al., 1999).

In a meta-analysis (Heine & Hamamura, 2007) of published cross-cultural studies on self-enhancement, pervasive and pronounced differences between East Asians and Westerners were revealed. Westerners demonstrated a clear self-serving bias, whereas East Asians did not (with Asian Americans falling in between). This evidence converges with other findings indicating that East Asians do not self-enhance.

Experimental studies bolster these cultural differences. Heine et al. (2001) examined self-enhancing and self-improving motivations in the Japanese and Americans by asking participants from each country to solve a challenging task where failure was a possibility. Americans who failed persisted less on a follow-up task compared to those who had succeeded, presumably because failure threatened their sense of competence. In contrast, Japanese who failed persisted longer than those who were successful. The investigators interpreted the pattern as evidence for a self-improving orientation among the Japanese, namely, that failures highlighted where corrective efforts were called for.

In an interesting twist, Muramoto (2003) conducted a study revealing that self-enhancement tendencies among the Japanese are more complex as well as more subtle. Consistent with the literature, participants tended to make self-effacing attributions for their success and failure. However, when asked, they revealed that they expected parents, siblings, and close friends to make internal attributions for their success, but not their failure. Thus, the Japanese would not enhance or protect their self-esteem explicitly, but they would do so indirectly, through the evaluative eyes of others.

The vast majority of cross-cultural analyses and studies on this topic have focused on the Japanese culture. However, others have addressed these issues in Korea and China. J. Kim et al. (2003) examined self-enhancing and self-effacing tendencies among Koreans. College students were read two scenarios, one in which the protagonist was bragging about positive accomplishments and a second in which the main character emphasized negative self-perceptions. The results revealed that the negative self-presentation was judged more favorably than the positive self-presentation, suggesting the role of self-effacement.

Y. Wang and Ollendick (2001) have reviewed literature revealing self-effacing tendencies observed in Chinese culture. Their perspective highlights the value that Chinese society places on modesty and harmonious social relationships. They argue that self-effacing behavior will be more likely to obtain favorable social responses from others that, in turn, will serve to maintain harmony. In contrast, the self-enhancing tendencies observed among European Americans functions to support an elevated sense of self-esteem.

Wirtz and Chiu (2008) recently offered an interesting perspective on the type of *ego* that differentiates those in Western and Eastern cultures. They describe the self-enhancing strategies and self-serving biases among Westerners in terms of Greenwald's (1980) concept of the "totalitarian ego." Greenwald has likened these self-protective and self-promotional tendencies to a controlling political state. Just as a totalitarian state exercises control of the media, relies on propaganda, and regulates political life, the self devotes effort toward information control and self-serving personal propaganda through a variety of self-enhancing cognitive biases. According to Greenwald, egocentrism, illusion of control, self-serving bias, confirmation bias, and manipulation of personal memory all operate to glorify the self. Wirtz and Chiu argue, as do other scholars, that this is but one conception of the self. They review literature suggesting the self in Eastern culture is more restrained or subdued. They suggest that the Eastern self, in contrast to the totalitarian ego, constitutes a more reserved representation that they label the "quiet ego." This theme is revisited in the concluding chapter.

Self-enhancement promotes positive feelings of self-esteem for Westerners, whereas self-effacement among Eastern societies undermines feelings of worth. However, what are the specific *sources* of self-esteem associated with independent and interdependent forms of self-construal? Within Western cultures, individual accomplishments and personal successes represent a critical pathway to high self-esteem. Pride is an appropriate emotional reaction in recognition for personal accomplishments. In contrast to Western culture, pride is viewed as a sign of arrogance as well as the failure to acknowledge the contributions of others (Cross & Gore, 2003; Stipek, 1998).

Although high self-esteem is not revered as a psychological commodity in Eastern cultures, harmonious relationships represent the primary sources of self-regard or self-respect (Diener & Diener, 2009; Kang, Shaver, Sue, Min, & Jing, 2003). Kang et al. have further reported that self-esteem predicted *life satisfaction* for European Americans, but not for Koreans and Chinese. Rather, *relationship quality* was found to be the path to life satisfaction for these Asian groups (but was not highly related for the Americans).

Cross-cultural differences in *autobiographical memory* parallel the distinctions raised above. For Americans with independent self-construals, the content of memory focuses on distinctive, personal accomplishment, whereas autobiographical memory in Eastern interdependent cultures emphasizes connectedness and interpersonal relationships. Leichtman, Wang, and Pillemer (2003) summarize findings that adults who have grown up in individualistic cultures recount earlier, lengthier, and more detailed childhood memories than do adults who have grown up in collectivistic cultures. Moreover, in their conversations with children, adults model the dominant narrative structure of their culture. Parental styles in individualistic cultures are more elaborative, encouraging children to embellish their narratives. As a result, American children's autobiographical accounts contain more description and more personal preferences, judgments, and opinions, compared to those of children from Korea and China. Their narratives also displayed a more autonomous orientation, reflected in the expression of personal needs, likes and dislikes, and personal control in the face of authority, as revealed in the research by Q. Wang and Leichtman (2000). These researchers further documented, in the stories of Chinese children, the greater orientation toward social engagement, concern with moral correctness, respect for authority, and themes of responsibility.

The Self as Unitary and Consistent versus Flexible and Variable across Situations

Western and Eastern conceptualizations of the self also differ with respect to whether the self is unitary or variable, respectively. Western thought is fashioned after models of Aristotelian logic that are linear and analytic. Clarity is emphasized, with little tolerance for ambiguity. Western formal reasoning requires that contradictions be resolved; only one argument can be logically correct (Nisbett, Peng, Choi, & Norenzayan, 2001). In contrast, East Asians are much more tolerant of inconsistency, ambiguity, and contradiction. Nisbett et al. refer to this form of Eastern thought as *naïve dialecticism*. When confronted with an apparent contradiction, Chinese participants will attempt to resolve the dilemma through compromise, reasoning that both positions have merit. This type of thinking can be traced to Eastern philosophical notions of *yin* and *yang* that are opposing, but also integrated, forces in the world.

This tolerance for contradiction generalizes to how the self is conceptualized in Eastern cultures. What would appear, on the surface, to be inconsistencies are attributed to the need to be flexible and to alter the self appropriately across different interpersonal situations. In contrast, Westerners have a strong need to view the self as an internal, stable structure that is consistent across situations. This *consistency motivation* or consistency "ethic" was first articulated by Lecky (1945) and has been a cornerstone of subsequent Western theories of self and motivation (see Cross & Gore, 2003; Heine, 2007).

There has been considerable documentation of this cultural distinction within the last decade. Spencer-Rodgers, Peng, Wang, and Hou (2004) have examined cultural differences in reasoning about psychological contradiction and the effects of naïve dialecticism on self-evaluations. Their research reveals differences between residents of mainland China and Westerners in their spontaneous self-descriptions. Chinese participants reported more evaluative contradictions, which the authors also refer to as "ambivalence." Spencer-Rodgers and colleagues have more recently replicated their findings with the Chinese and extended them to the Japanese who also apply naïve dialecticism, demonstrating the contradictory, changeable nature of the East Asian self-concept (Spencer-Rodgers, Boucher, Mori, Wang, & Peng, 2009). Others (see Hamamura, Heine, & Paulhus, 2008) have also documented the East Asian tendency toward dialectical thinking, manifest in a tolerance for contradictory beliefs. They also employ the term "ambivalence." Yet one needs to be cautious in applying such terminology because ambivalence can imply an emotional reaction, namely, that one is somehow troubled by contradiction. Such distress does *not* appear to be the case for East Asians.

Other treatments also focus on the situational specificity that is valued in Eastern cultures, where multiple selves are the norm. Suh (2002) makes explicit reference to the multiple selves that East Asian cultures conceptualize as comfortably coexisting realities. Suh's research questions the classic thesis in (Western) psychology that identity consistency is a prerequisite for psychological well-being. Koreans viewed themselves as more flexible across interpersonal contexts that predicted well-being and positive social evaluations, whereas identity consistency was a predictor for North Americans. Spencer-Rodgers et al., 2009 have further researched the naïve dialecticism (Nisbett et al., 2001) that defines East Asians' tolerance for contradiction and the expectation of situational change in the self.

A similar theme has been addressed by Nezlek et al. (2008), who have demonstrated that the self-esteem of Japanese participants changed more in reaction to daily social events (be they positive or negative) than it did for North Americans. Their findings highlight greater sensitivity of the Japanese to social context, compared to North Americans. A related study (Tafarodi, Lo, Yamaguchi, Lee, & Katsura, 2004) has revealed that East Asian cultures place more emphasis on the contextual adjustment of a person's behavior. Such an adjustment translates into greater variation in the outwardly presented self across contexts. These differences were manifest in comparisons of Canadian adults with Chinese and Japanese participants.

English and Chen (2007) have demonstrated a more complex pattern among Asian *Americans*. Like the studies cited above, they found that Asian Americans were less consistent in their self-descriptions across relationship contexts than were European Americans. However, their findings also revealed that whereas the Asian American self is variable across relationships, it is *stable within* a given interpersonal context. Moreover, the variations across relationships did not compromise the Asian Americans' sense of *authenticity*. This issue has also been addressed by Kashima et al. (2004) in two East Asian cultures (Japan and Korea) and three Western cultures (Australia, Germany, and the United Kingdom). The context sensitivity of the self was greater in the Eastern countries. Moreover, in the Western countries a stable, *context-invariant* self was identified as the true self. In contrast, in Japan it was the context-sensitive, variable self that was considered to be the true self.

This body of evidence converges with our own research on the construction of multiple selves within samples of American adolescents (Harter, 2006a; Harter, Bresnick, et al., 1997). Our work extends the findings for Westerners in documenting the perceived psychological *conflict* that contradictions produce, as well as the overt concern over true- versus false-self behaviors. As described in Chapter 3, we have designed a procedure in which we first ask adolescents to spontaneously generate self-descriptors across various relational contexts, for example, self with parents, with a best friend, with a group of classmates or casual friends, and with a romantic other. Participants then identify whether any of the pairs of descriptors reflect *opposites*, and then indicate if any of the opposing pairs of attributes produce internal, psychological *conflict* where the attributes are experienced as clashing within their personality.

The fact that American adolescents see themselves differently in different relational contexts sets the stage for attributes to be perceived as potentially contradictory as well as conflictual. Indeed, as noted in earlier chapters, William James (1890) first identified this phenomenon, coining it *the conflict of the different Me's*. Our participants identify such conflicts that peak in midadolescence. Thus, a certain level of conflict over the identified opposing attributes in their self-portrait is normative, as revealed by our findings across several studies (Harter, Bresnick, et al., 1997). We have speculated that the *consistency ethic* that has been identified as a value in Western culture (see Chapter 1) contributes to this concern in the face of identified contradictions.

One can hypothesize that in Eastern Asian countries, adolescents would report far fewer *conflicts* between opposing attributes. Such opposites, themselves, are to be expected given cultural role prescriptions dictating that one behave differently in different interpersonal contexts. The studies reviewed above clearly reveal that this is the normative pattern among East Asians. Presumably, because multiple selves are the cultural norm, conflict would *not* be experienced, particularly given the greater tolerance for contradiction. This is an interesting hypothesis worthy of examination.

Among our American samples of adolescents, the construction of multiple selves in which different attributes are perceived as contradictory should understandably also provoke concern over which of the opposing attributes in a given pair reflects one's *true self*. Our own research has revealed that the proliferation of selves during adolescence does engender problematic and soul-searching questions about which is the "real me," particularly when attributes in different roles appear contradictory (e.g., cheerful with friends but depressed with parents). During our multiple-selves procedure, a number of adolescents have spontaneously agonized over which of the contradictory self-characteristics represented their "true" self.

The Western view that the self should be stable or consistent across interpersonal contexts should not only give American adolescents cause for concern about contradictions between self-attributes but also lead to consternation given the identification of certain characteristics as false-self behavior. In contrast, the Eastern tolerance for contradiction should render opposing attributes as mere manifestations of their true self, as two studies reviewed above have revealed (English & Chen, 2007; Kashima et al., 2004).

A personal, professional experience supports these conclusions. In consulting with Professor Catherine Cooper, a faculty colleague in the psychology department at the University of Santa Cruz, I was introduced to a well-known visiting Japanese scholar, Professor Hiroshi Azuma, with whom she was collaborating. Each asked me to describe prototypical features of the adolescent self-portrait in the United States, as revealed in our own research. On a blackboard, I visually depicted the structure of the American self-structure (see the drawing on the left of Figure 8.1). I described how our adolescents report different selves across contexts, attributes that can be contradictory, and that part of each relational self contains true-self attributes but also personal characteristics that are perceived as false. Both contradictions and false-self behaviors are experienced as distressing.

To contrast the American self-structure with the Japanese self-structure, Professor Azuma very politely picked up a blackboard eraser

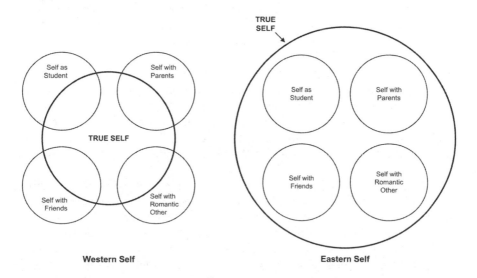

FIGURE 8.1. Depictions of the Western versus Eastern self among adolescents.

and systematically deleted the larger of my circles that separated true-from false-self attributes. He then drew a single circle around the entire configuration of multiple selves (see the depiction on the right, in Figure 8.1). He convincingly described how in Japan, adolescents clearly possess multiple selves that conform to normative cultural expectations and role prescriptions. He went on, however, to explain that in contrast to my portrayal of the American adolescent self-structure, Japanese teenagers do *not* consider attributes of their context-related selves to be in conflict, nor are they false. All attributes, though seemingly contradictory, comfortably coexist and are viewed as one's *true* self. His demonstration made the distinction between the Western and Eastern self compellingly clear.

Two years later, I had the opportunity to make a presentation on the self to Chinese scholars in Beijing. I described my encounter with Professor Azuma, who had distinguished between the self as construed in the United States and in Japan. I replicated the figure on the blackboard, as a visual aid that I hoped would help to cut through the language barrier. I was careful not to imply that the Japanese model necessarily mapped onto the Chinese conceptualization of the self. I asked how they would depict the Chinese self. They basically acknowledged that the Chinese self was much closer to the Japanese model than was the American characterization, suggesting some generalizability across two Eastern cultures.

More recently, a colleague of mine (see Waters, 2011) has collected relevant data from a sample of Taiwanese youth. From a cross-cultural perspective, one can ask whether they manifest *commonalities* in the self-differentiation process or whether the dynamics are *different*, compared to American adolescents. Waters argues that this should not be an either-or question but that thoughtful cross-cultural research should examine both. Asian youth may well demonstrate both developmental commonalities in the self-differentiation process as well as differences, consistent with cultural expectations about how the self should be displayed across relational contests. In Taiwan, the Confucian philosophical system encourages *interdependent*, differentiated, and role-appropriate self-expression rather than consistency across roles (Markus & Kitayama, 1991). Taiwanese youth (137 males, 173 females) completed an adaptation of Harter's multiple-selves procedure.

With regard to cultural commonalities, the proportion of opposing self attributes in conflict systematically declined over the high school years and into college, similar to the pattern for American youth, reflecting more universal cognitive-developmental processes. With regard to cultural differences, Taiwanese youth reported fewer opposites in conflict than American youth in Harter's samples. Moreover, when older Taiwanese adolescents were asked why seemingly contradictory attributes in different roles did *not* produce conflict, a popular explanation (not offered by American youth) emphasized the interdependent cultural obligation and appropriateness of displaying different selves across relationships. Waters argues that in Taiwanese culture, this represents healthy self-differentiation.

Assessment of Independent versus Interdependent Self-Construals

A conceptual analysis of cultural differences between independent versus interdependent construals have been described in the preceding section. However, how are these various self-construals best assessed? Researchers have developed instruments that capture each of the two types of self-construals. For example, Singelis (1994) has developed a two-subscale instrument containing 12 independent and 12 interdependent factors that yield an acceptable two-factor solution. This instrument has served as the major cross-cultural measure for identifying these two opposing forms of self-construal. A decade later, Hardin, Leong, and Bhagwat (2004) reexamined the factor structure of this instrument, to determine if a more multidimensional approach was warranted. Their psychometric analyses identified six factors. Four subscales defined dimensions of the *independent* self: (1) autonomy/assertiveness, (2) individualism, (3) behavioral consistency, and (4) primacy of the self. The remaining two *interdependent* subscales were labeled (1) esteem for the group, and (2) relational interdependence. The authors acknowledge that the relative usefulness of this six-factor approach has yet to be demonstrated. Thus, the jury is still out with regard to whether this multidimensional instrument furthers our understanding of cultural self-construals and associated psychological correlates. Until then, the two-dimensional model is still viable and is valued for its parsimony.

Cultural Differences in Child-Rearing Practices and School Experiences

Parent–child rearing practices and schooling influences are important mechanisms through which cultural values are assumed to impact self-construals and their associated psychological correlates. A large body of research now demonstrates that individualistic and collectivistic cultures differ in their child-rearing goals and related parenting behaviors (see Trommsdorff & Kornadt, 2003). These investigators have reported that Japanese mothers place more emphasis on cooperation, indulgence, thoughtfulness, and empathy than do German mothers, who represent the values of an individualistic culture. Good manners and politeness are also touted as child-rearing goals in collectivistic cultures (see B. Schwartz, Schafermeier, & Trommsdorff, 2005). In contrast, individualistic cultures emphasize independence, autonomy, self-reliance, and self-realization as child-rearing goals.

B. Schwartz et al. (2005) compared the child-rearing practices of Korean and German mothers. Rather than merely treating country as a proxy for cultural orientation, these researchers directly assessed individualism and collectivism, as a first step. As predicted, they demonstrated that Korean mothers were more collectivistic than German mothers, who were more individualistic than the Korean mothers. Individualistic orientations were positively associated with the goal of fostering the child's independence, whereas collectivistic orientations were associated with the goals of instilling children's obedience to their parents as well as the importance of academic success.

Other comparisons have targeted child-rearing practices in Japan and the United States, where variations in mother–child interactions have been observed (Kitayama et al., 2007). Bornstein et al. (1992) have reported differences in maternal speech to infants. Japanese mothers were more likely to employ "affect-salient" expressive speech (e.g., "The ball makes you happy!"), whereas American mothers gave more "information-salient" utterances (e.g., "The ball is red") and asked more information-seeking questions. Moreover, Fernald and Morikawa (1993) have reported that the infant-directed speech of Japanese mothers contains fewer words but a greater number of affect-laden, nonverbal vocalizations, compared to their American counterparts. On another child-rearing dimension, Bornstein and colleagues found that Japanese mothers employ emotional facial expressions to direct their infant's attention to themselves, whereas American mothers direct their infant's attention to objects and events in the environment.

Kitayama et al. (2007) point to further child-rearing differences between Japanese and American mothers. Japanese mothers spend more time in close proximity to their infants, including more physical contact. American mothers are more prone to distance their toddler, directing his/her attention to goal-relevant objects. An interesting finding by Barrett (1995) reveals that Japanese infants receive only about 2 hours a week in *nonmaternal* care, whereas American infants receive, on average, 23 hours. These cultural child-rearing differences have implications for how infants perform during the separation phase in the strange situation paradigm designed to assess attachment status (see Miyake, Chen, & Campos, 1985). Japanese infants show a higher level of anxiety than do American babies, leading to their greater classification as "C" babies who display an anxious–ambivalent demeanor.

This classification paradigm was developed for Western infants and mothers, where autonomous exploration of the environment and the acceptance of strangers is a reflection of secure attachment, leading to a B-baby classification (Ainsworth, 1979). However, one must be careful not to infer that Japanese infants are insecurely attached. As Markus and Kitayama (2003) caution, patterns of infant behavior that are normative in certain cultural settings outside of North America should not be categorized as insecurely attached, according to the Western criteria identified in attachment theory. Morelli and Rothbaum (2007) further note that Japanese attachment scholars are less likely to endorse the Western perspective of individualism and independence. One can conjecture that the behavior of Japanese infants reflects culture-specific child-rearing practices that may ultimately be adaptive in their subsequent adult environment of work and family where connectedness is valued over autonomy.

Japanese parenting also emphasizes the importance of fitting in, as well as empathy and the self-regulation of negative emotions (Morelli & Rothbaum, 2007). Children living in East Asian countries are typically described by Western observers as overregulated and more behaviorally inhibited, compared to children in the United States. These characteristics are lauded by Asian parents, who offer praise and acceptance for these behaviors. Compliance is also rewarded by parents in collectivistic societies. Each of these behavioral tendencies eventually contributes to the cultural goal of harmony for adults within the family and work-group contexts.

Collectivistic cultures perceive the use of controlling child-rearing techniques as sensitive parenting (see V. Carlson & Harwood, 2003). These findings stand in sharp contrast to the Western model of attachment in which responsive but nonintrusive maternal practices are considered to be sensitive caregiving techniques that give rise to the security of attachment (see Morelli & Rothbaum, 2007). Parental control, strictness, and directiveness are more highly valued in collectivistic cultures, as is conformity to clearly prescribed role expectations for children. Moreover, control is combined with warmth and closeness. These are thought to cement the parent–child relationship and foster the security of attachment.

Filial piety, in collectivistic cultures such as China, demands obedience to parents as well as respect for one's elders including the importance of honoring ancestors (Y. Wang & Ollendick, 2001). The need to foster filial piety in children justifies absolute parental authority. Moreover, obedience to parents constitutes a *moral* imperative and serves to instill in children a general fear of authority figures. For example, within the Korean community, the control exercised by parents is considered a moral duty to be responsible for protecting their children and for promoting the family welfare and honor (J. Miller, 2003).

Western psychologists, viewing these practices through the lens of American child-rearing values, would interpret them as *authoritarian* parenting (Baumrind, 1971) that is typically associated with parental hostility and rejection. McCrae (2001) contends that Westerners misinterpret the parental control exercised in collectivistic cultures. Moreover, Western attachment theorists maintain that efforts to physically control and directly shape infants' behavior interfere with their autonomous activity and reflect parental insensitivity that compromises the security of attachment (Morelli & Rothbaum, 2007). Authoritarian parenting, which includes harsh punishment, is viewed by Baumrind (1996) as the path to childhood aggression and other antisocial behaviors, based on her research with American families.

She also decries the overly *permissive*, indulgent style of parenting as fraught, given that it will undermine the child's respect for parents, preclude a clear sense of identity, and weaken the commitment to fulfill adaptive goals. She favors what she has termed *authoritative* parenting, rejecting the false polarity between a child-rearing ideology of indulgence and one of tyranny. She argues for a style of child rearing that balances appropriate control with warmth, open communication between child and parent, democratic decision making, clear enforceable expectations, and the encouragement of the child's individuality.

Baumrind's (1996) model of parenting shares certain tenets with self-determination theory as put forth by Deci and Ryan (1991), another Western approach with implications for child rearing. Its goal is to foster the child's *internalization* of the values of caregivers, such that behavior is no longer viewed by the child as due to external constraints that result from coercive parenting. One comes gradually to "own" the values of caregivers and the culture, perceiving one's behavior as self-determined, as a function of personal choice. This outcome would best be produced by the authoritative parenting style urged by Baumrind. These arguments are revisited in a subsequent treatment of how agency cannot be commandeered as a characteristic unique to Western cultures. Agency is alive and well in Eastern societies, albeit defined differently in keeping with the overarching goals and philosophical foundations of the culture.

The Cultural Value of Childhood Achievement in Child-Rearing Practices

One might be tempted to conclude that the Western emphasis on the development of independence and autonomy, on the need to compete and be superior, with a focus on self-accomplishments, might all dictate that academic strivings toward success would be more pronounced in Western cultures. However, sociocultural analyses and the pattern of findings do not support this expectation (see B. Schwartz et al., 2005). Asian parents actually place more emphasis on achievement as a child-rearing goal than do parents from Western cultures. C. H. Cooper (2011) also challenges the contention that school achievement is hampered in collectivist cultures. Rather, academic achievement is a pathway to personal advancement, higher social status, wealth, and respect for the individual as well as one's family and in-group.

As a result, Chinese parents actively pressure their children to achieve at school (Y. Wang & Ollendick, 2001).

This emphasis on achievement can be linked, in part, to historic cultural values and the impact of Confucianism. Ideologically, learning and achievement are central to Confucian thinking. Respect for an accumulation of knowledge, including past knowledge that reflects ancient wisdom, is an essential educational goal (Q. Wang & Ross, 2007). The acquisition of knowledge also includes the moral tenets of Confucianism. Moral self-cultivation is an essential cultural striving. These values stem in part from the central principle of "ren," stressing that qualities such as sincerity, kindness, and altruism are to be cultivated. Ren has also been referred to as the supreme virtue that translates as a sensitive concern for others, including connection to others and harmony in relationships (Cross & Gore, 2003). Achievement motivation, in particular, is also highly intertwined with filial piety that promotes and ensures strong ties to the family. From this perspective, moral self-cultivation is an essential cultural striving. In their academic pursuits, students attempt to enhance the social standing of the family by gaining admission to top universities and then securing employment at a prestigious company (see Markus & Kitayama, 1991, whose observations are primarily from Japan).

The child in collectivistic cultures that honor Confucianism develops an inner self that includes self-reliance, individual responsibility for learning, and the drive to achieve success, based on his/her personal capabilities. As such, J. Li and Yue (2004) argue that those who conclude that Confucian cultures only impose hierarchical, social roles on their people may propose arguments that are simplistic and one-sided (see also Meredith, Wang, & Zheng, 1993).

J. Li and Yue (2004) cite other scholars who have documented that Chinese children believe strongly in personal *effort*, a construct that clearly denotes a sense of individual agency. They suggest that such concepts have been overlooked in previous research and have sought to redress this cultural misperception. In their own investigation, they begin with the essential role that learning plays in the upbringing of Chinese children. They also invoke the principle of ren, which involves a lifelong striving for self-perfection that demands the development of the person's individual control. For the Chinese, learning is not merely a narrow academic pursuit but involves the individual's moral strivings. Learning virtues extend to the development of diligence, resolve, perseverance, and concentration. These virtues constitute the core of Chinese personal agency. Thus, learning consists of both individual *and* moral goals, countering certain claims about collectivist cultures.

This framework led J. Li and Yue (2004) to investigate, through open-ended interviews, both individual and social goals of learning among Chinese adolescents. Examples of *individual goals* included the development of one's skills and competence, aspirations and ambitions for the self, and the need to foster moral and spiritual wisdom. *Social goals of learning* focused on contributions to society, the importance of honoring parents and teachers, and the development of social relationships. Findings revealed there were significantly more (not fewer) types of individual than social goals for learning among these Chinese students. The authors concluded that findings portraying that individual goals of learning and agency "reflect the Chinese cultural value system regarding learning, which is largely Confucian" (J. Li & Yue, 2004, p. 37). They also caution that reducing these documented goals to the individualistic–collectivistic dichotomy does a gross injustice to the complexity of the self-concepts among the Chinese. A related study of perceived school climate, comparing Chinese and American adolescents, has recently revealed that Chinese students not only perceived more teacher and student support but more opportunities for autonomy in the classroom (Jia et al., 2009). Thus, in the academic realm, signs of individualism and autonomy are quite evident in Chinese culture, contrary to the stereotype. J. Li and Yue have cogently argued that no matter how educators structure the social context for learning, the individual is the agent who must be actively engaged for learning to occur. Toward these learning goals their findings also revealed, consistent with other evidence, that Asian adults and children emphasize personal *effort* more than intellectual *ability* (see also Stevenson & Stigler, 1992). The message is that everyone can achieve, if they put forth the effort. In contrast, the American educational system focuses more on individual differences in intellectual ability as the cause of success and teachers communicate this to their students, accordingly. East Asian children are urged to work harder both by parents and school teachers to become the best they can be (see Morelli & Rothbaum, 2007). Koreans codify this ethos in a phrase that translates as "No matter how hard you work, you can always work harder" (Grant & Dweck, 2001, p. 207).

As part of this constellation of achievement-related motives, Eastern Asians engage in the practice of *self-criticism*, from an early age. Thus, there is a focus on personal shortcomings toward the goal of overcoming these limitations. Chinese mothers engage their children in storytelling that critically highlights the child's transgressions (Morelli & Rothbaum, 2007). In Japanese schools, children are given a special period of time each day to reflect on their shortcomings and to address how they can improve their performance in the future. Thus, self-criticism is intimately linked to the importance of *self-correction* in Eastern Asian cultures.

American Mothers' Emphasis on Promoting Their Child's Self-Esteem

A primary child-rearing goal of American mothers targets high self-esteem as a psychological commodity to be fostered in their children, in contrast to the goals of effort, self-correction, and self-improvement among Asian mothers. Chao's (1996) research has documented that European American mothers identify self-esteem, social skills, and the importance of having fun as the critical goals that will lead to their children's success in preschool. In contrast, their Chinese American counterparts named hard work as the most important attitude for their children to develop. A more recent study (Chao, 2000) revealed that mothers of Chinese American adolescents expected that their teenage students be fully self-reliant with regard to their schoolwork. P. J. Miller, Wang, Sandel, and Cho (2002) have found that American mothers spoke at length about the importance of building their children's self-esteem. In contrast, few Taiwanese mothers talked about the importance of attending to their child's self-respect (a Chinese term that approximates self-esteem; there is no term for self-esteem in the Chinese language).

Other research within the United States also reveals the high priority that European American parents place on fostering their children's self-esteem (see Owens, 1995). In keeping with the self-enhancement techniques that were identified as common among Western adults, Forehand and Long (1995) have provided a telling list of child-rearing techniques that American parents should employ to enhance their child's self-esteem. Parents are encouraged to (1) offer frequent praise and limit negative feedback; (2) acknowledge and highlight the child's achievements, abilities, and interests; (3) avoid demands of perfection; (4) reward independent decision making; (5) encourage positive self-evaluations; (6) teach social and problem-solving skills; and (7) display acceptance of the child for who he/she is as a unique individual.

Forehand and Long (1995) view these American child-rearing techniques as indispensable in fostering the child's self-esteem. Two points are noteworthy. First, these techniques cast in bold relief the differences between Western and Eastern Asian child-rearing goals and practices. As described above, Eastern Asian mothers emphasize effort, self-criticism, and self-correction. Second, they highlight concerns that American parents are primarily intent on merely promoting *high* self-esteem rather than encouraging *realistic* self-appraisals (see Chapter 9, which explores the implications of each focus).

Critiques of the Dichotomous Characterization of Cultures

In recent years, cross-cultural theorists and research scholars have questioned the rather sharp distinctions between individualistic and collectivist cultures. As a reminder, Oyserman and Sorensen (2009) make a cogent argument for why a nation or country should not simply be equated with "culture" (e.g., equating China or Japan with collectivist cultures).

Treating a country as a proxy for culture masks important differences between nations. Moreover, it creates an artificial picture of culture as a stable entity and assumes that all members of a nation share one culture (McCrae, 2001). In addition, it blurs the fact that within a given country, there are demonstrable individual differences in values and self-construals. Furthermore, it ignores differences between countries assumed to share a cultural orientation, for example, treating China and African countries as highly similar in values and self-construals. Oyserman and Sorenson also observe that countries vary in their level of individualism and collectivism, and that every country possesses some degree of each.

Tsui, Nifadkar, and Ou (2009) make a similar point, namely, that nation and culture do not completely overlap, given that nations or countries differ in many respects beyond cultural values. As a result, they argue, the findings from studies that have employed nation as a proxy, without directly assessing the dimensions of culture, are difficult to interpret for two reasons. First, such studies do not take into account potential within-nation variability in cultural values. Second, they do not identify the many other factors in addition to culture that might be responsible for differences in behavior across nations. Mascolo and Li (2004) also point to limitations when nation is treated as the operational definition of culture. Unfortunately, the majority of studies in the cross-cultural literature *do* make comparisons between countries assumed to be individualistic versus collectivistic, without examining these dimensions directly.

Mascolo and Li (2004) have edited an entire volume devoted to this issue, which they titled *Culture and Developing Selves: Beyond Dichotomization*. They begin with the observation that the reduction of culture to the simplistic distinction between individualistic and collectivistic characterizations runs the perennial risk of treating cultures and associated self-construals as *monolithic* entities. Such a demarcation, they argue, ignores the many textured ways in which individualism and collectivism can be manifested in a given culture, as well as how a given culture reflects both elements simultaneously. Thus, they urge that research move beyond the dichotomous model. Similarly, they argue that the sweeping claims about the purportedly independent versus interdependent self-construals associated with each cultural orientation be reexamined with an eye toward a more complex and nuanced treatment of culture and the self. In a similar vein, Kitayama et al. (2007) argue that forcing individuals into such a dichotomization of self-construals leads to a caricature of people that ignores the complexity of their self-representations. Such a framework reduces to stereotypes that misrepresent the psychological makeup of individuals within a given culture. Oyserman et al. (2002) have also taken issue with those researchers who conceptualize individualism as the opposite of collectivism.

Markus and Kitayama (2003) take to task those who selectively attribute a sense of purposeful *agency* to members of individualistic cultures who possess independent representations of self. They argue that it is not the case that those from collectivistic cultures with interdependent self-construals lack agency (see also Kagitcibasi, 2005). Rather, they distinguish between different *models* of agency that parallel independent versus interdependent self-representations. For those who affirm the self as independent, the model of agency is predicated on the *disconnection* from others, where a sense of agency resides within the individual. Markus and Kitayama label this a "disjoint" model. Such a style is not, however, asocial. Such an individual actively attempts to control and influence others while expressing his/her independent self. In contrast, those with an interdependent representation of self are observed to actively adjust to others where the stance is purposeful receptiveness or responsiveness to the needs and wishes of others. They label this a "conjoint" model.

Those operating according to the disconnected or disjoint model experience a sense of agency that includes feelings of positive self-esteem, self-efficacy, and power. Actions are freely chosen and are viewed as contingent upon one's own preferences, goals, intentions, and motives. Moreover, the individual takes responsibility for the consequences of these actions. In contrast, those who adhere to the conjoint model experience agentic feelings that include connectedness to others, solidarity within the in-group, and sympathy for its members. Actions are consciously performed in response to the obligations and expectations of others and are thus interpersonally determined. Responsibility for the consequences of actions is shared among group members. The conclusion, from Markus and Kitayama (2003), is that agency is not the property of the independent perspective but rather differs in content and purpose when displayed within an interdependent relational context.

Turiel (2004) raises a different consideration in deeming the dichotomy between individualistic and collectivist cultures to be patently false. Here, he specifically speaks to the universality of *hierarchy* within cultures. He observes that most societies or cultures are structured hierarchically, often in response to distributions of power that are typically defined by socioeconomic class and/or gender. Critical to his analysis is the observation that people in positions of power and authority in such hierarchies are often highly individualistic. Turiel goes on to explain that men in patriarchal cultures possess a strong sense of autonomy, independence, personal entitlement, and freedom of choice. Men in such cultures are especially likely to assert their autonomy and control in relationships with women and other societal subordinates where they exert their dominance financially, socially, and sexually. The critical insight is that this type of hierarchical structure is rampant in many cultures that have been labeled as collectivistic. Neff (2001), a colleague of Turiel, has explored the implications of power and hierarchy in studying spousal relations in India (see also Turiel & Wainryb, 1994).

Horizontal and Vertical Dimensions of Culture

In addition to the distinction between individualistic and collectivist cultures, cross-cultural scholars have also differentiated vertical versus horizontal dimensions (see Markus & Hamedani, 2007; Triandis, 2009). The vertical dimension defines cultures in terms of whether there is a clear status *hierarchy* that defines the network of relationships. In horizontal cultures, there is more *equality* among group members where social relations are more egalitarian. Adding to the complexity, in moving beyond the dual conceptualization of cultures, is the contention that the vertical–horizontal dimension can be conceptualized as orthogonal to the individualistic versus collectivist dimension. Thus, there exist vertical as well as horizontal individualistic cultures and vertical as well as horizontal collectivistic cultures (see Triandis, 2009).

The United States is a prototype of *vertical individualism*. In such a culture, individuals are motivated to "be the best," to rise to the top of the hierarchy and in so doing to outshine others by virtue of their skills and accomplishments. To stand out is the goal of social comparison. Competition is key; in fact, it is viewed as a law of nature. *Horizontal individualism*, in contrast, is exemplified by the cultures of Sweden and Australia; the focus is on *uniqueness* but without standing out. Power, through competition, is *not* a major motivation.

India exemplifies *vertical connectionism*, defined by the importance of *hierarchy*. One seeks status as well as power and those at the top attempt to stand out and to bask in public recognition, if not glory. The task for those of lower status is to conform to the demands of the authorities at the top of the hierarchy. *Horizontal collectivism*, exemplified by Chinese culture, is characterized by cooperation, a critical motivator. Group members are high in their need for affiliation and display modesty in their interactions with others. This twofold classification scheme is welcome because it brings more complexity and clarity to our understanding of cultural differences. However, the field lacks empirical documentation of the behavioral and psychological consequences resulting from the intersection of these two dimensions.

The Co-Occurrence of Autonomy and Connectedness

Just as theorists have shifted away from the dichotomous characterization of cultures, these themes have been reconsidered within American culture. This literature has highlighted the limitations of contrasts between *autonomy* (linked to independent self-construals) and connectedness (the hallmark of interdependence). This distinction has been applied to the presumed primary orientations of males versus females. Many contemporary American psychologists now argue that a combination of autonomy and connectedness represents the most appropriate pathway to healthy outcomes, across the lifespan (see Harter, Waters, Whitesell, Kofkin, & Jordan, 1997; Neff & Harter, 2002; Raeff, 2004).

Several theorists have explored the broader cross-cultural implications of this shift in emphasis. For example, Kagitcibasi (2005) has developed a model of the intersection of the dimensions of autonomy and connectedness. He has concluded that the "autonomous-related" self, defined as high in both autonomy and connectedness, is the healthiest of the potential combinations because it recognizes the two basic needs for autonomy and relatedness. Moreover, Kagitcibasi has contended that in our postmodern world, this combination may be universally adaptive. He makes two noteworthy observations. First, he suggests that relatedness may be more common in Western societies, including the United States, than is assumed, consistent with our own findings. Second, he cites the "cultural diffusion" of the Western values (i.e., individualism and independence) that are now surfacing in many Eastern cultures. Globalization has thus led to the infiltration of Western influences, especially American values, as portrayed in the mass media (e.g., movies, television, and advertising). "Modern" is often equated with "Western," he notes, and as a result those in Eastern cultures are eager to emulate the standards of the West.

In reviewing recent cross-cultural research, Kagitcibasi (2005) finds evidence that certain Eastern countries are now embracing a model that combines relatedness, thought to be the traditional model, with greater autonomy. He cites a Korean sample, studied by Y. Kim, Butzel, and Ryan (1998), that displays independent agency and personal autonomy. He reviews another study of Chinese parents in Taiwan, who emphasized control, while also granted greater autonomy to their children in their parenting practices. A complete review of these cross-cultural findings is beyond the scope of this chapter. The interested reader is referred to Kagitcibasi's review of research that documents an increasing tendency for non-Western countries and cultures to embrace the values of individuation and autonomy, combined with traditional values of control and connectedness.

Misra (2001) has also addressed the cultural balance of autonomy and relatedness, pointing to implications for psychopathology. People in non-Western collectivistic cultures, Misra argued, require high levels of relatedness and moderate levels of autonomy to maintain positive mental health. In contrast, those in Western individualistic cultures require high levels of autonomy and moderate levels of relatedness to achieve a healthy state of mind.

K. Yang (2003) has developed an interesting cross-cultural thesis that stems, initially, from Maslow's (1943) seminal theory of motivation in which he identified a hierarchy of needs. Maslow's hierarchy, a Western conceptualization, begins with basic physiological and safety needs; above these are belongingness needs and the desire for esteem; finally, there is the ultimate need for self-actualization.

In K. Yang's (2003) more revisionist conceptualization, he acknowledges that both individualistic and collectivist cultures each aspire to the goal of self-actualization, albeit defined differently. The pathways to *esteem* also differ. Moreover, both cultural orientations have clear, though different, interpersonal or belongingness needs. Cutting through an overly simplistic, dichotomous characterization of Western versus Eastern cultures, K. Yang explores the complexity of these different need systems, as follows.

In collectivistic, Eastern cultures, self-actualization evolves through the process of socially oriented self-cultivation and self-improvement. This process involves the proper performance of roles, commitments, and responsibilities within the group. In individualistic Western cultures, the self is actualized through individual effort that includes self-enhancement and the full expression of personal talents and abilities, primarily in nonsocial life domains. *Belongingness* needs in collectivistic cultures are primarily guided by group interests wherein the person's desire for a social identity is stronger than individual identity. In addition, the psychological boundary between the person and the group is highly permeable and flexible. In Western cultures, actions are primarily guided by personal interests that are stronger than group interests. The boundary between the person and the group is firm if not psychologically impenetrable. Needs are considered from the vantage point of a contractual commitment to social obligations. Finally, in collectivist cultures, *esteem* is derived from successfully pursuing social and relational goals, what K. Yang (2003) refers to as social-relational esteem. Western esteem derives from the attainment of personal and internally defined goals, thus the term personal–internal esteem.

Methodological Critiques
of Cross-Cultural Research on the Self

A major methodological criticism of cross-cultural research involves the administration of measures designed in the West, primarily in the United States, to participants in other countries such as in Southeastern Asia. Here, there are numerous pitfalls. In addressing this issue for research in China, Y. Wang and Ollendick (2001) begin with the very basic observation that in the Chinese language, there is no equivalent term for "self-esteem." The same is true for Japanese. Yet the majority of studies investigating self-esteem among the Chinese (and other Asian cultures) have employed Western measures, assuming that such instruments are appropriate and therefore useful. Y. Wang and Ollendick suggest that this strategy is problematic because investigators assume that the construct of self-esteem has the same meaning in China, compared to the United States, leading to findings that are potentially misleading and inaccurate. This conclusion was borne out by a colleague, Professor Lee C. Lee (personal communication, April 15, 1987) who employed our global self-esteem subscale with first-generation Chinese immigrant children in New York. She indicated to me that these items lacked meaning for her sample, concluding that the concept of global self-esteem, as defined in American culture, was not appropriate to include on an instrument administered to Chinese children.

Others have found the psychometric properties to be inadequate. For example, Meredith, Abbott, and Zheng (1991) have reported that only 20 of the 36 items on our Self-Perception Profile for Children (Harter, 1985) factored appropriately in a Chinese sample. Moreover, in both this and another Chinese sample employed by Stigler, Smith, and Mao (1985), the reliabilities were unacceptably low (ranging from .44 to .61). The Global Self-Esteem scale was particularly problematic in both studies. Culturally inappropriate *content* on a given instrument, therefore, will invariably lead to an inadequate scale *structure* and unacceptable reliabilities.

A further concern inheres in the fact that for Chinese (Meredith et al., 1991; Stigler et al., 1985), Japanese (Maeda, 1997; Sakura, 1983), and Korean (U. Rhee, 1993) samples, the mean domain-specific self-concept scores, as well as the Global Self-Esteem ratings were considerably lower than scores in United States, Canadian, Australian, and European samples. There are several interpretations for this pattern. First, the Chinese self-effacing style, linked to the penchant for modesty (noted earlier in this chapter), would predictably lead to lower scores. In Japan, the salience of self-criticism would also lead to more negative self-evaluations. The contrasting American style of self-enhancement would ensure relatively high scores.

Another explanation for the more negative self-evaluations of Asian samples can be traced to our structured-alternative question format (Harter, 1985). Participants are presented with contrasting statements about children, one of which is positive and one negative. Consider the following sample item: SOME KIDS are very good at their schoolwork but OTHER KIDS have trouble doing their schoolwork. The child respondent is asked first to identify which kids he/she is more like, and then to indicate whether that description is Really True for you or Sort of True for you. This question format, therefore, requires *social comparison* with other children in his/her peer group. Stigler et al. (1985) indicate that social comparison is frowned upon in Chinese culture, where individual differences in competence or ability are downplayed. Thus, Chinese children's unwillingness to report that they may be superior to others should lead to a pattern of low scores that may not reveal their private perceptions of personal competence.

Thus, the inappropriate content of a Western instrument, the potential lack of meaningful items, a problematic question format (with our measures that pull for social comparison), self-effacing or self-critical response tendencies, and inadequate psychometric properties all conspire to make these measures methodologically inappropriate and culturally insensitive.

McCrae (2001) raises additional methodological concerns. One involves translation. Even if recommendations for back translation are followed (the scale is translated into the foreign language and a second linguistically capable researcher independently translates the scale back into English), there can be problems. Subtle differences in word choice and phrasing may lead to greater or lesser endorsement of items that, in turn, can lead to higher or lower mean subscale scores. Other factors may preclude true equivalence across cultures. Members of a given culture may be prone to use extreme categories. Moreover, as suggested above, respondents in different cultures may have self-presentational styles that can impact the positivity or negativity of the scores.

Others (e.g., Tsui et al., 2009) urge that we go beyond back-translation procedures, arguing that they are no longer sufficient to ensure the validity of measures across cultures. Bolstering points made above, they add that translations may not carry the same meaning in different cultures. One solution to the problem, they suggest, is to develop a new measure that contains only culture-specific items. Another suggestion is derived from Berry's (1969) efforts. Berry contends that an instrument designed for more than one culture should contain items that are meaningfully common across cultures, as well as items that are more culture-specific with regard to content. For example, Meredith et al. (1993), in administering our Self-Perception Profile for Children (Harter, 1985), have made the point that there are additional domains of relevance to Chinese children that are not included on American instruments. These include willingness to help others, respect for parental and teacher authority, and the display of behaviors that will meet with peer and adult approval and will avoid shame.

In a similar vein, Watkins and Regmi (1999) provide evidence that the content of Western instruments is inappropriate for children from impoverished villages high in the mountains of Nepal. They suggest that items about satisfying basic physical needs may be more appropriate for assessing the self-esteem of such children. From the perspective of Maslow's (1943) hierarchy, concerns with basic physical needs and safety may well be the most salient in these children's lives. One can question whether the concept of self-esteem is even relevant. A preoccupation with one's worth as a person, a more elevated concern on Maslow's hierarchy, is unlikely to even be on the radar screen of these Nepalese children.

At the time of this writing, in 2011, the world was witnessing tremendous upheaval in countries such as Tunisia, Egypt, and Libya. I received an e-mail from a Tunisian student, desperate for a self-esteem measure to administer to children in his country. I first cited the many reasons why an American instrument would be inappropriate. I then invited him to thoughtfully consider whether he really believed that self-esteem was the most pressing priority in the lives of Tunisian children, under the circumstances.

While useful, these criticisms about content do not deal with issues related to scale structure, psychometric properties, and concerns over question formats that are problematic. Nor do they address the problem of response tendencies (e.g., self-enhancing, self-effacing, self-critical) that may well impact the mean level of self-evaluative scores, leading to a misinterpretation of the findings. I recently received an e-mail from a student who, with naïve enthusiasm, wanted to administer our instruments to the Maori, the indigenous people of New Zealand. I attempted to make these arguments as persuasively as possible, suggesting that one should begin with a more culturally sensitive perspective.

The need for alternative assessment strategies in China is particularly pressing. The intellectual vacuum created by the Chinese Cultural Revolution has impacted the field of psychology, where, for several decades, progress and productivity were effectively halted. This vacuum has exacerbated the current search for methods, measures, and paradigms from Western countries. As I observed at a conference in Beijing, many American psychologists were more than eager to hawk their theoretical and methodological wares with Chinese psychologists. However, in our zeal to be benevolent (or to manifest our less than benevolent quest for fame!), we need to guard against the practice of imposing our parochial frameworks and related instruments that may be inappropriate for a given culture. Inappropriateness can stem from content that does not reflect cultural values, from the fact that the construct may not be that critical to the functioning of individuals within that culture, or both. That said, it has been heartening, as I have reviewed the last decade of research, to note that many genuine and productive collaborations between American and Asian scholars are now the norm, appreciating the need for cultural sensitivity.

Self-report measures may be deemed inappropriate in other cultures, for the reasons articulated above. As a result, several investigators have argued for the use of *implicit* measures as an alternative (see Oyserman & Lee, 2008; Oyserman & Sorensen; 2009). Indirect laboratory procedures, it is argued, can reveal dimensions of culture-specific attitudes and self-evaluations that are not accessible through the use of instruments that directly tap self-perceptions on questionnaires or with interviews. The indirect, experimental paradigms that have been developed are very clever and compelling. However, we need further studies that employ both types of approaches in order to determine the relative usefulness of explicit versus implicit measures in predicting culturally meaningful *outcomes*.

Another class of methodological criticism is devoted to limitations in the sampling procedures employed by cross-cultural researchers. Samples of convenience typically consist of university students rather than more representative community samples. As McCrae (2001) thoughtfully points out, undergraduates may not be accurate proxies for more nationally appropriate samples that are representative of age and experience in the culture. McCrae argues that if we are truly interested in the effects of culture, we should include those members who have clearly adopted the beliefs, attitudes, values, and practices of the culture, and not simply those whose citizenship or ethnic ancestry gives them nominal membership. Watkins, Mortazavi, and Trofimova (2000) echo this concern. The danger of generalizing about a country from a single group such as college students became evident in their own cross-cultural research where they consistently found differences between adult and student samples. McCrae makes another critical observation. University students around the globe have been westernized in many respects, and thus they constitute a poor choice when examining cultural comparisons, because they are not representative of the culture at large.

Oyserman et al. (2002) have offered a similar and equally trenchant critique, pointing to another important confound in the use of university students, namely, their higher socioeconomic status (SES). They concur that reliance on student participants is problematic because students may not accurately represent the values within a culture or reflect relevant differences between societies. More specifically, students, by virtue of their advanced educational level and higher SES, may not share the attitudes and values of the mainstream population. These differences, in turn, may attenuate observed cultural differences, which they suspect was true in their cross-cultural meta-analysis (see Triandis, McCusker, & Hui, 1990).

Thus, there are clear challenges in the assessment of constructs across cultures. The field must attend to these critiques and seek solutions to the problems plaguing assessment procedures as well as the selection of representative cultural participants. Solving these two dilemmas is critical, in order to provide a window through which we can observe cultural differences that are both accurate and meaningful.

Acculturation and Bicultural Adaptation

We can set the stage by asking the following questions. What are the consequences of moving from one culture to another? What is the impact on the self-concept if one inhabits more than one culture? To what extent can self-construals change? Does one develop multiple culture-bound selves or identities? Western theories of self are predicated on the assumption that consistency or stability of the self across situations is valued. What is the impact on self-appraisals when situation is defined as culture or country and the cultural context then changes dramatically? How does a self, shaped by one culture, adapt to a new culture that may have very different traditions, customs, values, attitudes, and practices? Given the greater flexibility of the self in Asian cultures, might an Eastern Asian immigrant or a student coming to the United States, adapt more readily to change given the culturally conditioned penchant for the greater flexibility of the self that can accommodate seemingly apparent contradictions? These questions are particularly apt, given the exploding globalization of the 21st century and increasing intercultural migration.

Cross and Gore (2003) have summarized the literature that reveals that individuals who experience more than one culture display new self-representations that come to coexist with the self-representations in their culture of origin. Where two cultural forms of self-appraisal may alternately be triggered in everyday life, individuals have been observed to engage in "cultural frame switching" (Hong, Morris, Chiu, & Benet-Martinez, 2000). The person selects behaviors appropriate for a given cultural context. This flexible application of cultural knowledge results in adaptive responses to the shifting bicultural milieus. Ng and Han (2009) have taken an exciting new step in their studies of the "bicultural brain." Their functional magnetic resonance imaging (fMRI) studies have revealed the power of culture in shaping the neural representations of self and others, which differ for Chinese and U.S. participants.

The process through which people adapt in the face of cultural change is generally referred to as *acculturation*. Originally, "transfer" models were proposed whereby an individual would transfer his/her identification with a single ethnic, racial, or cultural group to a new identification with the values and customs of Euro-American society, as one example. These models (see Gordon, 1964) were both unidimensional and unidirectional, conceptualized along a single continuum. They were unidimensional because the individual was forced to make a choice between his/her culture of origin and the majority dominant culture. They were unidirectional in that the only "healthy" movement was toward the assimilation of the values and customs of the dominant host culture.

More recently, cultural models have been reconfigured to address the typologies that may arise when the two dimensions of cultural values are viewed as *orthogonal* (Berry, 1980, 2005; Cross & Gore, 2003). These models are particularly applicable for those immigrating to the United States. Four typologies reflect differences in the willingness to shift values or retain the values of one's culture of origin. Descriptively, an individual's values can be (1) high on both dimensions, (2) low on both, (3) high for one's culture of origin but low on Anglo-American values, and (4) low for one's culture of origin but high on Anglo-American values. (See also Ryder, Alden, & Paulhus, 2000, who have also concluded that a bidimensional model has greater validity and is a more useful operationalization of acculturation.)

These four styles, or acculturation strategies, as Berry (2005) refers to them, have each been given interpretive labels that capture the dynamics of combining the two dimensions. The designations most recently assigned by Berry are labeled integration, assimilation, separation, and marginalization.

Integration defines those high on both the values of one's culture of origin and European American culture. There is a commitment to maintain one's original cultural customs as well as to adopt European American values and customs. The individual makes an effort to retain the integrity of the values of his/her country of origin while at the same time seeking to behave in accordance with the values of the dominant European American culture.

The *assimilation* strategy is displayed by those who choose not to maintain the values of their original culture but who vigorously embrace the tenets of the new host country by displaying European American values. The *separation* strategy reflects the opposite pattern. Individuals place a psychological premium on maintaining their original culture and attempt to reject European American values. They seek to avoid interaction with others from the mainstream culture, whenever possible. In previous treatments of this topic, this quadrant has alternatively been referred to as "rejection" and "traditional."

Finally, *marginalization* defines the "low–low" quadrant where the individual denies any interest in either set of cultural values. Berry (2005) observes that some who adopt this orientation may experience enforced cultural loss. These individuals show little desire to interact with others, often in response to exclusion or discrimination. In previous labeling schemes, this quadrant has been called "deculturation."

In a dissertation by Mehta (2005) with older adolescents of South-Eastern Indian heritage who had lived in the United States for at least 10 years, we challenged the label "integration" for those who reported that they were high on both cultural sets of values. They clearly endorsed the values of each culture. However, we questioned whether these values were truly integrated or, alternatively, coexisted comfortably but represented parallel orientations that were displayed appropriately in each separate cultural context analogous to "frame switching" (Hong et al., 2007), described above.

To examine this hypothesis, Mehta and I provided these young adult respondents (originally from India) with four written options, each of which was accompanied by a puzzlelike drawing that visually depicted that choice (see Figure 8.2). We sought to tap four different orientations: (1) *true integration*, (2) *unhealthy fragmentation*, (3) *healthy differentiation*, and (4) *no interest/reflection*. The first option, to tap "true integration," read: "How I am with different people *all fits together nicely* into a single me; it adds up to my sense of myself as a whole person." The second option was designed to reflect a less healthy form that implies fragmentation. It read: "How I am with different people does not all fit together into one piece, and that feels *uncomfortable or distressing to me.*" The third option

1. Read each statement and look at the puzzle next to it. Check the box that best descibes how you really are.

(A) How I am with different people all <u>fits together</u> nicely into a single me, it adds up to a sense of my self as a whole person.

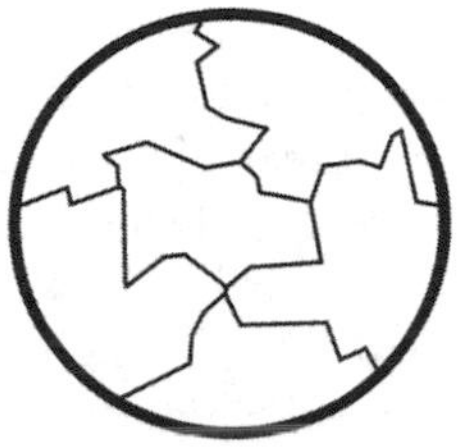

(B) How I am with different people doesn't all fit together in one piece, and that <u>feels uncomfortable</u> or <u>distressing</u> to me.

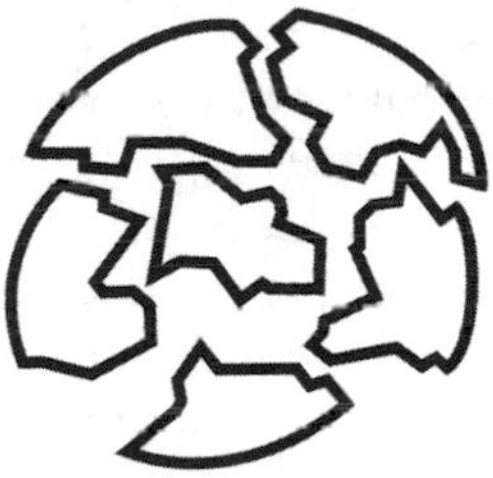

(C) How I am with different people doesn't all fit together in one piece, but that <u>feels OK</u> to me.

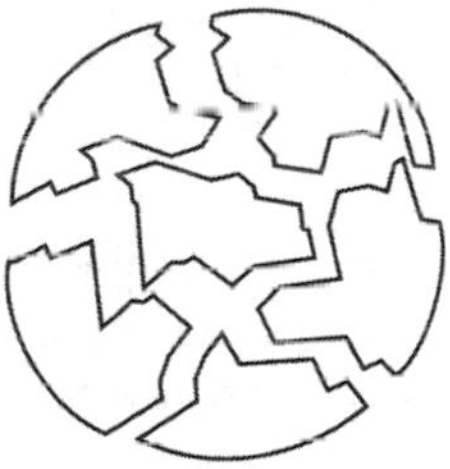

(D) I don't think a lot about how I am with different people or how it fits together.

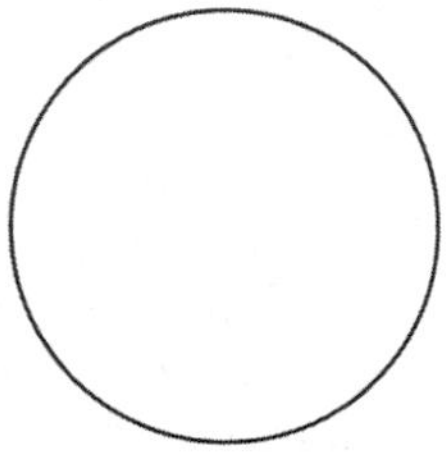

FIGURE 8.2. Measure to assess nature of multiple selves.

was designed to assess nonintegration but the comfortable coexistence of each acculturation style or strategy. It read: "How I am with different people does not all fit together into one piece, but that feels OK to me." We viewed this as healthy differentiation. A fourth option tapped little interest or reflection on this topic. It read: "I don't think a lot about how I am with different people or how it fits together."

Mehta (2005) and I predicted that the majority of East-Asian Indian participants would select the "healthy differentiation" option and that relatively few would endorse the "integrated" choice. These predictions were supported in that 70% did select the healthy differentiation option, whereas only 13% selected the "integrated" choice. Another 13% chose the "unhealthy fragmentation" option, with only 4% selecting the fourth "no interest, no reflection" choice. Based on this pattern of findings, we suggested that the high–high quadrant, where both sets of cultural values are endorsed, should not be conceptualized as "integration" given that this label did not capture most respondents' psychological experience. Rather, "bicultural" appears to be a more appropriate designation, because almost three-fourths of respondents indicated that each set of values could appropriately coexist. Integration, we feel, implies a different psychological process that is not borne out by our results. Our conclusion is consistent with the perspective of Friedman and Liu (2009), who define biculturalism as the ability *to comfortably understand and act in accordance with* the norms, ways of thinking, and attitudes of two cultural systems. The bicultural individual also has the ability to *shift* between these two systems appropriately, as the situation demands.

To return to the four quadrants, independent of slightly different labels, Berry (2005) has made the point that the adoption of these different acculturation strategies assumes that ethnic-minority individuals coming to the dominant culture have the freedom to choose how they want to acculturate. However, he thoughtfully observes that immigrants' success in realizing their acculturation goal will depend upon the attitudes of members in the dominant culture. Thus, an *integration* strategy will only be successful if the dominant culture is open and inclusive, where cultural diversity is valued (what Berry calls an atmosphere of *"multiculturalism"*). The desire for ethnic minorities to *assimilate* can only be achieved if the dominant culture displays a *melting-pot* mentality; in the extreme, if the dominant culture demands assimilation, the result is a "pressure-cooker" model. When the dominant culture forces *separation* on the ethnic minority group, it is operating from the vantage point of *segregation*. If *marginalization* is imposed by the dominant group, they are exercising their right of *exclusion*.

Evidence reveals that those who are able to develop a bicultural orientation report more positive manifestations of psychological adjustment, including higher self-esteem, greater self-efficacy, and more life satisfaction (see Sedikides, Wildschut, Routledge, Arndt, & Zhou, 2009). Consistent with Berry's (2005) analysis, these authors note that immigrants are most likely to successfully pursue biculturalism when the dominant culture endorses diversity. In contrast, immigrants are more likely to pursue separation and marginalization, and least likely to attempt assimilation, when the host culture favors discrimination.

In the multicultural literature, studies primarily compare immigrant groups (e.g., Asian Americans, Hispanic Americans) to European

Americans, the dominant cultural group, and do not assess cultural orientation directly. That is, they do not identify immigrants in terms of the four acculturation strategies identified by Berry (2005). These styles may well impact any outcome measures of interest. Nor do studies typically assess the generational status of the immigrant groups. Attempts at cultural adaptation will undoubtedly differ depending upon one's generation. A first-generation immigrant who has recently arrived in the United States will necessarily experience challenges and stressors that will not be the case for someone born in the country to parents, also born in the United States, whose ancestors came to this country several generations ago.

These two limitations were addressed in a dissertation by Guzman (1986), who was personally sensitized to such issues as a first-generation immigrant whose parents moved from Cuba to the United States when she was a child. Her study focused on Mexican American high school students where she identified three generational subgroups. First-generation youth were born in Mexico, as were their parents, before immigrating to the United States. Second-generation teenagers were born in the United States, with at least one parent who was born in Mexico. Third-generation adolescents were born in the United States, as were their parents. Her sample was drawn from a large high school in the city of Denver, where participants were sufficiently fluent to respond to questionnaires in English. This high school, like many such urban school environments, where the majority of students were European American, supported the endorsement of European American attitudes, though did not necessarily discourage the retention of Mexican American values. That is, there was an atmosphere of diversity and multiculturalism that, according to Berry (2005), should foster a bicultural adaptation. Thus, Guzman predicted that most student participants would endorse such an orientation.

Guzman (1986) first developed her Dual Acculturation Scale that tapped the level of endorsement of European American culture as well as Mexican American culture. This self-report instrument addressed everyday behaviors such as participants' choices of food, music, friendship patterns, language use, and celebration of holidays. Within each category, they rated both European American and Mexican American behaviors and preferences. Her scale, which displayed excellent psychometric properties, allowed her to operationalize Berry's (1980) model of the four acculturation strategies described above: *bicultural* (or potentially "integrated"), *assimilated* to American culture, *separated* (alternately labeled as traditional or rejecting of the dominant culture), and *marginalized* (no commitment to either culture).

As predicted, the majority of students, 74%, could be categorized as *bicultural*, endorsing both European American and Mexican American orientations. It was also expected that the assimilation quadrant would capture some portion of these adolescents, as it did, namely, 22%. It was anticipated that very few would endorse separation (or rejection of mainstream

American values), only 3.5%, and no students occupied the marginalization quadrant.

Generational differences were as expected for the two quadrants where there were sufficient numbers of participants to address this question. Those in the assimilation quadrant increased from 8%, for first-generation adolescents, to 16%, for second-generation students, to 32%, for the third-generational group. Given that the vast majority of Mexican American students fell, as expected, in the bicultural quadrant, generational differences were small but systematic. The trend was interpretable. Eighty-five percent of the first-generation, 77% of the second-generation, followed by 68% of the third-generation subgroups were identified as bicultural. The declining percentages can be attributed to the defection from the bicultural to the assimilation quadrant, as increasingly, a subgroup of adolescents came to primarily embrace European American values.

The findings of this groundbreaking study illustrate the importance of directly assessing acculturation orientations as well as taking generational differences into account. Consider the fact that generation has little meaning for most African Americans whose immigration can be traced to enforced slavery, beginning over three centuries ago. One's specific family heritage is clearly in question. The importance of generation is more central for those who have immigrated from Asian and Hispanic countries, and yet rarely is generation directly examined in multicultural research. One notable exception is the trenchant analysis of multicultural identities by Hong, Wan, No, and Chiu (2007), who highlight generation as a key consideration. Generational differences will, as Guzman's (1986) study reveals, predictably interact with acculturation status, enhancing our understanding of the bicultural self.

Hong et al. (2007) raise another interesting issue in discussing how the success of a bicultural identification will depend, in part, on how race is conceptualized. An individual will be more likely to succeed if race is viewed as a *socially constructed,* dynamic construct rather than an essentialist entity (i.e., a biologically constrained essence that is unalterable). Finally, Hong and colleagues make a compelling argument for how a multicultural *mind* and a multicultural *identity* are distinct. That is, one may have an in-depth *knowledge* of another culture, based on experiences in that culture, yet not identify with, or internalize, the values, traditions, and customs of that culture.

Studies of Race and Bicultural Adaptation in Predicting Self-Esteem

The most comprehensive and widely cited study is a meta-analysis by Twenge and Crocker (2002), who have examined race and self-esteem, comparing White Americans, Black Americans, Hispanic Americans,

Asian Americans, and American Indians. (These are the group designations employed by the authors who acknowledge that there is disagreement among scholars about the use of terms such as "race" and "ethnicity." They chose to employ the U.S. Census Bureau labels at the time.)

To set the stage, they identify different frameworks that would lead to predictions about potential racial differences in self-esteem. They review a long-standing hypothesis that the history of slavery, legalized segregation, prejudice, oppression, and discrimination experienced by Blacks should exact a psychological toll in the form of low self-esteem. Such a position can be derived from symbolic interactionist Mead (1934), who posited that the negative views of the "generalized other," in this case the White majority, will be incorporated into one's view of self, leading to the eventual internalization of stigma and unfavorable stereotypes by Blacks.

A competing hypothesis invokes "positive racial identity" as a factor that would lead to high self-esteem among Blacks, to the extent that they strive to achieve a positive in-group identity that emphasizes the favorable attributes of their group. Twenge and Crocker (2002) review previous studies that would support this hypothesis, given robust findings indicating that Blacks have higher self-esteem than Whites, when Black racial identity is central and positive. This interpretation can be derived from another symbolic interactionist, Cooley (1902), whose "looking-glass-self" formulation emphasized the internalization of the opinions of close significant others, namely, an in-group. In an earlier treatment of this issue (Harter, 1990), evidence revealed that the family and the Black American community (family, friends, neighbors, church groups) provide support that bolstered self-esteem. Moreover, not only was the community a positive source of self-esteem but it also served to filter out destructive racist messages, supplanting them with more positive feedback that enhanced self-esteem, what Twenge and Crocker highlight as the protective functions of the in-group.

Twenge and Crocker (2002) sought not only to examine Black versus White comparisons but to extend their meta-analysis to include Hispanic Americans, Asian Americans, and native American Indians. To explore a possible pattern of self-esteem based on stigmatization and prejudice, they first turned to literature examining the degree of negative stereotyping expressed toward each of these racial groups. Their review revealed a rank ordering in which Whites experienced the least negative stereotyping, followed by Asians, then Hispanics, and finally, Blacks at the low end of the prejudicial totem pole. (Data were not available for native American Indians). Based on this hierarchy of external levels of stigmatization, a model emphasizing the internalization of stigma would predict that self-esteem would follow this same pattern, from high to low esteem for the self.

However, the findings of their meta-analysis provided no support for such a model. Rather, Blacks were found to report significantly higher self-esteem than Whites, whose self-esteem was significantly higher than

Hispanics, Asians, and American Indians. Thus, there was no evidence for a model in which discrimination against racial minorities led to their internalization of the stigma or external prejudice expressed against them.

The impact of positive racial identity upon self-esteem, an alternative model, appeared to have some merit in explaining the highest level of self-esteem among Blacks, but not for other racial groups. Twenge and Crocker (2002) point to social movements and ideological shifts such as the civil rights, Black power, and other Black nationalistic movements that supported the development of positive racial identity and pride. In addition, I would submit that a growing emphasis on Black Is Beautiful could be observed in new media venues (e.g., magazines, movies, TV productions) devoted to the group's unique values and standards of appearance that elevated the status of African Americans, an emerging designation that traced Blacks to their original roots. These movements appeared more sweeping and dramatic than anything comparable for other minority groups that appeared a decade or two later, albeit smaller in scope and impact. For Blacks, a lag time was apparent in that the presumed effects on self-esteem did not appear until approximately 20 years later, in the 1990s. Twenge and Crocker speak to the developmental implications of this lag, arguing that youth are more impacted by social movements, in part because their sense of self is more malleable (compared to their elders). This pattern suggests the importance of taking both age and *generation* into account, although few of the subsequent studies to be reviewed seriously consider either.

I would add to the self-esteem advantage of Blacks the increasing acceptance and inclusion of Blacks into the realm of our high-profile national sports, where some athletes (e.g., Michael Jordan) have become bicultural icons. We see the dominance of Black men in football, basketball, and most recently, baseball. Black male athletes have become role models, if not idols for male Black youth. A similar, though less pervasive effect can be seen for certain women sports, most notably basketball. Moreover, tennis, long the bastion of White athletes, has also yielded to the infusion of Blacks, beginning with Arthur Ashe, and an increasing number of Black male tennis players. Among women, Althea Gibson broke the color barrier some decades ago and the Williams sisters, among others, are very much in the limelight, on the contemporary tennis scene for women.

Positive racial identity explanations suggest one possible path to the greater self-esteem of Blacks, compared to all other racial groups; however, they do not entirely account for this advantage. Nor do they provide a compelling interpretation for the lower self-esteem of other minority groups (i.e., Hispanics, Asians, and American Indians). Thus, to explain the overall pattern, Twenge and Crocker (2002) turned to broader *cultural* orientations harking back to the distinctions between individualism versus collectivism, with their respective parallels in independent versus interdependent self-construals.

Drawing upon a meta-analysis of individualism versus collectivism across nationalities by Oyserman et al. (2002), there are clear parallels between the pattern of self-esteem scores and the degree to which cultural groups display the psychological correlates, including self-esteem, of these two orientations. Blacks are observed to display the highest levels of individualism, followed by Whites, and then Asians and Hispanics (as well as American Indians where their collective orientation has been inferred from other observations rather than directly assessed in this meta-analysis). A cardinal correlate of individualism is an independent self-construal where distinctiveness and self-enhancement are paramount. These would appear to have increasingly characterized the mentality of Blacks in recent cohorts, in consort with racial pride.

Whites in the United States are a less homogeneous group, perhaps, but also endorse the individualistic orientation, including an independent, distinct, and self-enhancing self-style, leading to the next highest levels of self-esteem. Asians, Hispanics, and American Indians endorse a lower individualistic orientation with a higher collectivistic orientation, leading to a more modest or self-effacing presentation style that is associated with lower self-esteem. These interpretations provide a reasonable explanation for how *cultural patterns* established for the countries of origin might explain differences in racial groups once they are embedded in the United States. However, they do not speak to the importance of assessing directly the cultural orientations of these groups as well as to the issue of *generation*, as argued earlier in this chapter. That is, they do not address the dynamics of the bicultural self, in its different manifestations, as they apply to distinct cultural populations.

Finally, before reviewing additional single studies, it is notable that Twenge and Crocker (2002) address another dynamic that has also been articulated by Harter (1990). James (1890) first pointed to the role of discounting the importance of domains in which one is not competent. Thus, it has been argued that it may serve Blacks well to devalue the domain of academic competence in which they typically fare less well than Whites. It was suggested (Harter, 1990) that Black male youth, in particular, maintain a positive self-image by devaluing conventional White institutions and values, and by substituting compensatory values in areas where they can demonstrate competence. For example, athletic prowess, musical talent, acting ability, sexuality, and certain antisocial behaviors become more highly valued than academic success.

Within the last decade, single studies (in contrast to large-scale meta-analyses) have increasingly focused on the underlying processes impacting biracial adaptation within the United States. One constellation of studies includes Blacks or African Americans (terminology varies by study). Three such investigations are consistent with Twenge and Crocker's (2002) meta-analysis revealing the higher self-esteem of African Americans compared to other racial groups. For example, Negy, Shreve, Jensen, and Uddin (2003) have reported that African American university students obtained significantly higher self-esteem, as well as more positive ethnic identity, scores than did White and Hispanic students. In a second study, R. Yang and Blodgett (2000) surveyed Black and White young adults, finding that Blacks reported higher self-esteem than Whites, particularly if they cited positive reasons for leaving home (e.g., education, a job, or a significant relationship). In a third study with high school students (Greene & Way, 2005), Black students reported higher self-esteem than Latinos as well as Asian Americans (who viewed themselves least favorably).

In a related investigation, specifically addressing self-presentation style, Suzuki, Davis, and Greenfield (2008) demonstrated that European American and African American students in a multicultural high school shared a more self-enhancing perspective, whereas Asian American and Hispanic Americans adopted a more self-effacing style. As the earlier examination of the cross-cultural literature revealed, self-enhancement is associated with higher levels of self-esteem in Western cultures, whereas self-effacement, more common in Eastern Asian cultures, is linked to lower levels of self-esteem. Might this be related, however, to the generational status of the participants and their parents?

Two additional studies have addressed specific processes that were predicted to impact self-esteem in Blacks. In the first, Harris-Britt, Valrie, Kurtz-Costes, and Rowley (2007) demonstrated that the effects of racial discrimination were mitigated for youth who reported more parental messages about racial pride as well as greater preparation for the biases they experienced, leading to higher self-esteem. In a second study, Mahalik, Pierre, and Wan (2006) found that self-esteem was positively related to young adult Black males' internalization of racial identity attitudes. Interestingly, self-esteem was *negatively* associated with conformity to traditional masculine norms in the dominant White culture. (See also Schmader, Major, & Gramzow, 2001, for a discussion of psychological disengagement processes among negatively stereotyped ethnic-minority college students.)

Other researchers have focused on processes relevant to the self-esteem of East Asians who have immigrated to the United States. The pattern reviewed in cross-national studies has revealed that East Asians consistently report lower levels of self-esteem than those from Western nations. S. Rhee, Chang, and Rhee (2003) compared the self-esteem of Asian American and Caucasian American youth who grew up in the same neighborhood and found that self-esteem was significantly lower among the Asian Americans than for the Caucasian Americans. One factor implicated for the Asian American adolescents was their expressed difficulty in discussing problems with their parents when compared to their Caucasian counterparts. Here is an example of where it would be important to know whether there were generational differences between adolescents and their parents as well as in which acculturation quadrant they fell (see Berry, 1980; Guzman, 1986). For example, if the adolescent was born in the United States and was more bicultural, whereas the parents were born in their country of origin, there may well be a clash of values that would lead to parent–adolescent discord.

In a developmental study, Moneta, Schneider, and Csikszentmihalyi (2001) longitudinally tracked the self-esteem of sixth through twelfth graders, Whites, Hispanic Americans, and Asian Americans. Past research among White adolescents has revealed decreases in self-esteem from early to midadolescence followed by increases through late adolescence. Moneta et al. have reported a similar concave trend bottoming out around the tenth grade with a subsequent adaptive readjustment toward the end of adolescence. However, compared to White students, there were less positive developmental trends for the Hispanic American and Asian American adolescents. Possible explanations include perceived lack of academic success as well as the failure to live up to the associated expectations of self and others.

In research with Chinese American male and female university students, Tsai, Ying, and Lee (2001) sought to investigate the role of different facets of cultural orientation. An interesting pattern was observed. Pride in the Chinese culture was positively correlated with self-esteem; however, *affiliation* with Chinese people was *negatively* correlated with self-esteem. Moreover, gender differences revealed that pride was more important for females. For Chinese American males, self-esteem was primarily related to English and Chinese language proficiency.

A commendable study by Hyun (2001) addressed whether an independent construal of self is a prerequisite for Korean American well-being in the United States. Independent and interdependent self-construal levels were assessed directly. Individual differences revealed that an independent self-construal, commensurate with the expectations of contemporary American culture, contributed significantly to a variety of indices of psychological well-being (e.g., greater life satisfaction, fewer depressive symptoms). Of interest was the finding that Korean Americans who also acknowledged an *inter*dependent self-construal were not compromised, in terms of their psychological adjustment. This study profited from the direct assessment of self-construal style.

In a different approach to the prediction of adjustment among Chinese Asian American adults (ages 18 to 35), who had been born in the United States or lived here for at least 10 years, Kiang, Harter, and Whitesell (2007) employed a relational context framework. By this, they mean that the constructs of (1) support for one's ethnicity, (2) ethnic identity, (3) relationship quality, and (4) adjustment (a composite of self-esteem and affect, along a dimension of cheerful to depressed), can be separately assessed within three different relational contexts: Asian parents, Asian peers, and

Caucasian peers. Path analyses examined relationship-specific mediational models with support for one's ethnicity serving as a precursor to ethnic identity, with relationship quality and adjustment as sequelae.

Models for all three contexts revealed strong, significant paths (.59–.66) from ethnicity support to ethnic identity. Within one's same-ethnic identity contexts, namely, parents and Asian peers, ethnic identity, in turn, strongly predicted relationship quality that, in turn, was highly predictive of psychological adjustment. Support from parents and Asian peers also bore a significant, although more moderate, direct path to adjustment. The primary difference among models was that with Caucasian peers, one's ethnic identity did not predict the quality of that relationship, although support from Caucasian peers did impact relationship quality. We concluded with the interpretation that ethnic identity is more than a global, overarching construct. It is also flexible and can be differentiated across diverse, interpersonal contexts. Thus, mediational models may be most appropriate at the contextual level.

In contrast to the majority of researchers who have employed self-report measures, Devos (2006) studied *implicit* bicultural identity among Asian American and Mexican American college students. As noted earlier, implicit measures are assumed to assess cognitions that are not consciously controlled. Results revealed that both groups strongly identified with their own culture of origin as well as with American culture, revealing a strong bicultural pattern of identity. It would be of interest, in such studies, to include an explicit measure to determine whether they were similar and if not, which type of measure better predicted outcomes of interest.

Critique of Bicultural Research

There is a notable lag between the depth of thinking found in theoretical models of the bicultural self and the more perfunctory treatment of these issues observed in empirical studies. Within any field, this is understandable. Nevertheless, here is a wish list. There needs to be great precision with regard to the designations of participant populations. Labels such as Asian American or Hispanic currently carry little specific meaning given the broad number of cultures and countries of origin that are now represented under these outstretched umbrellas. Terms such as "race" and "ethnicity" need to be clarified. Most useful would be some agreement about a common terminology. As an outside observer to the field, I found the latest nomenclature troublesome, in its implications. Those formerly labeled Whites, aka Caucasians, were retroactively morphed into European Americans. Negroes became Blacks, only to be racially transformed into African Americans. The term "Asian Americans" encompasses multiple subgroups who, themselves, do not like to be so homogenized. The same is apparent for those herded into the generic Hispanic label.

Here is perhaps a personal idiosyncratic concern. The concept of immigrants does not really apply equally to either European Americans or African Americans in comparison to those designated as Asian Americans or Hispanic Americans. Here, the issue of *generation* appears relevant. As a now-designated European American, I can, if I wish, semisuccessfully trace my ancestral roots back many generations. Yes, I have been to Ellis Island, but I do not personally feel like an immigrant. African Americans supposedly gained a sense of pride and legitimacy with their new designation, despite the near impossibility of tracing their specific familial roots. I would doubt, however, that many of them actually feel like immigrants.

For those now designated as Asian Americans and Hispanic Americans, the issue of generation becomes very relevant to their status as immigrants. Terminology making reference to first-, second-, and third-generation Americans, the most common designations, is meaningful. Immigrant status is another consideration. That said, psychological researchers rarely take generation or immigrant status into account in their empirical studies. Some bicultural scholars do acknowledge the importance of generational and immigrant status. Those rare researchers who do examine generation as a potential cause of important cultural outcomes find predictable, interpretable differences of great psychological (and statistical) significance. This is a fertile field for young investigators who are devoted to these issues.

Certain bicultural researchers apply psychological constructs to cultures and countries of origin, although in my reading of this literature, these are infrequently operationalized. For example, how do concepts such as individualism and collectivism apply to immigrant subcultures, now broadly identified as Asian and Hispanic, who have been transported to the United States? How relevant are the associated self-construals identified in cross-cultural research, and relevant to what outcomes? Self-esteem, a focus of this chapter, is but one potential construct of interest and perhaps only a mediator of other outcomes of importance.

Bicultural theoretical models have also evolved into two-dimensional conceptualizations that recognize the intersection or othogonality of the values of the "host" country, typically the United States, and the values of the immigrant culture. This conceptualization, while acknowledging a dual-cultural model, does not directly dictate what these value systems entail. These values, and their relationship to the values of the culture or country of origin, must be determined. Guzman (1986) developed one such model and a related instrument for Mexican American youth. More such efforts are needed, in order to determine the links between the culture of origin and its subsequent manifestations in a new country and culture. To interpret similarities and differences is an interesting question in its own right.

As with cross-cultural studies, bicultural samples too often rely on university/college students, thereby questioning the generalizability of findings to adult community samples at large. As noted in the review of cross-cultural findings, these student samples differ not only in terms of educational level but often come from higher socioeconomic backgrounds, making their values unrepresentative of their racial/ethnic lower SES counterparts. Moreover, sample selectivity seems to have ignored the fact that among Hispanic groups, in particular, the issue of the *legality* of one's immigrant status has yet to be dealt with, in its vast complexity, from a sociopolitical perspective. Thus, in this subfield of multicultural studies, there is considerable work to be done in order to bring empirical efforts in line with increasingly rich conceptual frameworks.

Chapter 9

Reconsidering the Self

In Search of Authenticity

As the chapters in this volume have unfolded, a somewhat disturbing theme has gradually emerged, leading us to ask whether the self is an ally or the enemy. I concur with Leary (2004) that the self is a contemporary cause for concern. This chapter addresses one source of this concern, namely, how the *authenticity* of the self, the ability to act in accord with one's true inner self, can become compromised over the course of development. I first review what developmental factors during childhood and adolescence can contribute to a lack of authenticity.

After this developmental overview, the chapter turns to a larger canvas, painting a portrait of the potential costs of self-development that have been identified by Leary (2004) in his thought-provoking book *The Curse of the Self*. These can be observed in the form of self-enhancing strategies, self-serving biases, lack of self-awareness, the inflated self, and narcissistic tendencies that have been amply documented among adults. After reviewing this literature, I address further developmental considerations. At what ages or stages do children and adolescents develop both the *motives* and the specific *skills* to engage in these self-enhancement strategies, self-serving biases, and narcissistic behaviors that have negative personal consequences and can adversely impact interpersonal relationships? The authenticity of the self can also be compromised by the tendencies to inflate, becloud, and distort the real inner self, in seeking social approval and its presumed gains.

Discussion then turns to the issue of "optimal self-esteem" and the distinction between "true self-esteem" and "contingent self-esteem," highlighting the benefits of the former and the costs of the latter. Attention next focuses on an evaluation of the societal "self-esteem movement," where efforts to raise the self-esteem of our citizenry in general, and youth, in particular, were purported to cure many societal ills (e.g., crime, delinquency, teen pregnancy, school dropout). For youth, the school setting has represented the primary stage upon which this drama has been enacted. The controversy over educational interventions designed to enhance self-esteem is a major focus.

Issues involving a distortion of self are not merely the concerns of academic psychologists. As Leary (2004) discusses, various religious traditions speak to these issues, including Christianity, Judaism, and Buddhism. Despite certain differences across these religions, there are commonalities, for example, in their joint concern over an exaggerated and unhealthy preoccupation with the self. Buddhism is perhaps the most explicit in its emphasis on egolessness. In the contemporary literature, this theme is echoed in nonsecular treatment of the "quiet ego." Suggestions for moving beyond the ill-fated processes that preclude authenticity are the final focus of this chapter.

Developmental Precursors That Can Compromise Authenticity

In the earlier chapters on childhood and adolescence, the discussion of self-development devoted to the normative liabilities of selfhood and its pathological manifestations, reveals that self-development can go awry. The construction of the self, within the crucible of interpersonal relationships, where there is considerable dependence upon socialization within the family, is in large part responsible. These processes apply to the potential creation of a false self.

Childhood

The need for very young children to construct a positive self-narrative can be undermined by caregivers who can co-opt the story line. Caregivers' renditions of their child's narrative can distort the child's experiences, planting the seeds of an inauthentic self, if the child accepts the falsified version of his/her life story. In addition, the acquisition of *language* represents a double-edged sword (Stern, 1985), a co-conspirator, as it were, in the development of false-self behavior, because one can distort one's experiences and linguistically create a falsified construction of the self. The very capacity for objectifying the self through verbal representations allows one to transcend, and therefore potentially to distort, one's immediate experience and thereby create a falsified construction of the self.

During early to middle childhood, these processes continue. The self at this period is still a victim of all-or-none thinking, contributing to the continuation of unrealistic perceptions of virtuosity. In addition, overindulgent parents insistent on promoting inflated images of their child's virtues, parents whose mantra is that their child is "special," exceptional, and excels in comparison to peers, can lay the groundwork for the potential distortions in the self. Unrealistic views of the self can thus be promoted, supplanting perceptions of one's authentic self.

During middle to late childhood, among the many new cognitive acquisitions comes the capacity to make the distinction between one's real and one's ideal self, where the ideal self is more worthy. This realization can potentially lead to negative self-evaluations. One strategy for reducing this discrepancy is to distort the real self, inflating one's perceptions of competence or adequacy, bringing it more in line with the ideal self. Parents who conspire, promoting unrealistically positive views of their child's talents and abilities, can contribute to the inflation of the real self. As more trait-like perceptions of the self are normatively consolidated, and the need to stand out in a crowd is promoted, excessive, unrealistic praise from parents may contribute to a distortion that favors false-self behaviors.

Adolescence

During adolescence, there is increased concern with what *peers* think of the self (Harter, 2006a; M. Rosenberg, 1986). A preoccupation with what others think of them leads to the first serious efforts at *impression management*. However, because different significant others may hold divergent opinions of the self, it is difficult to develop a sense which of one's multiple selves is one's *true* self. Thus, the construction of a self that is too highly dependent upon the opinions of others can lead to the creation of a false self that does not mirror one's authentic experience. Our own research (see Harter, 2006a) reveals that it is not until early adolescence that the concept of acting as a false self becomes very salient in the consciousness of young teenagers. Although false-self behavior typically has its roots in childhood, the young adolescent now becomes painfully aware that he/she is being phony, which adds another level of distress at this developmental juncture, given the realization that one's sense of authenticity has been compromised.

Unhealthy levels of false-self behavior are particularly likely to emerge if caregivers make their approval contingent upon the young adolescent's attempts to live up to unrealistic, and therefore unattainable, standards that are dictated by parents (Ryan & Deci, 2000). Thus, the true self is co-opted. This "conditionality," as we have termed it (Harter & Marold,

1993), not only produces false-self behavior but lower self-esteem and feelings of depression.

During *middle* adolescence authenticity is made more difficult given the proliferation of roles that demand the creation of multiple selves that lead teenagers to experience conflict and confusion (see Harter, Bresnick, et al., 1997). These contradictory self-attributes contribute to unstable self-representations that cannot be integrated into a unified sense of self and exacerbate distress and doubt over which characteristics represent the true self. Moreover, in search of the true self, experimentation with one's self-presentation across roles may be identified as hypocrisy by peers and thus met with derision.

During late adolescence, the increasing internalization of standards and opinions that one comes to own as personal choices represents a double-edged sword. When the locus of self-knowledge shifts inward and older adolescents must now rely more on their own autonomous insights in order to reach conclusions, then the sense of self-certainty and authenticity can be compromised. These issues are not necessarily resolved with movement to the next stage of emerging adulthood where there are obvious individual differences in these processes. Shulman et al. (2005) identify one pattern in which certain young adults, unable to cope with the new developmental demands, adopt a competent guise that masks their underlying sense of authenticity. Thus, the lengths to which adults will go to deny and distort the self, a topic to which we now turn, have their roots in experiences during childhood and adolescence, and are made more understandable given the preceding developmental analysis.

The Prevalence of Self-Enhancement Strategies and Self-Serving Biases among Adults

In his thoughtful and provocative volume entitled *The Curse of the Self,* Leary (2004) begins with a description of how many of the features of the self would appear to render it a rather beneficial evolutionary adaptation. Among its benefits is the ability to think about the person we are or may become and to anticipate future contingencies that aid us in planning. The self also aids in the service of self-regulation and the control of our behavior, plus it allows us to cognitively adopt the perspectives of other people.

That said, Leary (2004) acknowledges that there is a dark side of the self; it is not an unmitigated blessing. He contends that the self is single-handedly responsible for many of the problems that human beings face today, as individuals and as a species. For example, the ability to self-reflect can produce distorted perceptions about ourselves, causing us to draw faulty conclusions that prompt bad decisions. The self also conjures up negative emotions that can produce great personal suffering (e.g., anger, anxiety, jealousy, and depression, including negative self-conscious emotions such as shame, guilt, and humiliation; see Chapter 6). It also permits us to ruminate unproductively about these affective states.

Moreover, "the inherently egocentric and egotistical manner in which the self processes information can blind us to our own shortcomings and undermine our relationships with other people" (Leary, 2004, p. 21). In addition, these processes may cause people to endanger their own well-being through egocentric risk taking that may jeopardize one's personal safety. On the social stage, the self can also be responsible for conflict with others, for example, by stereotyping people we dislike, warring with them at high costs, and perpetuating unthinkable acts of cruelty toward undesirable others. Leary concludes that the self is both our greatest ally and our fiercest enemy, the latter because it contributes to how we mismanage the struggles that confront us in our daily lives. What are some of the specific maladaptive self-processes, according to Leary, that get us into trouble?

A major concern is our constant *preoccupation* with the self. Although Leary (2004) contends that such self-focus and accompanying self-talk may, on occasion, be helpful, we are victimized by endless internal chatter that is both unnecessary and distracting. Inner monologues and dialogues, including excessive rumination, can be detrimental in that they divert our attention from the immediate sights and sounds of the real world within which we should be functioning. Leary concludes that when people are preoccupied with themselves, absorbed in "a cacophony of irrelevant self-generated thoughts" (p. 32), it leaves little cognitive room for other mental processes, including adaptive memory and attention to others.

As our developmental analysis has revealed (see Chapter 3), a preoccupation with the self rises dramatically in adolescence as new cognitive acquisitions promote intense *introspection*. The beacon turns both on the self as well as on the opinions that one envisages others hold about the self. Not only do adolescents engage in their own self-rumination but many, notably girls, extend this activity to *corumination*. They share with close friends their preoccupation with negative life events (e.g., not being invited to an important party) that have undesirable implications for the self.

Leary (2004) also argues that we hold multiple illusions that distort the truth about ourselves and he then proceeds to enumerate numerous specific self-enhancement strategies and self-serving biases. Perhaps the most common is the penchant for people to overestimate their positive qualities, to see themselves as more competent, socially skilled, and morally upstanding than, in fact, they truly are. That is, the majority of people lack a balanced perception of their strengths and weaknesses.

Leary (2004) cites Greenwald's (1980) concept of the "totalitarian ego" in this regard. Greenwald compared the self to a totalitarian political regime in which events are interpreted and history is rewritten to highlight the positive qualities of the dictator as well as the government. Ugly truths are squelched and accomplishments are embellished. Greenwald likens such a regime to the human ego that fabricates successes, ignores failures and weaknesses, and revises one's personal history to cast one in the best possible, albeit unrealistic, positive light. Another related mechanism was cited earlier in this book, namely, Greenwald's concept of "beneffectance," a self-protective strategy in which one's core or central attributes are viewed as uniformly positive, whereas any negative characteristics are relegated to the periphery of the self.

In identifying these phenomena as "shallow thoughts about the self," Gilovich, Epley, and Hanko (2005) describe how people's assessments of their own traits and ability have repeatedly been shown to be overly optimistic, far exceeding an objective analysis of their actual characteristics. Gilovich et al. argue that optimistic self-evaluations involve minimal self-reflection. Rather, they constitute snap judgments that arise automatically and lead to the favorable verdicts stemming from illusions of personal worth. They contend that people base their perceptions almost exclusively on rapid-fire, optimistically biased judgments, all but ignoring any negative self-attributes. Such evaluations do not originate in a reflective consideration of one's characteristics. Moreover, people seize upon their own good *intentions*, ignoring the fact that they may not act in accordance with such personal goals, which further contributes to overly optimistic self-assessments.

Gilovich et al. (2005) rightfully observe that not all individuals engage in these illusions of personal worth. Those who suffer from low self-esteem combined with depression are much less likely to exhibit such automatic, shallow, self-evaluations. Rather, many of the cognitions that accompany depression are more elaborated and very conscious deliberations that unfortunately can provoke self-destructive rumination (see Nolen-Hoeksema, 2000).

The overwhelming tendency for the majority of people to overestimate their competencies raises the question of whether they are at all aware of this penchant. Kruger and Dunning's (1999) research reveals that those who are the least competent on a variety of laboratory tasks do *not* manifest such self-awareness. Those in the lowest quartile greatly overestimated their abilities and failed to correct their self-assessments after they were given feedback and access to knowledge about the more superior performance of others. Hodges, Regehr, and Martin (2001) were intrigued by the implications that these findings might hold for a group of novice physicians who were family medicine residents in training. Their findings replicated those of Kruger and Dunning in that those at the lowest skill levels were most at risk for inaccurately assessing their ability. In contrast, those at higher levels of ability, when given feedback, were able to recalibrate their self-assessments more accurately. In reaction to these troublesome findings, Hodges et al. explore the implications for medical training.

The Better-Than-Average Effect

When asked, most people tend to judge themselves as better than the average person on virtually every dimension imaginable (Alicke, Klotz, Breitenbecher, Yurak, & Vredenburg, 1995; Leary, 2004). Alicke et al. have reported that college students rated themselves more positively than average on 38 of 40 traits. Hoorens (1993) has reported that most people rated themselves as safer than the average driver, more sexually adroit than the average lover, and more ethical than the average citizen. In another study, in which people were asked about the likelihood that they would go to heaven, 87% of respondents indicated that they were so destined, a greater likelihood than for others (Sheler, 1997). When asked to compare themselves to a list of well-known celebrities, these same participants indicated that they were more likely to go to heaven than anybody else on the list, including Mother Teresa!

Myers (1982) has reported on a survey asking high school seniors to indicate how they felt about themselves in various areas of ability, compared with other people their age. Judging from the responses, it would appear that America's high school seniors are not plagued by feelings of inferiority. Sixty percent reported that they were better than average in athletic ability; in terms of leadership ability, 70% rated themselves as above average. In rating the ability to get along with others, 0% rated themselves below average. Myers offers an egocentric paraphrase of Elizabeth Barrett Browning's poetic query: "How do I love me? Let me count the ways."

Downward Social Comparison

Another strategy, in an attempt to repair one's self-esteem in the face of failure, is to compare the self to others who are perceived to be less competent (Tesser, 1988). The conclusion that one is superior to others functions to temporarily enhance self-esteem, although it simply reflects another distortion about how one fares in the wider social world. Tesser also reviews a considerable body of literature revealing that people avoid interpersonal closeness to those who outperform them in those domains on which their own self-esteem is predicated. Some individuals even resort to tactics to interfere or subvert the goal strivings of others who display superior performance or success in their own ego-relevant domains.

Attributional Biases

Self-serving biases can also be observed in the *attributions* that people make for events in their lives. A convincing number of studies now reveal that the attributions that people provide as explanations for their behavior are biased by portraying the self in a favorable light (see review in Blaine

& Crocker, 1993). These self-serving biases are demonstrated in laboratory studies where research participants indicate that if they do well on a task, it results from their being smart or skilled in that arena. In contrast, when people perform poorly, they attribute their performance to an unfair or excessively difficult task, distracting testing conditions, or bad luck. Thus, individuals claim too much credit for their successes and provide excuses for doing poorly.

Another self-serving bias can be observed in the tendency for people to underestimate the prevalence of their positive characteristics in the population, thereby concluding that their personal strengths and capabilities exceed those of others and are relatively unique or unusual (Mullen & Goethals, 1990). This *false uniqueness* effect allows people to feel superior to others as they bask in the glow of their desirable competencies. Another telling bias is the tendency for people to judge the positive characteristics that they personally possess and value as more important and desirable than potentially favorable attributes that they do not possess (Dunning, 2003).

Leary (2004) describes how self-serving biases also operate among those in group work environments, such as on committees or teams. When the group is successful, the individual feels that he/she was more responsible for the positive outcome, compared to other group members. However, when the group performs poorly, each member feels less responsible for the outcome than the average member (Schlenker & Miller, 1977). If group members are made aware of others' attributions, then social conflict can erupt in the face of a successful outcome. Each member may feel that others are claiming more responsibility than they deserve, while not giving them the personal credit they feel is their due (Leary & Forsyth, 1987).

Leary (2004) describes another rather astonishing phenomenon, namely, that people are biased in their belief that they are not biased! For example, in a study by Pronin, Lin, and Ross (2002), 87% of the participants rated themselves as better than the average student at their university, thus demonstrating the above-average effect. However, after debriefing these participants, explaining the better-than-average bias, they were asked whether they themselves felt that they might have been susceptible. The vast majority of students did not recognize or acknowledge any personal bias, even though they had just fallen prey to the better-than-average effect. Thus, people are relatively blind to their very own demonstrable biases.

Interestingly, people are much more likely to acknowledge biases in *others* (see Leary, 2004). In general, we tend to believe that we have more insights into our own and other people's psyches and behavior than do others. Moreover, Leary reports that there is a tendency for people to believe that they have a greater ability to respond rationally, compared to others. For example, individuals will report that they are less influenced by advertising, propaganda, and other calculated efforts to impact their behavior than are other people. Thus, we interpret *others'* behavior as irrational, but deny that we might be so victimized.

It would appear that the various self-enhancement strategies and self-serving biases are designed to maintain high self-esteem, project a consistent self-image, and expand the self, in order to manage the impression that the self is creating. However, Leary and colleagues (Leary, 2008; Leary & MacDonald, 2003) challenge this assumption. They contend that such strategies actually operate in the service of *interpersonal* rather than intrapsychic goals. They argue that the various self-enhancement strategies, what they term the so-called "self-motives," primarily function to facilitate people's social effectiveness, reflecting efforts to be valued and accepted by others. Thus, one's social currency is at stake, given a basic need to *belong*.

Developmental Considerations

In Chapter 2 (on childhood) and Chapter 3 (on adolescence) I raised two developmental questions. To what extent do those at the various stages identified have the *motives* to engage in the self-enhancement that has been demonstrated for adults? Second, at what point in development do they have the requisite *skills* to enact such strategies?

Very young children have an unrealistically positive sense of sense that serves a self-protective function and promotes a sense of confidence that fuels early mastery attempts. However, I have argued that the motives are *not* comparable to the self-serving biases of adults that defensively protect fragile and negative self-views. Young children naturally have an inflated perception of their competencies, and thus there is no such defensive need to enhance their virtues even further. Moreover, they do not possess the *skills*—for example, social comparison—that underlie so many of the self-serving biases that adults exhibit.

Among older children, the developing ability to more accurately assess the opinions of others can normatively lead many to lower their self-evaluations, including their global self-esteem. This period is critical, from a developmental perspective, because those children with negative self-views now begin to possess a *motive* to engage in self-protective strategies. In addition, older children can rely on budding cognitive skills that allow them, albeit at rudimentary levels, to enact certain strategies that are observed in adults. For example, they can begin to utilize downward social comparison to enhance and protect the self.

For adolescents, negative perceptions of self, not only provoked within the peer culture but supported by the comparative environment of school culture, provide further motivation to engage in strategies to protect the self. Moreover, they now have a repertoire of skills to enhance and protect the self. For example, they can fully engage in social comparison, view themselves as better than average, make stable, internal attributes for success (blaming failures on external factors), and emphasize their positive characteristics as central, while relegating failures to the periphery of the self. Impression management is critical, although all of these skills may still be a bit shaky, requiring practice and feedback with regard to their success, as one moves forward to adulthood.

The Cost–Benefit Ratio of Self-Serving Biases and Self-Enhancement Strategies

Upon the review of these self-serving distortions of reality and concomitant self-enhancement strategies to defend against potentially negative self-evaluations, an obvious question arises: Are such illusions beneficial or detrimental to the individual's well-being? Opinion is sharply divided on this issue. There are some who tout the benefits, whereas others argue that the misrepresentation of the self has detrimental effects, particularly in the long run.

Taylor and Brown (1988) are among those proponents who have argued that certain positive illusions, which overestimate one's abilities and are overly optimistic, nevertheless contribute to an individual's mental health and general well-being. They identify three potential benefits. Rose-colored glasses can produce a reduction of negative emotions and lead to enhanced perceptions of control that promote a more positive mood. Illusions may also enhance one's motivation, leading to increased effort and persistence on life tasks, given the expectation of eventual success. People with positive self-views are also likely to feel more charitable toward others, leading to benevolent acts that can enhance relations with others. Moreover, romantic relationships may be temporarily enhanced to the extent that positivity biases extend to the illusion that one's partner is deeply caring.

Others are more likely to focus on the costs of such illusions. For example, Leary (2004), in his exploration of the curses of the self, acknowledges that such unrealistic self-perceptions cause people to feel better about themselves, may have motivational benefits, and lead to greater sociability, but only in the short run. He questions the long-range benefits of perceiving the self and others inaccurately. He thoughtfully concludes that we will make better life decisions if we clearly take into account accurate information about ourselves that is untainted by self-serving illusions.

Leary (2004) elaborates on some of the liabilities of maintaining such self-serving illusions. He suggests that adopting overly flattering perceptions of the self can lead to bad decision making. Moreover, self-serving illusions blind people to their shortcomings that will, in turn, interfere with their motivation to confront and improve upon their less than desirable characteristics. While rose-colored, ego-enhancing glasses may promote a temporary sense of well-being, Leary agrees with Rogers (1951) that, in the long run, such distortions eventually lead to anxiety and unhappiness. Leary observes that most theories and mental health practitioners consider an accurate view of reality to be the hallmark of psychological adjustment.

Why, then, Leary (2004) asks, do self-serving biases continue to persist? He argues that one motivation lies in the fact that human beings can cognitively reduce fears and anxieties on a temporary basis by reinterpreting, and thereby minimizing, threat to the self. However, in the long run, such illusions eventually break down, exposing the self and compromising one's ability to deal effectively with the challenges of life. Nowhere is this more obvious than in the case of narcissism, which seems to be an increasingly prevalent feature of contemporary psychological life.

Narcissism

From a clinical perspective, the central characteristics of adult narcissism include a grandiose sense of self-importance, an inordinate need for the admiration of others, a sense of overwhelming uniqueness and entitlement, a lack of empathy, excessive jealously or envy, and a tendency to exploit others (American Psychiatric Association, 2000).

Manifestations of Narcissism in Childhood and Adolescence

Here, too, it is necessary to adopt a developmental perspective, asking when these adult characteristics emerge, and whether less mature forms of narcissism prevail at younger ages. Among very young children, Freud (1914) first identified "primary, normative" narcissism in which omnipotent illusions served to aid in self-preservation. Others (e.g., Erikson, 1963; Kohut, 1986; Winnicott, 1965) considered these illusions to be critical precursors of positive feelings about the self. Others (Bleiberg, 1984; Kernberg, 1975) have viewed early normative narcissism as primitive mechanisms that protect the infant/toddler from separation anxiety, frustration, and disappointment. The desire to be the center of attention and resulting exhibitionism is engaging among healthy young children, whereas in pathological narcissism the demands for constant admiration are excessive, defensive, and unrealistic.

During early to middle childhood, the normative narcissistic demand for attention becomes tempered as children become more aware of the social reactions of others. The need to be admired is tempered by genuine expressions of gratitude toward the caring adults in their lives. Thus, they display a sense of reciprocity in giving back affection (Kernberg, 1975). Although fantasies about their future success and fame are less than realistic, they share their visionary goals with peers and siblings. In contrast, children with pathological narcissistic tendencies are likely to be envious and resentful.

During late childhood, earlier normative manifestations begin to fade. However, new *pathological manifestations* of narcissism emerge. The older narcissistic child lacks empathy for others (Kohut, 1977). Grandiosity, a seriously inflated sense of self, and impulsivity all preclude a tolerance for outcomes that are not immediately successful. Others are blamed for one's personal deficits, compromising peer relationships. Feelings of superiority and entitlement lead to the manipulation and exploitation of peers. Preoccupied with protecting a fragile sense of self, these narcissistic children devalue others and if criticized, display rage.

In early adolescence, the specific features of narcissistic personality disorders become more evident and can begin to crystallize (Bleiberg, 1984; Bukowski et al., 2009). These include an omnipotent sense of self, refusal to acknowledge one's shortcomings, and unrealistic demands for public affirmation. Narcissists' inflated sense of self is revealed in their perception of themselves as far more intellectually or socially competent than is warranted by objective criteria. The defense against threats to their fragile and unrealistic self-views often takes the form of aggression. Moreover, narcissistic distortions of the self, related to defensive forms of peer aggression, become quite stable during early adolescence (Bukowski et al., 2009).

During midadolescence, feelings of excessive omnipotence among pathological narcissists clearly interfere with their ability to achieve realistic competence goals enabling them to be effective. Omnipotence defensively expands into even more extreme grandiosity that provokes desperate maneuvers to protect very precarious self-esteem and an illusory sense of control. These attempts are typically unsuccessful, provoking shame and humiliation. Lapsley and Stey (in press) argue that narcissistic dysfunction is defined by excessive forms of omnipotent, uniqueness, and vulnerability compared to "normative narcissistic" manifestations.

Lapsley and Stey (in press) provide a psychodynamic perspective on narcissism that emphasizes how if normative *separation–individuation* demands are not well handled, older adolescents can fall prey to pathological narcissistic symptoms during late adolescence, particularly if they plan to leave home for college or job-related transitions. Excessive separation anxiety for some can lead to maladaptive narcissism that provokes rage at parents who are perceived as the perpetrators. These older adolescents fit Bleiberg's (1994) description of the "histrionic exhibitionist" type of narcissism for those especially troubled over separation issues that accompany impending adulthood.

Further Distinctions and Dynamics That Apply to Adult Narcissism

There are those (see Raskin & Terry, 1988) who have argued that, among adults, there are "normal" or subclinical forms of narcissism that represent milder manifestations, as assessed by their Narcissistic Personality Inventory (see also arguments by W. K. Campbell & Green, 2008). On this instrument, certain subscales tap "maladaptive" or unhealthy forms of narcissism (i.e., exaggerated entitlement, exhibitionism, vanity, and exploitativeness). Healthier or more adaptive manifestations include a sense of *authority*, which reflects confidence in one's leadership abilities, and *self-sufficiency*, which reflects a sense of responsibility for making one's own life decisions. With regard to the more maladaptive features of sufficient magnitude, Baumeister and Vohs (2001) have argued that narcissism represents a pattern of *self-esteem addiction*, characterized by unstable and inflated perceptions of one's worth as a person. Thus, the individual inconsistently vacillates between highs and lows in evaluating the self.

When narcissists fail to sustain a grandiose sense of their self-esteem, they can become angry and aggressive, Baumeister and Vohs (2001) point out. Short-term highs may bring temporary gratification in feelings of excessive pride or hubris, as well as euphoria that can foster extraversion. Narcissism is also associated with reduced anxiety and depression (W. K. Campbell & Buffardi, 2008). However, as these latter authors observe, narcissism represents a social trap. Long-term egocentrism does damage to interpersonal relationships and ultimately results in self-destructive outcomes.

Some (e.g., Wink, 1991) have argued for another distinction that is essential in considering the forms that narcissism can take, namely, the contrast between *overt* and *covert* narcissism. The overt narcissist displays the characteristics that have been identified in the official clinical syndrome, namely, in someone who is a grandiose exhibitionist, self-indulgent, manipulative, and with an overwhelming need to be admired. The covert narcissist, in contrast, is insecure, hypersensitive to criticism, and vulnerable in the face of threats that will promote feelings of inferiority. This contrast has led others (see Pincus & Lukowitsky, 2010) to argue that the narcissism phenotype is comprised of two primary components, grandiosity and vulnerability, although the DSM-IV (American Psychiatric Association, 2000) only identifies behaviors associated with grandiosity as the cardinal clinical features (e.g., entitlement, an inflated sense of self not borne out by real accomplishments, and fantasies of power, superiority, and perfection). The vulnerability component, Wink argues, is marked by hypersensitivity, humiliation in response to narcissistic injury, and a pattern of shameful reactivity.

Certain theorists (e.g., Morf & Rhodewalt, 2001) have made an argument for the *self-regulatory* functions of narcissistic manifestations. That is, a grandiose yet vulnerable self appears to underlie the continual need for external affirmation from others. W. K. Campbell and Green (2008) elaborate, contending that self-regulatory strategies that keep narcissists looking good often require that (1) one replace others in his/her social world who no long serve this purpose, and (2) one escalate narcissistic behaviors (e.g., overestimating intellectual abilities and attractiveness and ensuring that one is entertaining and colorful) in order to capture and maintain the attention and admiration of others.

There is evidence for the increasing prevalence of overt, grandiose narcissism. A meta-analysis of 85 samples of U.S. college students has recently revealed that egos have gradually but significantly become inflated over time (Twenge et al., 2008). Almost two-thirds of contemporary college students reported scores reflecting an increase in narcissism of 30% between 1982 and 2006. The researchers ask whether this substantial rise in narcissism has positive or negative implications. They cite literature revealing that narcissism has many costs to the self such as distorted images of one's abilities (see Paulhus, Harms, Bruce, & Lysy, 2004) and risky decision making (see W. K. Campbell, Goodie, et al., 2004).

Twenge et al. (2008) observe that many of the costs of narcissism are unfortunately borne by other people. These liabilities include troubled romantic relationships (see Foster, Shrira, & Campbell, 2006) and aggression (see Bushman & Baumeister, 1998). Thus, narcissism may have positive transient effects in the short run for those who have unrealistically inflated their egos but negative outcomes for other people, society, and eventually the individual, in the long run (see also W. K. Campbell & Buffardi, 2008). An example of narcissistic overconfidence is reflected in findings that today's students have markedly higher and more unrealistic educational expectations and aspirations for success (W. K. Campbell, Goodie, et al., 2004). By way of illustration, they report that slightly more than half of recent high school students predicted that they would earn graduate or professional degrees, even though only 9% of 25- to 34-year-old high school graduates actually obtain such credentials.

Finally, in examining narcissism around the globe, Foster, Campbell, and Twenge (2003) have found that those from individualistic cultures report higher levels of narcissism, compared to those in collectivistic cultures. Thus, countries that emphasize independence, uniqueness or distinctiveness (e.g., standing out from the crowd), and the pursuit of individualistic goals that require societal success, are more likely to produce narcissists. Gender differences (greater narcissism among men) are interpreted as the greater emphasis that males place on these individualistic values and independent self-construals.

Another issue looms large in the literature on narcissism. There is controversy over the relationship between narcissism and self-esteem, including their role in promoting aggression and violence. There is agreement that the empirical correlation between self-esteem and narcissism is negligible (Barry, Frick, & Killian, 2003; R. P. Brown & Zeigler-Hill, 2004; Harter & McCarley, 2004). We have argued that these two constructs need to be distinguished theoretically, methodologically, and empirically (see Barry et al., 2003; Bushman & Baumeister, 1998). Theoretically, narcissism is characterized by grandiose evaluations of the self, an inflated sense of entitlement, and an exploitative stance toward others. In contrast, high self-esteem rests upon self-assurance and a positive sense of worth that does not have to be constantly questioned or socially validated. In our own research (Harter & McCarley, 2004), we have operationalized the two constructs accordingly. Empirically, we demonstrated that the correlation between narcissism and self-esteem was .03 in a sample of adolescents.

So what is the controversy? It involves the prediction of aggressive or violent behaviors. Central to this controversy are the claims of Baumeister et al. (1996), who have argued that there is a "dark side to high self-esteem" in that, if threatened, high self-esteem can provoke aggressive behavior. The findings of Thomaes, Bushman, Stegge, and Olthof (2008) indicate that *narcissism* in combination with high self-esteem lead to exceptionally high aggression in the face of threat, but only if the child participants had been *shamed*. These findings are of interest, given our own demonstration that humiliation, a cousin of shame, serves as a mediator between ego-threatening harassment at the hands of others and peer violence (Harter, Low, et al., 2003).

Others have argued that *low* self-esteem is a significant risk factor leading youth to engage in destructive violence. Barry et al. (2003) have reported that those with a combination of high levels of narcissism but *low* self-esteem manifested the greatest rates of conduct disorders. Further analyses of their data revealed that characteristics associated with maladaptive, but not adaptive, narcissism, a distinction raised earlier, predicted delinquency 3 years later. Adaptive narcissism was found to be correlated with positive parenting practices (e.g., positive reinforcement and caring parental involvement). Maladaptive narcissism was associated with negative parenting practices (e.g., poor monitoring or supervision and harsh discipline). Findings indicated that the combination of maladaptive narcissism and negative parenting predicted the highest levels of delinquency.

In our own research (Harter & McCarley, 2004), we have examined the claims of Baumeister and colleagues (1996) that narcissism, *high* self-esteem, and lack of empathy, in the face of a threat to the ego, would be predictive of violent ideation. We (see Harter, Low, et al., 2003) have found evidence for a model in which *low* self-esteem, in combination with its predictors (e.g., social rejection and perceptions of incompetence), predicted violent ideation as well as self-reported depression. We found, consistent with Baumeister et al.'s claims, that narcissism, lack of empathy, and the frequency of threats to the ego were all significant predictors of violent tendencies. What differed from the position put forth by Baumeister et al. was the clear finding that *low* (not high) self-esteem was part of the predictive constellation of variables.

How can these seemingly disparate claims and findings be reconciled? There are several possible explanations. Consider the implication of the evidence revealing that the correlation between self-esteem and narcissism is negligible. As a result, there are four possible combinations or quadrants, the most relevant of which are those with *high* self-esteem coupled with high narcissism, and those with *low* self-esteem coupled with high narcissism. (Those with high self-esteem and low narcissism would appear to represent a healthier adaptation and those with low self-esteem and low narcissism are less theoretically relevant, although a cause for clinical concern).

First consider those with high self-esteem coupled with high narcissism. These individuals may well be at risk for violent thoughts and behaviors for a variety of reasons that concern the nature of their high self-esteem. Four potential features of such high self-esteem that may conspire with narcissism to provoke violence could be problematic: (1) self-esteem could be unrealistically high and therefore result in a defensive stance; (2) high self-esteem could be unstable or fragile in the face of threat; (3) it may be too highly dependent on the unpredictable external evaluations of significant others, provoking resentment; and (4) it may be associated with the more maladaptive features of narcissism such as anger that can accompany grandiosity. Any or all of these combinations may be likely to spawn aggressive thoughts and tendencies toward violence.

Now consider the combination or quadrant in which *low* self-esteem is associated with high narcissism. These individuals may be more likely to experience features of narcissism that have been identified as *vulnerability*, associated with hypersensitivity to the criticism of others, provoking humiliation in the face of narcissistic injury. As our own research has revealed, a common response to humiliation in the face of harassment and threats to the self, is violent thought and action (Elison & Harter, 2007; Harter, Low, et al., 2003). Moreover, those with low self-esteem who are of the vulnerable type could also harbor jealousy and envy that provoke anger and aggression toward others. Thus, the overall argument is consistent with the notion of *equifinality*, common in the clinical literature (see Cicchetti & Rogosch, 1996), namely, that there can be different pathways to any given form of pathology such as conduct-disordered behavior that results in violence.

Consistent with such an approach, we can ask whether there are different developmental antecedents of narcissistic personality traits in childhood. For example, Thomaes et al. (2009) explore how temperamental factors contribute to narcissism. Those "approach" traits such as high-intensity pleasure, high activity level, impulsivity, and risk taking have been implicated. However, Thomaes et al. also identify two different socialization pathways that involve early interactions with parents that can result in narcissistic behavior. In one such pathway, parents shower the child with excessive unconditional praise coupled with overindulgence. These parents communicate the message that their child is "special" or "deserving," above and beyond his/her peers. Thus, such children are raised to display grandiose self-perceptions from an early age that must be maintained by dependence on continuous external validation.

An alternative theory holds that harsh parental coldness, unrealistically high expectations, and lack of genuine support represent the antecedents of narcissism (a position held by such psychoanalytic proponents as Kernberg, 1975, and Kohut, 1977). According to their formulations, children create inflated, narcissistic perceptions of themselves as a defense against feelings of parental rejection that imply worthlessness. Their continual cravings for attention and approval represent an attempt to compensate for the lack of parental warmth. Thomaes et al. (2009) cite evidence for both developmental pathways to narcissism.

In considering Kernberg's (1975) contention, Lapsley and Stey (in press) observe that the child, subject to the latter parenting practices, approaches life challenges with feelings of depletion and perceptions of inadequacy. The child resorts to narcissistic grandiosity as a defense against frustration and rage over the caregivers' failure to meet his/her needs. Lapsley and Stey describe Kernberg's criteria by which one can distinguish normal from pathological manifestations of narcissism in children. Among pathologically narcissistic children, grandiose fantasies are more unrealistic. Narcissistically prone children overreact to criticism, and to the demands of parents that are excessive and cannot be met. Relationships with parents are cold and aloof, vacillating between the idealization and the devaluation of caregivers that can readily result in destructive behaviors. Citing Sarnoff (1987), Lapsley and Stey observe that the defensive maneuvers to cope with feelings of emptiness and low self-worth lead to attempts to restore the ego by adopting a heightened sense of uniqueness, indestructibility, and personal agency. It was Blos's (1962) contention that such narcissistic ideation impairs one's judgment and is therefore a problematic aspect of ego development, despite its defensive function.

Lapsley and Stey (in press) make an interesting developmental observation, pointing to the normative adolescent penchant for constructing a "personal fable" of their experiences (Elkind, 1967), which typically involves themes of *invulnerability, omnipotence,* and *personal uniqueness.* Among adolescents, these are normative and transient manifestations that, in part, reflect certain cognitive limitations of this period (see Harter, 2006a). For example, the inability to control newfound abstractions leads the adolescent to overdifferentiate concepts of self and others, leading to the conclusion that others could never imagine the uniqueness of one's own experiences. In normative adolescent development, further cognitive development and support from significant others allow one to confront reality, leading to the abatement of such perceptions. However, for the child who has been socialized in ways that support a narcissistic view of the self, this penchant can become entrenched as a personality style with all of the costs that have been described, such as exaggerated self-enhancement and self-serving biases.

Optimal or True Self-Esteem versus Contingent or Conditional Self-Esteem

Many contemporary theorists have argued that too much research attention has been paid to the *level* of self-esteem, ignoring other qualitative features that define the nature of one's worth as a person. For example, Crocker and colleagues (see J. Crocker & Park, 2004; J. Crocker & Wolfe, 2001) have identified "optimal self-esteem," contrasting it to self-serving strivings that are deliberately designed to obtain and maintain high levels of self-esteem. Optimal self-esteem is achieved, paradoxically, when it is not a concern in one's daily life, when it is not a conscious and relentless pursuit (see also J. Crocker, 2006a). Too often, Crocker argues, when an individual is preoccupied with the goal of establishing and sustaining high self-esteem, the liabilities associated with unrealistic illusions about the self take their toll. As described earlier in this chapter, these include multiple self-enhancement strategies and self-serving biases that lack veracity that will, in turn, compromise interpersonal relationships and are ultimately damaging to the self. Optimal self-esteem is grounded in reality, in that the individual has adopted a balanced perspective on his/her strengths and weaknesses including the search for learning opportunities that will further self-understanding and avoid future failures.

As Crocker and colleagues (J. Crocker & Park, 2004; J. Crocker & Wolfe, 2001) conclude, optimal self-esteem is best characterized by the absence of a preoccupation with one's personal worth or value. Paradoxically, therefore, it is best achieved by individuals who do not actively pursue high self-esteem as a goal, when there is not a relentless quest that will divert time and energy from more appropriate learning goals. Appropriate learning and mastery aspirations can serve to foster self-confidence and may contribute to optimal self-esteem that is grounded in realistic appraisals of one's strengths and weaknesses.

J. Crocker and Wolfe (2001) also consider the downside of "*contingent self-esteem*" in which for some people feelings of self-worth are overly dependent upon positive *social* evaluations. Other people may stake their self-esteem entirely upon their academic or *professional* success. As described earlier (see Chapter 6), still others concentrate on meeting the punishing standards of physical *attractiveness*. Crocker and colleagues (J. Crocker & Park, 2004; J. Crocker & Wolfe, 2001) argue that basing one's self-esteem on external sources inherently provokes greater costs and liabilities. Because the outcomes in these domains are at the mercy of others, people's evaluations and environmental events are typically beyond one's control. Feedback from external sources of self-worth may shift over time or differ across relationships and situations. Any significant vacillations can lead to greater self-esteem instability that, in turn, has been linked to depression and hostility (see Kernis & Goldman, 2003, 2006; Mruk, 2006).

A relentless quest for high self-esteem will divert time and energy from more appropriate learning goals. This active and energy-draining pursuit can take its toll in many life arenas (J. Crocker, 2006b). Failures can lead to intense negative emotions (e.g., depression and anger) that, in turn, can provoke withdrawal or aggression, respectively. Lack of success can suggest to people that they are worthless, leading to crippling anxiety that interferes with motivation in the service of self-improvement. When the goal primarily targets self-validation, then opportunities to learn from mistakes and failures are precluded. Moreover, the preoccupation with regaining one's self-esteem can hinder interpersonal relatedness, given the intense self-focus on meeting one's own needs, ignoring those of others.

Thus, a preoccupation with high self-esteem diverts people from fulfilling their fundamental needs for competence, autonomy, and relatedness (see Deci & Ryan, 2000; Ryan & Brown, 2006). J. Crocker (2006b) also points to costs for both one's mental and physical health. The instability associated with contingent self-esteem can lead to depression as well as to stress levels that can compromise immune system functioning as well as increase the risk for coronary disease.

Rhodewalt (2006) presents a complementary analysis in describing the costs of contingent self-esteem. When the possession of high self-esteem becomes a goal in and of itself, dependent upon external contingencies imposed by others, it may well produce failure experiences that can backfire, leading to a major devaluation of the self. Moreover, such a preoccupation can readily result in self-esteem uncertainty and instability (Kernis & Goldman, 2003) and provoke defensive and often hostile efforts to protect and repair one's fragile self-esteem (see Baumeister et al., 1996). Rhodewalt observes that contingent self-esteem requires a "high maintenance" personal effort given that one of the costs of fragile self-esteem is that it requires chronic attention. Often the pursuit is accompanied by the self-aggrandizing illusions that were observed in the lives of narcissists who typically display fragile and unstable self-esteem. Like J. Crocker (2006b), Rhodewalt concludes that *possessing* a secure sense of self-esteem does not require that one must relentlessly *strive* for it.

Ryan and Brown (2006), in building upon self-determination theory (see also Deci & Ryan, 2000; Ryan & Deci, 2000), distinguish *contingent self-esteem* from *true self-esteem*. Contingent self-esteem arises whenever a person's global evaluation of worth is grounded in meeting goals established by others. This can include rather desperate attempts to gain others' admiration and approval because the individual requires constant validation. Like the observations of J. Crocker (2006b), Kernis and Gold-man (2003), and Rhodewalt (2006), Ryan, Deci, and colleagues observe that contingent self-esteem is unstable and invariably very fragile. Thus, in the face of a setback, it can plummet and/or lead to desperate attempts to regain favor in the eyes of evaluating others.

In contrast, *true self-esteem* is a sense of self as worthy, not by virtue of external trappings or specific accomplishments, but because one experiences self-worth as inherent (Ryan & Brown, 2006). Thus, true self-esteem is noncontingent and relatively stable. It does not become inflated when one succeeds, nor does it crumble in the face of failure. Moreover, people with true self-esteem exhibit greater personal integrity and authenticity because they do not base their self-worth on achieving goals established for the self by others. Thus, individuals are free to pursue learning and mastery goals, as well as the basic developmental needs for competence, autonomy, and relatedness.

Self-determination theory finds the roots of contingent self-esteem, as the label implies, in the contingent feedback of parents or caregivers (Deci & Ryan, 2000; Ryan & Deci, 2000). When parents are heavily invested in specific child outcomes, they often purposely or unwittingly convey love, regard, or support that is contingent upon the child attaining often unrealistic, socially implanted goals. Thus the child only garners favor if he/she meets the parents' explicit expectations such as being smart, athletic, and attractive.

As discussed in an earlier chapter, we labeled a related construct "conditional positive regard" given that parents set the conditions under which they will provide approval. However, we learned, in interviews with adolescents, that they clearly did not experience conditionality as approval, from their perspective. Rather, it specifies the psychological hoops through which they must jump in order to please demanding parents whose expectations are typically unattainable. We have demonstrated that high conditionality, coupled with low levels of approval, leads to hopelessness about ever garnering positive support from parents, which in turn leads to false-self behavior as a last resort, as adolescents distort the self in order to obtain approval (Harter, Marold, et al., 1996). We have demonstrated the same dynamics within the realm of peer relationships.

Kernis and colleagues (see Kernis & Goldman, 2006) pursue this theme, observing that individuals who are forced to seek contingent self-esteem are preoccupied with their standings on the evaluative dimensions deemed critical by significant others. Thus, children, as well as adults, continually recalibrate their behaviors in the face of these external evaluative standards, in an attempt to validate their self-worth in the eyes of these others. As such, contingent self-esteem is necessarily fragile because it can only remain high if one successfully meets these unrealistic expectations, which for children typically involve the domains of academic success, physical attractiveness, and peer social approval. Moreover, the strong need for continual external validation drives the child or adult to seek more and more success that, if not achieved, will cause contingent self-esteem to plummet.

In our own research, described in Chapter 5, we have addressed the extent to which young adolescents contingently base their self-esteem on their physical appearance or derive their global feelings of self-worth from perceived peer approval (Harter, Stocker, et al., 1996). We discovered that those basing their self-esteem on their appearance reported more markedly lower self-perceptions of appearance, markedly lower self-esteem, and greater depression. These liabilities were not reported by those who indicated that if they first liked themselves as a person, then they valued their appearance, even if it did not totally measure up to cultural standards of attractiveness. Basing one's self-esteem (one's inner self) on perceptions of one's looks (one's outer self) is by far the more pernicious directionality orientation.

Liabilities also emerge for those who remain drawn like a magnet to the social mirror as another major source of self-evaluation. This issue becomes particularly relevant during the period of early adolescence because at this stage of development, teenagers begin to form metatheories about the perceived causal links between constructs that involve the self and others. Moreover, these metatheories, for example, about the directionality of peer approval and self-esteem, have implications for several correlates, including actual behavior.

We devised a methodology in which we developed questions asking young adolescents to endorse one of two orientations: (1) If others my age approve of me first, then I will like myself as a person, or (2) If I first like myself as a person, then others my age will like and approve of me (Harter, Stocker, et al., 1996). The findings revealed that 59% selected what we have called the *looking-glass-self orientation*, selecting the first choice, basing their self-esteem on perceived approval, whereas the remaining 41% opted for the second sequence of events. That more endorsed the "peer approval precedes self-esteem" orientation was not surprising, given that at this stage of development, most adolescents are highly preoccupied with the opinions of others and are extremely self-conscious (Elkind, 1967; Erikson, 1968; Harter, 1990; M. Rosenberg, 1986).

Our faith in the validity of participants' selections was bolstered by the explanations for their response choices. For example, those endorsing the looking-glass-self orientation offered the following justifications: "If other people my age don't like me as a person, then I wonder if I *am* a good person. I care about what people think and say about me," "If no one liked you, you probably wouldn't like yourself very much," and "If other kids approve of me and say good things about me, then I look at myself and think I'm not so bad and I start liking myself."

In contrast, those who reversed the sequence, placing opinions of self (i.e., self-esteem) as causally prior to the opinions of others, gave the following kinds of justifications for their stance: "In seventh grade, I didn't like myself as a person, so there weren't many people that liked me, but in eighth grade, I felt more confident about myself and then I found that I had many more friends that liked me," "You have to appreciate yourself first, as a person. If you wait for other people to make you feel good, you could be waiting a long time!" and "The way I figure it, if you can't like the person you are first, then how do you expect other people to like you?"

Moreover, there was a predictable pattern of correlates revealing liabilities for those who endorsed the looking-glass-self orientation:

1. Looking-glass-self adolescents reported a significantly greater *preoccupation* with approval compared to those who endorsed the other directionality.
2. Looking-glass-self adolescents reported greater *fluctuations in approval*, which we predicted, given that they would be more likely to detect real or imagined vacillations in peer acceptance.
3. Looking-glass-self adolescents also reported greater *fluctuations in self-esteem*, which was expected. To the extent that they are basing their self-esteem on fluctuating peer approval, their self-esteem should vacillate, in tandem.
4. We also found that looking-glass-self adolescents reported *lower levels of peer approval*, which we predicted. In their preoccupation with approval, looking-glass-self adolescents may engage in behaviors that do not garner the desired peer support. They may try too hard to win acceptance or employ inappropriate social strategies that may annoy or alienate their classmates.
5. Looking-glass-self adolescents also reported lower levels of self-esteem. Given that they base their feelings of worth on peer approval, which was low, then it was expected that their self-esteem would suffer, as a result.
6. Finally, and importantly, our last measure was an objective teacher rating of *social distractibility within the classroom (not* a self-report measure).

Teachers, blind to the purpose of the study, provided objective ratings, confirming our expectation that the looking-glass-self adolescents would be more socially distracted, given their greater preoccupation with peer approval. Their excessive concern with social validation interfered with their ability to attend to class work and to concentrate on learning and mastery goals. This last finding provides behavioral evidence for the costs of a preoccupation with approval as the basis for one's self-esteem, clearly a liability that interfered with classroom learning.

It was noted earlier in this chapter that others (e.g., J. Crocker, 2006b;

Ryan & Brown, 2006) have also observed that the pursuit of high self-esteem, often predicated on self-validation goals, can compromise learning and mastery (see also Covington, 1984). One's mistakes, failures, criticism, and negative feedback represent self-threats that preclude opportunities to learn and to improve the self. Self-determination theory (Deci & Ryan, 2000; Ryan & Deci, 2000) also places considerable emphasis on mastery goals, as children strive for both competence and autonomy. These theorists argue that contingent self-esteem, in its preoccupation with meeting external goals established by significant others, will compromise these normative and necessary developmental strivings.

In a recent creative integration of attachment theory and goal orientation theory, Rusk and Rothbaum (2010) pursue these themes. From each of these theoretical perspectives, they argue that following setbacks and failures, learning goals (in contrast to the pursuit of self-validation) are much more likely to lead to cognitive openness, mastery, effective problem solving, appropriate support seeking, and adaptive emotion regulation. They focus on the theorizing of Mikulincer (1997, 1998), an attachment theorist, and Dweck (1986, 1999), a major proponent of goal orientation theory.

Within attachment theory, learning about the environment is facilitated by caregivers who provide a secure base from which the infant can explore the environment, but return for comfort, if he/she encounters environmental stressors. From this perspective, those who are compromised by negative attachment styles (e.g., anxious–ambivalent or avoidant) that stem from lack of parental responsiveness or attunement, will employ strategies that lead to an underlying concern with approval and self-worth, rather than a focus on mastery and learning goals. For goal-oriented theorists, a major distinction is drawn between *self-validation* and *learning* goals that are also referred to by some as mastery goals (see Kaplan & Maehr, 2007). Self-validation strategies are clearly handicapping.

From both perspectives, despite differences in their theoretical origins, mastery or learning goals are viewed as adaptive, whereas seeking to validate one's self-esteem is viewed as maladaptive, as summarized by Rusk and Rothbaum (2010). From the viewpoint of attachment theory, those with an avoidant pattern engage in defensive self-enhancement, seeking to convince others of their self-sufficiency and superior abilities. Those with an anxious–ambivalent pattern seek the approval of others to defend against perceptions that the self is not worthy of others' attention, approval, and nurturant care (Mikulincer & Shaver, 2007). Thus, both insecure attachment styles are associated with preoccupying self-validation goals that interfere with effective learning.

Dweck's (1986, 1999) theory is particularly relevant in that those who adopt an *entity* theory of their characteristics (e.g., intelligence) view attributes as fixed and therefore immutable. Those labeled as *incremental* theorists, in contrast, see the promise of improvement and change, due to their own personal effort. The entity perspective has much in common with self-validation tendencies, whereas incremental perspectives are more aligned with mastery goals. A complete discussion of the integration of attachment theory and goal orientation theory is beyond the scope of this chapter. However, each perspective is consistent with the message of those formulations reviewed thus far in this chapter, namely, that a preoccupation with the validation from others, in the pursuit of enhanced self-esteem, will interfere with the more adaptive goals of mastery and learning. Another major theme that has characterized the discussion, thus far, has focused on the extent to which self-evaluations are *realistic*. With these issues as a segue, attention now turns to those efforts to raise self-esteem at a societal level, as reflected in the interventions within the "Self-esteem movement," and among those proposing self-enhancement strategies within the educational establishment.

To Raise or Not to Raise Self-Esteem within Both Society and Our Schools?

For two decades, considerable debate and controversy has surrounded this question. Initiatives have been proposed to raise self-esteem at the national and state level, as a cure-all for many societal ills. Parallel interventions at the classroom level have been urged by some educators who presume that self-esteem enhancement should motivate students to attain higher levels of academic achievement. The initiative adopted by the state of California, in 1990, reflects one of the most ambitious efforts to tackle this issue at a legislative level (California Task Force to Promote Self-Esteem and Personal and Social Responsibility, 1990). This particular initiative became a public marker of the "self-esteem movement." Its message was also a subtext in the playbooks of many educators.

California state legislators expressed their conviction that by raising the self-esteem of its citizenry, many social ills would be significantly reduced, for example, crime, teen pregnancy, delinquency, drug abuse, and school underachievement. Such a widespread intervention would lead to better societal, as well as personal, outcomes. The California initiative vaulted the topic of self-esteem into the national limelight, as the media scrambled to cover the frenzied efforts to alter self-perceptions in the service of the greater cultural good. Swann (1996) likens the quest for high self-esteem to the search for the Holy Grail, pointing to the dizzying array of programs that proliferated. Unfortunately, these efforts did not have their intended effects, based upon very disappointing findings that did not produce the desired outcomes. Self-esteem did not represent the anticipated panacea that would cure our social ills (see Swann, Chang-Schneider, & McClarty, 2007). The quick fixes proposed not only failed to enhance self-esteem but raised false hopes that only added to the anguish of the victims of low self-esteem (Swann, 1996).

As I have argued elsewhere in this volume, attempts to enhance self-esteem will be misguided unless the targets for intervention are the theoretically based and empirically demonstrated *causes*. My argument also emphasizes the need to address *realistic* self-appraisals. The interventions enacted in the California initiative addressed neither the issue of demonstrated causes nor the accuracy of self-evaluations (see California Task Force to Promote Self-Esteem and Personal and Social Responsibility, 1990).

How the self-esteem movement played out on the stage of America's classrooms, as an educational microcosm of society, is of particular relevance to this volume on self-processes and their implications for our youth. A major focus of many educational interventions has been the enhancement of self-esteem, given the argument that student achievement would improve, as a result. These contentions have fueled an intense debate that is reflected within the educational and psychological literatures. Proponents have touted the advantages of enhanced self-esteem, whereas opponents have vociferously argued that such efforts are not only misguided and useless, at best, but destructive, at worst. What are the primary arguments, pro and con?

The claims of the proponents are perhaps the most straightforward, given the belief and insistence that raising the self-esteem of students will produce higher levels of achievement and foster academic success, primarily measured by grades and test scores (see Beane, 1994; Tice & Gailliot, 2006, for thoughtful reviews of the dispute). Two issues, in particular, seem to loom large on the controversial landscape, one of which hinges on the magnitude of the empirical relationship between self-reported global self-esteem and objective indices of achievement. The second concerns the interpretation of the causal links, or the directionality of effects, between these two constructs.

First, those who believe in the value of enhancing self-esteem among our students argue that while admittedly modest, the correlation between these two constructs is sufficient to warrant educational intervention. Second, these proponents also contend that the enhancement of self-esteem will *produce* educational benefits, that is, global perceptions of one's worth as a person act causally to promote gains in academic achievement.

Opponents of educational interventions first point out that the magnitude of the correlation between self-esteem and academic achievements is relatively trivial and thus without serious implications. (One person's effect size is another person's error term!) Second, they challenge the presumed directionality of effects. That is, although the two constructs may bear a modest correlation to one another, it is just as likely that successful achievement in the classroom (as indexed by good grades and high standardized test scores) represents the *cause* of higher self-esteem, not the effect. These are the general arguments that define each position. Next we turn to the more nuanced considerations, identifying the key players in this debate.

A major concern addressed by many opponents is that seeking to boost self-esteem can *artificially* destroy any incentives for students to devote *effort* toward scholastic goals (Tice & Gailliot, 2006). This observation is consistent with the theme of the liabilities of unrealistic self-evaluations that were discussed earlier in this chapter. Inflated self-esteem provides no incentive for self-improvement (see also J. Crocker, 2006a, 2006b). Moreover, the practice of inviting students to make unconfirmed self-affirmations as to their worth ("I am smart," "I am wonderful") do not appear to be effective (Beane, 1994).

Damon (1995) was also among the first to be critical of what he considered an overemphasis by educators on promoting high self-esteem, particularly when these efforts lead to an inflated sense of one's self-worth. Damon has viewed such efforts as not only misguided but potentially detrimental, arguing that they divert educators from the active teaching of skills and deprive students of the thrill that results from personal accomplishment. It has been Damon's contention that self-esteem has become an overrated commodity and that the effusive praise that parents and teachers heap on children to make them feel good about themselves is often met with suspicion by the children, themselves. Moreover, it interferes with their attention to the goal of building specific skills in the service of genuine achievement. As Covington (2006) maintains, it does a grave educational injustice to encourage children to think well of themselves without having earned it. Cote (2009) has joined the ranks of opponents, decrying the "cult of self-esteem" that has gripped schools in this country.

"Feel-good activities," a mainstay of many of the self-esteem interventions to emerge in the 1980s, have produced few gains, despite the widespread commercial packaging of programs designed to enhance self-esteem. They demand that teachers suspend corrective feedback and remove challenging material, dumbing down the curriculum (Damon, 1995). Such activities divorce self-esteem from palpable achievements that result from realistic attributions to the student's personal effort. As a result, they confound self-esteem with egocentrism, arrogance, and conceit (see Beane, 1994; Mruk, 2006). That said, proponents of these packaged programs claim that the self-affirming affective exercises and techniques will extend, not only to heightened school performance but to broader societal goals to help curb such teenage social ills as pregnancy, drug use, and delinquency. However, there is little evidence to warrant these claims (see Covington, 2006). Moreover, given my own experience in the schools over the years, many teachers who were forced to administer what they called touchy-feely exercises complained that this was not their job definition, rendering them less than effective if they attempted to mouth the self-esteem mantra.

Opponents' concerns resonate with the earlier conclusions of those who have argued (e.g., Dweck, 1986, 1999; Mikulincer, 1997, 1998, as described in Rusk & Rothbaum, 2010) that self-validation goals interfere with the educational goals of learning and mastery. As Covington (2006) observes, enhanced achievement is more likely if children are motivated to learn for the sake of learning, stimulate their own curiosity, challenge themselves, and set personal goals that involve skill improvement. If the reasons behind school performance are more self-promotional and defensive in nature, for example, striving to succeed in order to avoid failure with its implication that one is incompetent, academic motivation will wane because of the fear that one cannot succeed.

Although *effort* has been identified as a handmaiden of mastery, effort represents a double-edged psychological sword for the student wanting to project an image of competence. In this context, Covington (2009) raises the question of why students don't try harder in order to succeed. Paradoxically, effort does not compensate for the onus of failure. As Nichols (1984) cogently pointed out some years ago, older children come to develop a realistic understanding of the perceived relationship between effort and ability. Failure, in the face of enhanced effort, signifies lack of *ability*. Furthermore, social comparison contributes to this interpretation; for example, "If I have to work that much harder and longer on my assignments compared to my classmates, then I must really be stupid." To the extent that personal competence contributes to enhanced self-worth, the student will strive to protect perceptions of ability by avoiding effortful attempts that may result in failure that signifies inadequacy.

Thus, students are placed in a motivational dilemma, one that has emotional consequences, as well. In accordance with the arguments put forth in Chapter 6, the acknowledgment that one lacks ability, making an attribution about one's personal deficiencies or fundamental flaws, will produce shame. An attribution for failure that results from lack of effort, on the other hand, is more likely to produce guilt, a less painful affect that is attached to more specific behaviors (e.g., "I was too busy at sports practice to complete the teacher's homework assignment").

As Covington (2009) observes, this motivational dilemma promotes an arsenal of *excuses*. In wrestling with the conflict surrounding the implications of effort and ability, "excuses allow students to repackage otherwise questionable actions, like not trying, in a more flattering, less blameworthy form" (p. 145). Thus, to suggest a well-worn example, the scenario in which "the dog ate my homework" may, in the short run, engender some empathy from the teacher and classmates. However, Covington notes that chronic excuse making (e.g., if the dog subsists on a steady diet of homework) can take a dangerous personal turn. Rather than mere attributions to hapless unpreparedness, the student must now struggle to escape the perception in the eyes of others, and therefore the self, that he/she is basically stupid. Affirmations to the contrary, urged by proponents of self-esteem enhancement (e.g., "You are really special and smart"), are deceptively simple and therefore ineffective solutions, leading down an eventual path of self-delusion.

Perhaps one of the strongest and most vocal opponents of self-esteem enhancement programs within the school system is Baumeister and colleagues (Baumeister, 1996; Baumeister, Campbell, Krueger, & Vohs, 2005). Baumeister's devastating critique is captured by this assertion: "At worst, the pursuit of high self-esteem is a foolish, wasteful, and self-destructive enterprise that may end up doing more harm than good" (1996, p. 120). What is the basis for his contentions?

To begin with, Baumeister (1996) is critical of the California initiative to promote self-esteem, which professed to represent a social vaccine to cure or hopefully inoculate citizens against the evils of "crime, violence, substance abuse, teen pregnancy, child abuse, chronic welfare dependency, and educational failure" (California Task Force to Promote Self-Esteem and Personal and Social Responsibility, 1990, p. 4). He rightfully asserts, consistent with the evidence presented in the previous section on narcissism, that for many in this country, self-esteem is already inflated. He also observes, as noted earlier, that the correlations between self-esteem and its hoped-for consequences are mixed; they are either entirely absent or modest, in some cases statistically insignificant and therefore of little practical relevance. He notes, appropriately, that where the correlations are moderate, many researchers who have attempted the challenge of unraveling issues of causality have concluded that self-esteem is more likely to be an *outcome* of achievement rather than a cause. That is, school success, or conversely school failure, will *result* in correspondingly positive or negative feelings of self-esteem; they are the cause, rather than the effect, countering the claims of those who argue for self-esteem enhancement.

Baumeister (1996) is also well aware of the literature on the negative correlates and consequences of inflated self-esteem. Thus, he rightfully observes that inflated self-esteem, fragile self-esteem, unrealistic and distorted self-perceptions, and other indicators of egotism and narcissism, including lack of empathy, can contribute to violence. In developing this theme, he cites literature supporting the view that bullies, delinquents, and gang members typically have very high self-esteem, given that they derive their sense of worth from like-minded peers who share their values. However, let the reader recall that the high-profile school shooters who were the *victims* of bullying, expressed *low* self-esteem and yet engaged in the most heinous acts of violence, namely, the indiscriminant shooting and murder of classmates. As noted earlier, there is more than one pathway to violent ideation and action.

Where Baumeister (1996) goes awry is in his implicit equation or conflation of high self-esteem with those characteristics that define narcissism, which he does with great insistence (see also Baumeister et al., 2003). While at one point in his treatment of the topic, he seems to appreciate that high self-esteem can reflect confident and secure assessments of the self, he too quickly moves to the assumption that it can also mean conceited, arrogant, narcissistic, and egotistical behavior. This latter observation is not the manner in which high self-esteem has been defined or characterized in the mainstream literature. There, it reflects security, confidence, stability, and self-awareness but without preoccupation. Swann et al. (2007) are also critical of Baumeister's seeming equation of the defensively self-protective statements of narcissists with those of people with true and secure high self-esteem.

As argued earlier in this chapter, there is a minority of individuals for whom high self-esteem *accompanies* the more negative aspects of narcissism, but high self-esteem should not be *equated* with these characteristics as Baumeister's (1996) argument too often glibly implies. His rhetoric too readily and frequently slips into such language. As such, he undermines his own arguments. The "dark side of self-esteem," his catchphrase, only applies to those in the minority who display unstable, inflated, and therefore unrealistically high and fragile self-esteem; these are the individuals who are threatened by challenges to their sense of self.

That said, Baumeister (1996) makes a number of excellent arguments about school interventions that apply to those who already possess inflated perceptions of their self-esteem. He suggests that one should not attempt to further inflate their overly unrealistic positive views of self. Rather, educators should seek to support accurate perceptions of abilities and talent. Thus, a realistic appreciation for one's strengths and weaknesses should be the goal. Thus, in agreement with others, Baumeister argues that educators should not provide positive feedback that has not been earned.

Perhaps a more controversial point, in my opinion, is Baumeister's (1996) contention that self-esteem should not be boosted when it is already within an accurate range. As an illustration, he suggests that a student who believes that math is not his/her strong suit should not be given exaggerated notions of what he/she can accomplish, because this could lead to eventual failure and heartbreak. One can immediately counter this argument in the case of an N of 1, namely, Einstein, who purportedly failed math! Facetiousness aside, in my experience as a university professor as well as a clinician, I have encountered students with sincere aspirations to enter into fields for which they did not have the requisite skills. Rather than dash their professional hopes to the rocks, I worked with them to find skill-training opportunities that would boost their levels of competence and, in turn, confidence, and eventually enhance their self-esteem, realistically.

In contrast to Baumeister's (1996) stance, others (e.g., Swann et al., 2007) have been more sanguine about the possibility of enrichment opportunities that may improve the self-perceptions of our youth. In prefacing their arguments, Swann et al. are critical of Baumeister and colleagues

(2003), who seem to assume that self-esteem is an "affective" construct, whereas domain-specific self-concepts are primarily "cognitive" in nature. The implication of such an assumption is that of the two, self-esteem should theoretically be more likely to predict outcomes of psychological significance. Swann et al. rightfully point out that both global self-esteem and domain-specific self-concepts are, at the same time, cognitive appraisals *and* affectively laden judgments.

Swann et al. (2007) also cogently argue for the principle of *specificity matching*. That is, in examining the relationship between self-perceptions and behavioral outcomes, there should be a match between the *level* of self-evaluations and the behavior to be predicted. They give, as an illustration, the prediction of math performance, pointing out that one should employ a domain-specific measure of perceived math proficiency, *not* a measure of global self-esteem. They make a parallel argument for examining the correlates of global self-esteem, arguing that one should look to related constructs that are defined by "bundles of behaviors" that are at the same level of generality, for example, depression. Depression, defined clinically, as well as in nonclinical assessments such as our own measure of the dimensions of depression (Harter, Nowakowski, & Marold, 1988), represents at least five symptoms or manifestations. We found very strong correlations between global self-esteem and depression so defined (r's ranging from .55 to .70).

Swann et al. (2007) review literature indicating that as the specificity of the predictor and corresponding criterion variable increases, so too does the strength of the empirical relationship between them. By way of illustration, they cite a meta-analysis by Hansford and Hattie (1982) revealing that measures of academic self-concept better predicted academic ability than self-esteem. Marsh and Craven (2006) have come to the same conclusion. In their own work, math self-concept was substantially correlated with math grades ($r = .71$) and standardized math achievement scores ($r = .59$), whereas global self-esteem was not (r's of $-.03$ to .05). Swann et al. claim that Baumeister and colleagues (2003) have violated the specificity principle by erroneously focusing on the ability of global measures of self-esteem to predict specific outcomes (e.g., Does self-esteem predict grades in a math class?). It is thus not surprising, Swann et al. conclude, that researchers find few empirical links between global self-esteem and specific outcomes.

With these caveats as a backdrop, Swann et al. (2007) ask whether it is worthwhile to attempt improvements in the evaluative self-views of youth and adults (see also Swann, Chang-Schneider, & Angulo, 2008). Here there is obvious controversy. Critics of self-esteem interventions report that there is no evidence that "boosting self-esteem (by therapeutic interventions or school programs) causes benefits" (Baumeister et al., 2003, p. 1). Swann et al., to the contrary, summarize evidence suggesting that certain programs designed to enhance self-esteem also improve standardized test scores, reduce school disciplinary problems, and lead to declines in the use of drugs and alcohol (DuBois & Flay, 2004; Haney & Durlak, 1998). However, don't such efforts violate the specificity matching principle?

The arguments are more complex. Most intervention programs contain many components and associated goals. For example, there may be program features designed not only to elevate self-esteem but to enhance self-efficacy, promote social skills and positive interpersonal relationships, improve academic achievement, reduce behavioral conduct problems, increase self-control, and so forth. While some may argue that such multifaceted programs *confound* the contribution of multiple predictors, I would suggest a semantic alternative, namely, that they *compound* the effects of such predictors. If positive results are obtained with these omnibus interventions, then it behooves the researcher, through further investigation, to determine which of the many independent variables packed into a program are responsible for demonstrated gains in both specific and general outcomes. Swann et al. (2007) similarly observe that such programs are likely to contain a mix of effective and ineffective strategies. They cite DuBois and Tevendale (1999), who contend that the benefits of programs could be enhanced still further by bolstering the effective components and eliminating those features that are ineffective. Of course, the difficult work must be done in the form of research to tease apart the influential components of a program from those that do not contribute to the intended gains.

Elsewhere in this volume, I have suggested the usefulness of distinguishing between the *goal* of a program (e.g., enhanced self-esteem) and the *target* of one's interventions (i.e., its causes). Although self-esteem enhancement may be a goal, intervention strategies should be directed at its *determinants* that are ideally theory driven and have been empirically documented. Thus, the specific causes need first to be identified, after which interventions can be designed to modify these causes (be they poor academic competencies, inadequate social skills, or conduct problems). In the 1960s and 1970s, an earlier movement that invoked simplistic attempts to enhance self-esteem was unsuccessful. These urged general self-affirmations (e.g., "I'm OK, you're OK" messages) and affective feel-good exercises that were designed to impact self-esteem directly. They did not attend to the *causes* of low self-esteem, which should be the proximal targets of an intervention.

The issue of causality is key. If, as Swann et al. (2007) entertain, the multiple features of a program target changes in several behavioral domains, as illustrated above, then self-esteem enhancement could well be the *result* of these interventions that lead to improved academic achievement, for example, and not the cause of specific behavioral change. Leary (2008) concurs, citing evidence suggesting that positive and negative outcomes appear to be the causes rather than the effects of self-esteem. This contention is consistent with our own view that program evaluators need to identify the determinants of self-esteem as the focus of an intervention, not attempt to impact self-esteem directly. Swann et al. are in agreement with our own thinking, in arguing that programs organized around simplistic interventions such as self-affirmations are fanciful and ephemeral (see also J. Crocker & Park, 2004; Swann, 1996). Effective strategies must be designed to "alter the raw materials that provide the basis for healthy, sustainable self-esteem" (Swann et al., 2007, p. 90). Moreover, programs should cultivate behaviors that produce self-views that are both *realistic* (i.e., based on objective evidence) and *adaptive* (i.e., promote activities that predict long-term adjustment to the demands of society).

Swann et al. (2007) also raise another critical point in their observation that certain strategies may be effective for some but ineffective for others. Previously, I have made a similar claim (see Harter, 2006a) in arguing that "one program does not fit all." For example, our own research demonstrates that for older children and adolescents there are multiple pathways or causes to low self-esteem and its correlates, primarily depression and hopelessness (see Harter, 1999). Thus, intervention efforts need to first target, and then be tailored to, the particular pathways for a given individual or subgroup of those who share common pathways, a staggering mission, to be sure. Of course, this is what sensitive clinicians do on a daily basis. However, an appropriate diagnosis is often more readily accomplished than is the design and implementation of an effective intervention strategy, particularly given the typical challenging need to work with both the family and the school.

On a broader scale, Twenge et al. (2008) relate these various observations to their findings that demonstrate how narcissism has systematically increased over the past three decades, in speculating about what societal trends may be responsible. They suggest that the media, in general, and schools, in particular, have perpetuated messages and practices that promote narcissism. Affirmations of "specialness" and educational practices such as grade inflation and dumbing down the curriculum prompt unrealistic views of competence and provoke narcisstic self-promotion among today's students.

Authenticity and the Potential Threat of Multiple Selves

An underlying theme in this chapter has been the importance not only of realistic self-evaluations but a sense of *authenticity*. As observed earlier, there are potential liabilities associated with the construction of a self that is so highly dependent upon interpersonal socializing influences that can cause self-development to go awry. One such liability is the construction of a false self that does not mirror one's authentic experiences. As has become evident in our previous developmental analysis, the creation of a self designed to conform to the wishes and dictates of significant others whom one feels obligated to please may not only compromise the true self, but can also lead to associated negative outcomes such as low self-esteem and depression.

The preoccupation with authenticity in our culture can be observed in the vast vocabulary we have developed to describe its absence, namely, deceit, as Lerner (1993) points out in her book entitled *The Dance of Deception*. Verb forms make reference to fabricating, withholding, concealing, distorting, falsifying, pulling the wool over someone's eyes, posturing, charading, faking, and hiding behind a façade. Adjectives include evasive, elusive, wily, phony, fake, artificial, two-faced, hypocritical, manipulative, calculating, pretentious, crafty, conniving, duplicitous, deceitful, and dishonest. Noun forms include charlatan, chameleon, impostor, hypocrite, a fake, and a fraud.

In our own developmental research, we have discovered that it is not until adolescence that an awareness of the false-self behaviors of others, and eventually the self, becomes particularly acute (Harter, Bresnick, et al., 1997). Many of the linguistic forms highlighted by Lerner (1993) begin to emerge at this point in development, as if adolescents had spawned attenae to detect hypocrisy. When asked for a description, they define false-self behavior as concealing what you really think or feel and saying things that you don't really believe. Our earlier analysis has pointed to child-rearing practices, such as conditionality and contingent support as the precursors of false-self behavior (see Chapter 2).

In the introductory chapter I presented Gergen's (1991) perspective on how false-self behavior has become a contemporary societal problem. Authenticity was a major commodity during the era of *modernism*. However, it is his belief that certain features of *postmodernistic* society has compromised the true self. Gergen marks the explosion of *technology* available to the layperson (e.g., easy access to air travel, computers, electronic and express mail, fax machines, cell phones, beepers, answering machines, the Internet) as critical sociocultural causes. He contends that these advances have dramatically accelerated our social connectedness and thrust us into a dizzying swirl of relationships, creating the "saturated" or "populated" self. For Gergen, the demands of multiple relationships split the individual into a multiplicity of self-investments, leading to a "cacophony of potential selves" across different relationships.

Kernis and Goldman (2003) echo this scenario, describing how the proliferation of selves has been exponentially expanded by the diversity of self-relevant information available through an ever-increasing array of communication technologies (Internet chat, e-mail, blogs, BlackBerry phones, Facebook, iPods, digital photography, computer-based conferences, and so forth). These may help in meeting the demands of a pluralistic *postmodern* society. However, Kernis and Goldman observe that these technologies "allow for self-relevant information to be instantaneously accessed, refined, indeed, even fabricated before being assimilated into the self-system" (p. 112).

These new technologies have implications for the self-images of society's citizens. The enormity of self-relevant information may, consistent with Gergen's (1991, 1996) analysis, give rise to uncertainty about the self and can therefore lead to its destabilization. As Weber (2000) has also argued, the demands of contemporary life necessarily create tension between the need to continually redefine the self and the conflicting need to somehow stabilize the boundaries of the self, in all of its multiple manifestations.

Kernis and Goldman (2003) also point to a critical feature of contemporary cultural technology, namely, that one's *anonymity* can be preserved, for example, through Internet chat rooms and online dating services. They emphasize the relevance to explorations of self among our youth. This feature would appear particularly relevant to our discussion of authenticity. Consider the following question: Does anonymity permit the protective license to express one's *true* self or, conversely, does it provide the implicit permission to fabricate a *false* self to garner the approval of one's communication partners, where deception may go undetected? Just who is the "Internet self?"

Several investigators have addressed the issue of Internet identity, concluding that anonymous online communication provides youth with a safe environment in which to explore, express, and expand upon their psychological selves. Turkle's (1995, 2005) extensive work on this topic reveals how the Internet, with its optional anonymity and multiple opportunities for social interaction, provides individuals with a virtual laboratory within which to explore and experiment with alternative conceptions of the self. Thus, she argues that the Internet affords one a forum for self-expression that allows one to express those aspects of the self that one so strongly yearns to reveal, namely, self-attributes that reflect the true self, features that are not often expressed in the reality of daily life.

Maczewski (2002), a youth case worker, heard complaints from many at-risk adolescents that there were not listened to within the community; their voices were not being heard. He arranged an opportunity for them to express themselves anonymously on the Internet where they could interact with others online. Subsequent interviews with the adolescents revealed three primary benefits. These youth (1) experienced excitement and self-expansion; they (2) felt the freedom to be who they really were, as well as to experience power and connection; and (3) were able to explore their potential identities through these virtual relationships.

Of particular interest to me, in light of the concerns about the cultural overemphasis on unattainable standards of attractiveness (see Chapter 5) were adolescents' comments about the irrelevance of appearance, given this type of online communication. One interviewee indicated that she gained self-esteem because "you are judged by your brain online and not your looks." Another teenager, who in reality was self-conscious about glasses, buck teeth, and a bad haircut, offered the observation that "Well, no one knows what you look like online, you make tons of friends, even people who normally wouldn't be friends with you in real life, because they don't see you or prejudge you first on how you look. So I felt much more comfortable to be myself, I felt accepted."

Another group of researchers (Bargh, McKenna, & Fitzsimons, 2002) explicitly asked whether the Internet activates the disclosure of the true self (as revealed in the title of their article, "Can You See the Real Me?"). They observed that first and foremost, the anonymity of Internet interactions avoids the typical expectations and constraints that arise with those who know us. It greatly reduced the risks and costs of everyday social sanctions. Thus, one is more likely to disclose the qualities of one's true self, which further facilitates empathy and mutual understanding. Their findings with college students supported these contentions in demonstrating that more of the true self was revealed through Internet communication than in actual face-to-face encounters. These investigators also concluded that not being aware of each other's physical features, in the online condition, contributed to their ability to express their true selves. This, in turn, allowed Internet partners to better like and admire each other. Thus, across these research endeavors, there is consensus that online anonymous communication is most likely to bring out self-disclosure that reflects the true self, along with opportunities to explore new and different identities (see also Valkenburg, Schouten, & Peter, 2005, who document adolescents' Internet identity experimentation). How this transfers to actual, real-life relationships is an interesting topic for further research.

Within the social psychological literature, authenticity, the sense that one is being one's true self, has been linked to high self-esteem (see Goldman, 2006). Those features that define secure or optimal self-esteem (e.g., stability and genuineness) are particularly relevant to psychological authenticity. The individual who pursues authentic goals that resonate with his/her true sense of self will invariably report optimal self-esteem. Goldman also links authenticity to a greater sense of self-*clarity* about who one is as a person (see J. D. Campbell et al., 1996). Campbell et al. report that lack of clarity about the self is associated with low self-esteem and high levels of depression and neuroticism, as well as low agreeableness, low conscientiousness, and ruminative self-focus.

Goldman and Kernis (Goldman, 2006; Goldman & Kernis, 2002; Kernis & Goldman, 2003) further describe the components of what they label as "dispositional authenticity." These include (1) *self-awareness* in the form of self-understanding; (2) *unbiased or realistic self-appraisals*; (3) *congruence* between one's values, needs, and actions; and (4) a *relational orientation*, being open, honest, and genuine in close relationships. Dispositional authenticity is positively correlated with greater life satisfaction and positive affect and negatively correlated with negative affect such as depression, consistent with our findings (see Harter, 1999). They also found that authenticity correlated positively with secure self-esteem but was negatively correlated with contingent and fragile self-esteem.

Wood, Linley, Maltby, Baliousis, and Joseph (2008) have recently published their successful efforts to develop a measure of dispositional authenticity. Three distinct but moderately correlated factors emerged: (1) self-alienation, which reflects the lack of recognition for the true self; (2) authentic living, which refers to behaving consistently with the true self; and (3) accepting external influence, which taps conformity to expectations of others (the antithesis of true-self behavior). Greater authenticity was predictive of higher self-esteem, more positive affect, and life satisfaction.

The Role of the Multiplicity of Selves

From a historical perspective, there has been controversy over the role of multiple selves. For James (1890), multiplicity was the rule and not the exception, as he concluded in his observation that "A man has as many social selves as there are individuals who recognize him and carry an image of him in their mind" (p. 190). Thus, James set the stage for the more contemporary perspective that selves will vary across relational contexts. Moreover, his observations scooped recent theorizing with his insight that multiple selves may not always speak with the same voice, ushering in his concept of "the conflict of the different me's" which could be observed in the potential incompatibility of self-expression across different roles.

Theoreticians in the first half of the 20th century did not embrace James' (1890) pluralistic contentions. There was historical resistance in the form of a "consistency" ethic. Many scholars, in the tradition of *modernism*, heralded the integrated, unified, and rational self (Allport, 1961; Horney, 1950; C. J. Jung, 1928; Lecky, 1945; Maslow, 1954; Rogers, 1951). For example, Allport emphasized the importance of a sense of *inward unity*. Lecky highlighted the theme of self-consistency and the need to maintain the integrity and unity of the self. As late as 1973 and 1981, Epstein argued that one's self-theory must meet the criterion of *internal consistency*, which he formalized as the "unity principle," arguing that there is a basic need to ensure the unity and coherence of the conceptual system that defines the self.

The pendulum appears to have swung back to an emphasis on multiplicity, with increasing zeal for models depicting how the self varies across relational contexts. Yet a new controversy has emerged. The dispute centers on whether the multiplicity of the self, now a given, reflects a realistic and adaptive stance in the postmodern world or signals potential stress and conflict for those who cannot navigate these contradictory psychological pathways. For those adhering to the first, more optimistic perspective, multiplicity is a positive adaptation where the terrain may consist of only minor speed bumps. For those adhering to the second perspective on the perils of multiplicity, the landscape is a cluttered and potentially treacherous minefield.

Paulhus and Martin (1988) are among those who have endorsed the *functional flexibility* of multiple selves that can be called upon, confidently and adaptively, across different relational contexts. For others (e.g., Gergen, 1991, 1996), the multiplicity of the self, driven to its height by postmodernism, represents a threat to the self-system that can lead to conflict and paralysis in the face of contradictory social demands. Our own approach to the study of multiple selves has been to first document their existence in the lives of adolescents and then to demonstrate *individual differences* in the degree to which teenagers cope with this reality. That is, individuals are neither universally crippled by the challenges of their multiple selves nor can all readily resolve the potential contradictions that are embodied in such disparate selves.

I have adopted a developmental perspective, identifying three distinct periods of adolescence (early, middle, and late). As described in Chapter 3, it is not until middle adolescence that conflict over the recognition of seemingly contradictory selves emerges. Our interpretation, supported by Fischer's (1980) neo-Piagetian theory of cognitive development, hinges on findings that it is not until this period (ages 14 to 16) that adolescents can directly compare cognitively abstract representations of themselves in different relational contexts and so come to realize that there are contradictory attributes that define their different selves. This realization can provoke intrapsychic conflict and cause distress.

Contradictions within the self can be problematic. However, the important point is that conflict or its absence is *not* unilaterally experienced by everyone. We need to reframe the inquiry: For whom do opposing attributes within the self-portrait portend conflict and for whom can they be handled quite adaptively, as normative features of coping with the world? Those adolescent interviewees who wrestle uncomfortably with these contradictions will give us reasons such as "How can I switch so fast from being cheerful with my friends, and then getting frustrated and nasty to my parents? Which one is the real me?" In other studies (see Harter, Bresnick, et al. (1997), those who have adapted more successfully to their multiple selves will tell us, "You can't be expected to be the same with everyone, that wouldn't be normal, it would be weird!"

For whom *do* opposing attributes cause psychological grief? We have clearly demonstrated across several studies (see Harter, Bresnick, et al., 1997) that adolescent females consistently report more conflict and distress upon the developmental realization of contradictory attributes in their self-portrait. Earlier in this volume I have suggested several interpretations. We have fewer clues to explain individual differences within each gender. Thus, this is an important arena for future research, in order to understand the developmental and social underpinnings of critical individual differences in the reaction to one's multiple selves.

There is little research on the possible precursors of individual differences in those who report conflict versus those who report harmony across their multiple selves. However, the literature that has been reviewed may offer some suggestions. Perhaps those with less concern over multiplicity have more grounded perceptions of self within a given context, more optimal self-esteem, more unconditional support, more genuine relationships, greater self-certainty, and a stronger sense of their true self. The opposite pattern may exist for those reporting greater conflict.

One psychological opportunity for examining individual differences in the display and acceptance of multiple selves involves a comparison of the self-attributes reported by high and low self-monitors (M. Snyder, 1987). High self-monitors are concerned with the interpersonal appropriateness of their social behavior across different relational contexts. They are particularly sensitive to their self-presentation with others and adjust their behavioral and attitudes accordingly. Low self-monitors are less concerned with self-presentation; rather they are more interested in being themselves and in being consistent across situations. However, there is some dispute about just how these differences are to be interpreted. M. Snyder views the behaviors of high self-monitors as adaptive, allowing them to flexibly adjust their behavior to the relational demands of different social situations. Others (e.g., Gergen, 1991) are less sanguine, pointing out that in their role as social chameleons, high self-monitors may question the authenticity of their behavior.

We examined these differential expectations employing our multiple-selves procedure. College students were first identified as high and low self-monitors. They were then asked to generate different self-attributes in major relational contexts (Badanes & Harter, 2007b). Students also indicated the extent to which each attribute reflected their true self, as well as how much they liked each self-attribute. We found, as expected, that there was less overlap among the attributes in different relationships for the high self-monitors, that is, they defined themselves as more different across relational contexts. The high self-monitors also reported more false-self attributes, more conflict between seemingly contradictory attributes across relationships, and less liking of their attributes, compared to low self-monitors. Thus, there would seem to be liabilities for those who place a premium on displaying different characteristics in different relational contexts, in the service of self-presentation, and who go to great lengths to obtain the approval of others, defining features of high self-monitoring.

Religious Perspectives on the Preoccupation with the Self and Authenticity

The concerns, thus far, over the Western (primarily American) preoccupation with the self, including the costs of self-serving biases, self-enhancement strategies, unrealistic self-portrayals, and lack of authenticity, have been raised in the context of secular society. However, various religious traditions, notably, Christianity, Judaism, and Buddhism, have weighed in on these issues, as well. As Leary (2004) observes, most religions are in agreement that the self creates three problems that may interfere with desirable spirituality. First, a preoccupation with the self precludes spiritual insights that should derive from attentiveness to the divine. Mundane self-chatter and self-absorption drown out potential messages from one's divinity, obscuring accurate perceptions of ultimate reality.

Second, these religions assert that a preoccupation with the self can interfere with spiritual transformation (Leary, 2004). Most individuals tenaciously cling to their existing identities as comfortable, understandable, and predictable, as reliable bases for decisions about future actions. Thus, people are resistant to external pressures urging them to change their self-views, even when they are negative (see Swann's, 1996, arguments and evidence for self-verification theory). Thus, such resistance stifles any motivation to engage in personal, religious transformation.

Third, failure to devote time and effort to the demands of various religious practices (e.g., worship, meditation, the study of scriptures, the performance of rituals) can thwart spiritual insight into what is considered to be the true self. Alternative egoist concerns and self-centered hedonism will lead people to deviate from the righteous path. The goal of many religious practices is to divorce the desires of the highly packaged and defended ego from the true self, viewed as the spiritual route to salvation. Thus, from the perspective of most religions, ego enhancement is considered to be an impediment to spiritual growth and morality (see Leary, 2004).

To combat this compromising and debilitating investment in the ego, Christianity and Judaism have employed admonitions against such ego indulgences, emphasizing willpower and the need to exercise *self-control*. The transformation of one's sinful self requires sacrifice and behavioral discipline in order to sustain or renew one's faith. Thus, one must engage in intense devotion, unfailing adherence to religious rituals, and diligent obedience to moral directives (see Leary, 2004). Although moral rules and practices are defined differently in Christianity and Judaism, nonetheless the transformation of the self requires strict obedience to tenets that will ultimately ensure the approval of God. Eventually, religious adherence to dogma and ritual will allow one entry into the kingdom of heaven, however it is defined by one's version of the afterlife.

Buddhism shares certain concerns about the overindulging ego that can be distinguished from a person's spiritual center that reflects greater authenticity. As one contemporary Buddhist master explained, "Two people have been living in you all your life. One is the ego, garrulous, demanding, hysterical, calculating; the other is the hidden spiritual being, whose still voice of wisdom you have only rarely heard or attended to" (S. Rinpoche, 1993, p. 120). Thus, from each religious perspective, the self-centered desires of the ego serve as impediments to an appreciation of one's inherent spiritual nature, closely linked to personal authenticity. Those commonalities notwithstanding, Buddhism takes its adherents down a somewhat different path.

A Buddhist Perspective

Although Buddhism has traditionally been associated with Eastern cultures, certain Buddhist scholars (e.g., Trungpa Rinpoche, 1976, and Thich Nhat Hanh, 1995, 1999, as well as the Dalai Lama himself) have gone to great lengths to make Buddhism more palatable to the Western world, adapting some of its tenets and practices accordingly. A central thesis of Buddhism is the cultivation of *egolessness*, which involves the denial of those ego-enhancing strategies that dominate Western preoccupations with the self. Buddha initially referred to this aspiration as "no self." He proposed that much of human suffering stemmed from the fact that people desperately cling to the idea that they must protect and preserve the self that he claimed has no real permanence, no fixed existence. From his perspective, one merely fabricates a loose confederation of feelings, questionable concepts, and perceptions that temporarily define the self. Moreover, we invite others to share in these fantasies.

Consider the following observation from a Buddhist scholar (Tarthang Tulku, 1978) who would appear to *begin* with a looking-glass-self perspective, although the implications take a decidedly different turn:

> Each of us has a self-image that is based on who we think we are and how we think others see us. When we look in a mirror, we know that what we see there is only a reflection. Even though our self-image has the same illusory quality, we often believe it to be real. Our belief in this image draws us away from the true qualities of our nature. Because the self-image is based on how we wish we were, on what we fear we are, or how we would like the world to see us, it prevents us from seeing ourselves clearly. (pp. 102–103)

Another Buddhist scholar, Trungpa Rinpoche (1976), describes how we attempt to create the illusion that self and other are solid, continuous, and consistent. He writes: "We build up an idea, a preconception, that self and other are solid and continuous, and once we have this idea, we manipulate our thoughts to confirm it and are afraid of any contrary evidence" (p. 13). According to Trungpa Rinpoche, we create a *watcher*, which is actually a very complicated bureaucracy that we construct to seemingly protect and enhance the self. In applying James's (1890) distinction, the watcher represents the rather frenetic, encumbered, and at times desperate, I-self, preoccupied with strategies for managing the impression that the Me-self is making on the world.

However, from a Buddhist perspective, one must go beyond this form of self-observation, one must remove the complicated bureaucracy that is created to preserve the permanence of the self. As Trungpa Rinpoche (1976) observes, once we take away the watcher, there is a tremendous amount of space, since the watcher and the bureaucracy take up so much room. Thus, if one eliminates the role of the watcher, the space becomes sharp, precise, and intelligent. In fact, one does not really need the watcher or observer of the self at all.

One can see, in this brief comparative analysis of Western and Eastern perspectives, rather divergent views on how the I-self should be occupying its time. From the perspective of Western psychology, the I-self should be gainfully employed in protecting the Me-self, packaging it as a valued commodity in the social marketplace. From a Buddhist perspective, far more fringe benefits will accrue if the I-self averts its myopic gaze, which represents a distorted lens that obscures one's true nature. The I-self should direct its energies outward, exercising its capacity to enjoy life experiences openly, rather than turning inward in its preoccupation with the construction of a Me-self fitfully designed and distorted in order to be acceptable to the society at large.

How, from a Buddhist perspective, should the I-self achieve these lofty goals? A major answer lies in the cultivation of "mindfulness" that involves a thoughtful awareness of who and where one is "in the moment." Here, it is important to contrast the goal of living *in* the moment from more impulsive and thoughtless attempts to live *for* the moment. Living *in* the moment involves the complete awareness of the self in the present surroundings, be they sights, smells, an appreciation for other people, or just being one's true self. Living in the moment may not always be idyllic, it might call up an awareness that one has to wash the dishes and pay the bills! However, it contrasts with the reckless abandon of living *for* the moment (e.g., "Let's just get drunk tonight and forget about studying for the test"). Contemporary psychologists, bridging Eastern and Western perspectives, concur. Langer (1989, 2009) describes mindfulness as a flexible state of mind that sensitizes us to our context in the present and opens us up to novel ways of thinking. It is to be aware and attentive in the here and now; this is the essence of being mindful.

Buddhism also encourages us to drop the elaborate fabrication that represents an embellished "story line" of our life. Too often we create a

Cecil B. DeMille production in which we are simultaneously the director, the producer, and the protagonist: "This is my life, the second greatest story ever told!" Interestingly, our self-dramas typically focus on the past and the future, but not the present. We rarely stop to ask the more critical question, "What is going on *right now*?" This question is at the core of mindfulness. How, from a Buddhist perspective, can one achieve such mindfulness? The common answer is through *meditation* practice. By way of explanation, here is a story told by one of the Buddhist scholars in the Boulder, Colorado community.

Buddha realized that he was in the throes of a common human dilemma, caught in the negative cycle of *passion, aggression*, and *ignorance* that we all experience. Buddha was passionately distressed over his observations of the hunger, pain, and death that he saw all around him, and went dashing about, desperately and somewhat aimlessly, across the land, trying to prevent such suffering. He experienced frustration and anger, in his failed attempts, at times reacting aggressively but to no avail. He thus attempted to escape from this reality, to run from it, *ignoring* the causes and consequences, thereby completing the sequence of passion, aggression, and ignorance. Eventually, he could no longer be victimized by this recurring cycle. As our Buddhist scholar told the story, Buddha said to himself "Wait a minute, I have got to just stop frantically and aimlessly running from here to there and simply *sit down* for a while and rid myself of this unproductive rumination!" And that became the dawn of meditation!

A true or apocryphal story, notwithstanding, the name Buddha, we were told, derives from the word meaning "to be awake." The goal of mindfulness and the awareness of one's present surrounds, including an accurate perception of oneself. In the Buddhist tradition, meditation becomes the pathway to such realizations. There have been very thoughtful treatments of the meditation process by American psychologists (e.g., Benson, 1975, 1984; Langer, 2009; Leary, 2004; D. H. Shapiro, 1980; S. L. Shapiro, 2009; Walsh & Shapiro, 2006) exploring the benefits, many of which correspond to the Buddhist perspective.

A major goal of meditation is to promote mindfulness by, paradoxically, perhaps, reducing our constant mental chatter. We typically engage in considerable cluttered thinking that is reflected in our self-absorbed internal monologues as well as dialogues among our multiple selves. Not only do they dominate our waking moments but intrude upon our dream life, as well. Such thinking diverts our attention from a more mindful focus on the present that Eastern and Western scholars agree is more adaptive. Meditation helps to cut through the mental chatter by slowing down our rattled thought processes and preoccupations, allowing us to be alone with ourselves, ideally suspending our normal mode of thinking. This goal is not easily achieved, however. During meditation, intrusive thoughts often relentlessly knock on the door of our concentration. Typically, people grasp at evaluative perceptions of themselves or others in a very judgmental manner. They overanalyze their thoughts, foolishly convincing themselves that they have achieved great insight into their problems. They impose faulty logic that justifies their conclusions.

In meditation one is encouraged to suspend these thoughts, focusing on one's breath or a simple mantra that precludes unproductive rumination. Letting go of one's judgmental thoughts may seem to some as if the meditator is not being thoughtfully analytical or insightful. Meditation is not something that can be easily or logically explained; it has to be experienced. Simply sitting for some period of time, dropping one's self-protective armor, clearing out the underbrush of negative thoughts, of self-aggrandizing illusions, paving the way for the true self to make a visit, are all processes that are difficult to explicate. Meditation does not have to involve religious trappings (such as the tenets of Buddhism). It can be effectively employed as a secular technique to reduce mental chatter, freeing up cognitive space to authentically face the challenges of the day, to invite the true self to make a visit (see Benson, 1975, who has explored the benefits of nonreligious meditation techniques).

Quieting the Ego

A major goal of meditation and other techniques to remedy the excesses of the Western self is to quiet the ego (Leary, 2004; Wayment & Bauer, 2008). As observed, in reviewing self-enhancement techniques, the Western ego is quite "noisy," excessively so in the case of narcissism. The quiet ego, in contrast to Greenwald's (1980) characterization of the totalitarian ego, is far more subdued (see Wirtz & Chiu, 2008). Thus, the quiet ego has been amply contrasted to the noisy, self-aggrandizing ego that requires a self-serving megaphone aimed at audiences whom one hopes will be attentive. However, often the self-promoting proclamations eventually fall on deaf ears.

In their book devoted to explorations into the quiet ego, Bauer and Wayment (2008) observe that the very need to coin such a term stems from the realization of a core problem with contemporary egotism: the individual is screaming for attention to the self. That said, the more desirable quiet ego is not totally silent. Rather, it is quiet enough to hear others and to balance their concerns with those of the self. As a counterpoint to the characteristics of the noisy ego, Bauer and Wayment suggest four defining features of the quiet ego:

1. *Detached awareness,* in which the person's awareness of self and situation is nondefensively detached from egoistic appraisals.
2. *Interdependence,* which allows one to caringly understand others' perspectives without merely conforming to their point of

view; rather, the individual maintains his/her own perspective, as well.

3. *Compassion*, which includes empathy, acceptance, and a genuine desire to foster the well-being of others.

4. *Growth*, which allows space and opportunity for the future positive ego development of both the self and others.

Kernis and Heppner (2008) add to this constellation of features the authentic functioning of the true self, mindfulness, and secure self-esteem, qualities that have been described earlier in this chapter (see also Deci & Ryan, 2000; Niemiec, Ryan, & Brown, 2008).

Neff (2008) expands upon the third quality of compassion, suggesting that quieting the ego can also enhance personal well-being by developing the capacity for *self-compassion*. In contrast to the harsh self-condemnation that often accompanies reactions to personal failures, setbacks, or suffering, self-compassion allows us to be understanding, kind, and caring about ourselves. Self-compassion, Neff points out, requires mindfulness so that one is not swept away by a tidal wave of self-derogation that flows from negative rumination. Another feature reflects an appreciation for our *common humanity* when we encounter failure that leads to personal suffering. If such experiences are only interpreted from the perspective of a "separate self," in isolation, then there is little opportunity to appreciate the fact that others have also similarly suffered, that we share such common histories.

Thich Nhat Hanh (1987), a Buddhist scholar, pursues a similar theme in suggesting that if we recognize our essential interdependence and commonalities, life's failings do not have to be taken quite so personally. In appreciating the shared nature of the human condition, one can also extend kindness and compassion to others. Wirtz and Chiu (2008) further observe that Eastern cultures are more *inclusive* in their overlapping conceptualizations of self and other. Thus, in addition to self-compassion, Easterners are therefore more tolerant and accepting of negative experiences that are shared by significant others who have been incorporated into their self-definition (see Chapter 8).

Self-compassion, Neff (2008) observes, is quite distinct from self-pity in which one's plight and suffering are overdramatized, compared to others', and where the self is viewed as quite unique and therefore separate, leading to a potential breach in the relationship. Self-compassion can also be distinguished from self-esteem. If self-esteem is fragile, fluctuating, and lacks authenticity, it can be derailed in the face of failure, whereas self-compassion is available precisely at the moment that self-esteem is likely to falter.

Others, for example, Bauer and Wayment (2008), view *humility* as self-awareness tempered by self-compassion, a combination that also contributes to the quieting of the ego. Tangney (2009), in her thoughtful treatment of humility, highlights one feature that is directly related to the quiet ego. She describes humility as a "forgetting of the self," which is *not* the denial of the self. Rather, it requires the recognition that one is but part of the larger universe, putting the self into perspective as a small cog in a much larger world wheel. That said, Tangney is quick to assert that humility is *not* self-deprecation. It involves the acceptance of one's limitations, as well as strengths; it realizes that one has a certain degree of personal power but that one is not omnipotent. Exline (2008) concurs, suggesting that this acceptance represents a nondefensive willingness to evaluate the self accurately.

Moreover, humility requires a certain relinquishment of self-focus or self-preoccupation. As Tangney (2009) explains, "A person who has gained a sense of humility is no longer phenomenologically at the center of his or her world" (p. 484). Rather, there is a focus on the larger community of which one is a part. She develops this argument, observing that in relinquishing an egocentric focus, the person with humility becomes more open to recognizing the ability and potential worth of *others,* not just the self. One turns down the *volume* of the voice of the ego. Becoming "unselved" is Tangney's term, analogous to the quiet ego. A positive consequence is that persons no longer need to pronounce, defend, and enhance the all-important self by negatively evaluating others.

Certain theorists have addressed the issue of the quiet ego from the perspective of adult models of development (Bauer, 2008; McAdams, 2008). Bauer takes as his theoretical starting point Loevinger's (1976) theory of ego development. He navigates us through Loevinger's stages in an insightful excursion, highlighting how the noisy ego, a given in the early stages of childhood (e.g., loud demands prefaced by "Me, me!"), can become progressively quieted as one moves through the levels of ego development that encompass adulthood.

The processes that define a healthy progression include (1) the increasing cognitive capacity to take the perspectives of others, (2) the ability to make moral judgments that require an understanding of rights and principles, (3) the control of impulses, (4) the development of mature defenses that replace immature mechanisms that have been abandoned, (5) an increasing relatedness to others defined as a healthy sense of mutuality and interconnectedness, (6) an identification with broader social groups, and (7) a desire for psychological growth that respects the boundaries of ego development (without the compromising trappings of self-distortion and unrealistic illusions). Gradually, these processes can lead to squelching the transcendence of self-interest and will contribute to the gradual development of a quieter ego. (Unfortunately, as we have seen, for some this developmental process can become derailed.)

McAdams (2008), in his treatment of the quiet ego, adopts Erikson's (1963) perspective, focusing on the adult stage of *generativity.* He links this stage, which concerns itself with caring for future generations, to the concept of the quiet ego, in that attention shifts to the nurturance and the promotion of the well-being of one's juniors. From this perspective, the opposite of generativity is self-preoccupation that leads to eventual personal stagnation. In McAdams's translation of Erikson, the emergence and ascendancy of a quiet ego at this stage of life requires the prior consolidation of a clear, stable, and well-defined sense of one's adult sense of self (devoid of the compromising defensive processes that have been a major focus of this chapter).

Those who consistently display excessively noisy egos are unlikely to garner social approval or to elicit compassion from others, nor have they developed the maturity (see Bauer, 2008) to engage in self-compassion (Neff, 2008). The bullhorn that blasts public messages of self-importance eventually precludes the caring attention of others. It may initially drown out haunting perceptions of personal inadequacy, failure, social rejection, and lack of self-worth that play out in defensive strategies and self-serving ploys to pump up the self. Eventually, the unacceptable negative self-perceptions that lie dangerously close to the surface can, for some, no longer be denied, their intensity cannot be muted by the psychological armor that one has donned. For many, the painful subliminal awareness of inadequacy and social rejection becomes too difficult to suppress. The defensive and protective unconscious mechanisms can finally become overwhelmed by conscious reality.

Swann (1996), in his description of "self-traps," provides a complementary explanation for why the ego cannot successfully dip into the armamentarium of self-enhancing strategies that supposedly protect the self. The thesis of Swann's *self-verification theory* is that people seek evaluations that confirm or validate their self-perceptions, be they positive or negative. His argument hinges on the assumption that people do not welcome feedback that contradicts their existing identities that provide a needed psychological blueprint for action, namely, social guideposts for how to react and behave. As counterintuitive as this position may appear, Swann provides evidence that those with low self-esteem require the unfavorable evaluations of others that verify their own negative perceptions of self. However, such perceptions can become overbearing.

As a last resort, in order to escape from such painful self-perceptions, the beleaguered ego attempts to "shrink the self" (Baumeister & Boden, 1994). Intensely negative self-awareness becomes "burdensome, stressful, distressing, and troublesome" (p. 145). I would contend that shrinking the self is the antithesis of quieting the ego, it represents an act of desperation. Pervasive and powerful negative self-perceptions of one's incompetence, unattractiveness, and social inadequacy may, for some, become overwhelming. Baumeister and Boden observe that a realistic acknowledgment of one's deficiencies can provoke anxiety, shame, and humiliation. Consistent with evidence presented in Chapter 6, these negative self-conscious emotions are most likely to be intensely experienced if personal deficiencies are internally attributed to fundamental flaws in the self (as opposed to external factors beyond one's control, such as the actions of others or chance/fate).

High levels of aversive self-awareness can ensue, necessitating the need for escape. The mental narrowing or "cognitive destruction" required to escape from the self (Baumeister, 1991) can take a variety of forms that can lead to the abuse of alcohol, drugs, and, in the extreme, suicide. Baumeister and Boden (1994) point to several features of shrinking the self that facilitate these forms of escape. For one, normal inhibitions are neutralized, fostering impulsive actions that preclude sensible planning and responsible choices. There is also a frantic need to numb one's negative emotions, given painful anxiety and distress. All of these features that characterize shrinking of the self would facilitate alcohol and drug abuse. Pyszczynski (2006) also observes that individuals who are unable to maintain an acceptable level of self-esteem will turn to alcohol and drug abuse, in order to blot out or numb the effects of anxiety. In addition to reducing the distressing levels of self-awareness, alcohol and drug users may be attracted to a like-minded subculture that provides an alternative source of approval. Of course, as Baumeister and Boden point out, suicide is the ultimate escape, obliterating the self as we know it, entirely.

Concluding Perspectives

Although illusory self-enhancement strategies would appear to represent a Western staple of life, the last decade has witnessed a proliferation of efforts to counter the self-serving biases that compromise personal well-being and interpersonal functioning. Throughout this chapter, we have encountered those who argue for what they consider more promising human pursuits. Primary are the fostering of *realistic* self-perceptions, engagement in *mindfulness,* and the pursuit of one's *authentic self.* Consider a social experience, rare perhaps, where you come away from an interpersonal situation feeling great because you realize that "I was actually myself!" If such an experience, no matter how pleasurable, is rare, one may well ask, "Then just exactly who am I being the rest of the time?" Authenticity, for many, seems to be a lost art. Many argue that it needs to be revived and incorporated into our everyday lives, with caring and *compassion* toward ourselves and others.

An entire movement, entitled "positive psychology," has mushroomed in the last decade, to counteract the negativity that has dominated the field for over a century, including maladaptive psychological processes that implicate the self. Well-being has been the new focus, with an emphasis on such virtues as happiness, hope, optimism, resilience, altruism, and gratitude, in addition to the positive attributes that have just been reviewed, namely, mindfulness, authenticity, compassion, and humility (see Lopez & Snyder, 2009, whose handbook of positive psychology maps out the entire terrain of topics). Clearly, these efforts turn the field, broadly conceived, on its head. For example, after several publications on false-self behavior, I was asked to write a piece on authenticity, its antithesis, and it was refreshing to consider the more redeeming features of the human condition.

Obviously, a comprehensive review of the many features that define the positive psychology literature is beyond the scope of this volume, as it comes to a close. However, it is noteworthy that these contemporary antidotes to the negative characterization of the self-serving ego represent a breath of fresh air. They provide a needed sense of balance that should guide further inquiry and soften our indictment of the self. The accused is guilty on several counts, to be sure. However, perhaps as judges we should exercise some compassion and grant leniency, not life in prison, merely sentencing the ego to parole.

References

Adams, R., & Bukowski, W. (2008). Peer victimization as a predictor of depression and body mass in obese and non-obese adolescents. *Journal of Child Psychology and Psychiatry, 49*, 858–866.

Ainsworth, M. (1979). Infant–mother attachment. *American Psychologist, 34*, 932–937.

Alcohol, Drug Abuse, and Mental Health Administration. (1989) *Report of the Secretary's Task Force on Youth Suicide* (DHHS Publication No. ADM 89–1621). Washington, DC: U.S. Government Printing Office.

Alessandri, S. M., & Lewis, M. (1993). Parental evaluation and its relation to shame and pride in young children. *Sex Roles, 29*, 335–343.

Alicke, M. D., Klotz, M. L., Breitenbecher, D. L. Yurak, T. J., & Vredenburg, D. S. (1995). Personal contact, individuation, and the better-than-average effect. *Journal of Personality and Social Psychology, 68*, 804–825.

Allen, J. P. (2008). The attachment system in adolescence. In J. Cassidy & P. R. Shaver (Eds.), *Handbook of attachment: Theory, research, and clinical applications* (2nd ed., pp. 419–435). New York: Guilford Press.

Allen, J. P., Hauser, S. T., Bell, K. L., & O'Connor, T. G. (1994). Longitudinal assessment of autonomy and relatedness in adolescent–family interactions as predictors of adolescent ego development and self-esteem. *Child Development, 64*, 179–194.

Allen, J. P., Kuperminc, G., Philliber, S., & Herre, K. (1994). Programmatic prevention of adolescent problem behaviors: The role of autonomy, relatedness, and volunteer service in the Teen Outreach Program. *American Journal of Community Psychology, 22*, 617–638.

Allen, K., Byrne, S., Blair, E., & Davis, E. (2006). Why do some overweight children experience psychological problems? The role of weight and shape concern. *International Journal of Pediatric Obesity, 14*, 239–247.

Allport, G. W. (1961). *Pattern and growth in personality*. New York: Holt, Rinehart & Winston.

American Association of University Women. (1992). *How schools shortchange girls*. Washington, DC: American Association of University Women Educational Foundation.

American Psychiatric Association. (2000). *Diagnostic and statistical manual of mental disorders* (4th ed., text rev.). Washington, DC: Author.

American Society for Aesthetic Plastic Surgery. (2008). *2008 statistics*. Washington, DC: American Association of University Women Education Foundation. Available at *www.surgery.org/sites/default/files/2008stats.pdf*.

Amodio, D., Devine, P., & Harmon-Jones, E. (2007). A dynamic model of guilt: Implications for motivation and self-regulation in the context of prejudice. *Psychological Science, 18*, 524–530.

Anderson-Fye, E. (2004). A Coca-Cola shape: Cultural change, body image, and eating disorders in San Andres, Belize. *Culture, Medicine, and Psychiatry, 28*, 561–595.

Anderson-Fye, E. P., & Becker, A. E. (2004). Sociocultural aspects of eating disorders. In J. K. Thompson (Ed.), *Handbook of eating disorders and obesity* (pp. 565–589). New York: Wiley.

Arnett, J. J. (1997). Young people's conceptions of the transition to adulthood. *Youth and Society, 29*, 1–23.

Arnett, J. J. (2000). Emerging adulthood: A theory of development from the late teens through the twenties. *American Psychologist, 55*, 469–480.

Arnett, J. J. (2001). Conceptions of the transition to adulthood: Perspectives from adolescence to midlife. *Journal of Adult Development, 8*, 133–143.

Arnett, J. J. (2003). Conceptions of the transition to adulthood among emerging adults in American ethnic groups. In J. Arnett & N. Galambos (Eds.), *New directions for child and adolescent development: Cultural conceptions of the transition to adulthood* (pp. 63–75). Chichester, UK: Wiley.

Arnett, J. J. (2007). *Adolescence and emerging adulthood: A cultural approach* (3rd ed.) Upper Saddle River, NJ: Pearson/Prentice Hall.

Arnett, J. J. (2010). *Adolescence and emerging adulthood: A cultural approach* (4th ed.). Upper Saddle River, NJ: Pearson/Prentice Hall.

Arnett, J. J., Kloep, M., Hendry, L. B., & Tanner, J. L. (Eds.). (2011). *Debating emerging adulthood: Stage or process?* New York: Oxford University Press.

Arnett, J. J., & Tanner, J. L. (2011). Themes and variations in emerging adulthood across social class. In J. J.Arnett, M. Kloep, L. B. Hendry, & J. L. Tanner (Eds.), *Debating emerging adulthood: Stage or process?* (pp. 31–52). New York: Oxford University Press.

Aronfreed, J. (1976). Moral development from the standpoint of a general psychological theory. In J. Lickona (Ed.), *Moral development and behavior* (pp. 54–69). New York: Holt, Rinehart & Winston.

Asendorpf, J. B., & van Aken, M. A. G. (1993). Deutsche versionen der Selbstkonzeptskalen von Harter. *Zeitscrift für Entwicklungspychologie und Padagogische Psychologie, 25*, 64–86.

Ashmore, R. D., & Ogilvie, D. M. (1992). He's such a nice boy ... when he's with Grandma: Gender and evaluation in self-worth-other representations. In T. M. Brinthaupt & R. P. Lipka (Eds.), *The self: Definitional and methodological issues* (pp. 236–290). Albany: State University of New York Press.

Badanes, L., & Harter, S. (2007a, April). *Consistency of attachment styles across relational contexts: Implications for the self-system in college students.* Poster session at the biannual meeting of the Society for Research on Adolescence, San Francisco, CA.

Badanes, L., & Harter, S. (2007b, April). *Do high and low self-monitors differ with regard to the nature of their multiple selves?* Poster session at the biannual meeting of the Society for Research on Adolescence, San Francisco, CA.

Baile, G. (2006). The imitative self: The contribution of Rene Girard. In P. C. Vitz & S. M. Felch (Eds.), *The self: Beyond the postmodern crisis* (pp. 3–24). Wilmington, DE: ISI Books.

Baldwin, J. M. (1895). *Mental development of the child and the race: Methods and processes.* New York: Macmillan.

Baldwin, M. W., Keelan, J., Fehr, B., Enns, V., & Koh-Rangarajoo, E. (1996). Social-cognitive conceptualization of attachment working models: Availability and accessibility effects. *Journal of Personality and Social Psychology, 71,* 94–104.

Bandura, A. (1977). Self-efficacy: Toward a unifying theory of behavioral change. *Psychological Review, 84,* 191–215.

Bandura, A. (1991). Self-regulation of motivation through anticipatory and self-regulatory mechanisms. In R. A. Dienstbier (Ed.), *Nebraska Symposium on Motivation: Vol. 38. Perspectives on motivation* (pp. 79–94). Lincoln: University of Nebraska Press.

Bandura, A., Caprara, G. V., Barbaranelli, C., Gerbino, M., & Pastorelli, C. (2003). Role of affective self-regulatory efficacy in diverse spheres of psychosocial functioning. *Child Development, 74,* 769–782.

Bardenstein, K. K. (2009). The cracked mirror: Features of narcissistic personality disorder in children. *Psychiatric Annals, 39,* 147–155.

Bargh, J. A., McKenna, K. Y. A., & Fitzsimons, G. M. (2002). Can you see the real me? Activation and expression of the "true self" on the internet. *Journal of Social Issues, 58,* 33–48.

Barlett, C., & Harris, R. (2008). The impact of body-impacting video games on body image concerns in men and women. *Sex Roles, 59,* 586–601.

Barnett, D., Ganiban, J., & Cicchetti, D. (1999). Maltreatment, negative expressivity, and the development of type D attachments from 12 to 24 months of age. In J. Vondra & D. Barnett (Eds.), Atypical patterns of infant attachment: Theory, research, and current directions. *Monographs of the Society for Research in Child Development, 64*(3), 97–118.

Barrett, K. C. (1995). A functionalist approach to shame and guilt. In J. P. Tangney & K. F. Fischer (Eds.), *Self-conscious emotions: The psychology of shame, guilt, embarrassment, and pride* (pp. 25–63). New York: Guilford Press.

Barrett, K. C., & Campos, J. J. (1987). Perspectives on emotional development: II. A functionalist approach to emotions. In J. Osofsky (Ed.), *Handbook of infant development* (2nd ed., pp. 555–578). New York: Wiley.

Barry, C. T., Frick, P. J., Adler, K. K., & Grafeman, S. J. (2007). The predictive utility of narcissism among children and adolescents: Evidence for a distinction between adaptive and maladaptive narcissism. *Journal of Child and Family Studies, 16,* 508–521.

Barry, C. T., Frick, P. J., & Killian, A. L. (2003). The relation of narcissism and self-esteem to conduct problems in children: A preliminary investigation. *Journal of Clinical Child and Adolescent Psychology, 32,* 139–152.

Barry, C. T., & Malkin, M. L. (2010). The relation between adolescent narcissism and internalizing problems depends on the conceptualization of narcissism. *Journal of Research in Personality, 44,* 684–690.

Bassen, C., & Lamb, M. (2006). Gender differences in adolescents' self-concepts of assertion and affiliation. *European Journal of Developmental Psychology, 3,* 71–94.

Bates, E. (1990). Language about me and you: Pronominal reference and the emerging concept of self. In D. Cicchetti & M. Beeghly (Eds.), *The self in transition: Infancy to childhood* (pp. 1–15). Hillsdale, NJ: Erlbaum.

Bauer, J. J. (2008). How the ego quiets as it grows: Ego development, growth stories, and eudaimonic personality development. In H. A. Wayment & J. J. Bauer (Eds.), *Transcending self-interest: Psychological explorations of the quiet ego* (pp. 199–210). Washington, DC: American Psychological Association.

Bauer, J. J., & Wayment, H. A. (2008). The psychology of the quiet ego. In H. A. Wayment & J. J. Bauer (Eds.), *Transcending self-interest: Psychological explorations of the quiet ego* (pp. 7–20). Washington, DC: American Psychological Association.

Baumeister, R. F. (1987). How the self became a problem: A psychological review of historical research. *Journal of Personality and Social Psychology, 52,* 163–176.

Baumeister, R. F. (1991). *Escaping the self: Alcoholism, spirituality, masochism, and other flights from the burden of selfhood.* New York: Basic Books.

Baumeister, R. F. (1996). Should schools try to boost self-esteem? Beware the dark side. *American Educator, 43,* 14–19.

Baumeister, R. F., & Boden, J. M. (1994). Shrinking the self. In T. M. Brinthaupt & R. P. Lipka (Eds.), *Changing the self: Philosophies, techniques, and experiences.* Albany: State University of New York Press.

Baumeister, R. F., & Bushman, B. (2007). Angry emotions and aggressive behaviors. In G. Steffgen & M. Gollwitzer (Eds.), *Emotions and aggressive behavior* (pp. 61–75). Ashland, OH: Hogrefe & Huber.

Baumeister, R. F., Campbell, J. D., Krueger, J. I., & Vohs, K. D. (2003). Does high self-esteem cause better performance, interpersonal success, happiness, or healthier lifestyles? *Psychological Sciences in the Public Interest, 4,* 1–44.

Baumeister, R. F., Smart, L., & Boden, J. M. (1996). Relation of threatened egotism to violence and aggression: The dark side of self-esteem. *Psychological Review, 103,* 5–33.

Baumeister, R. F., Stillwell, A. M., & Heatherton, T. F. (1994). Guilt: An interpersonal approach. *Psychological Bulletin, 115,* 243–267.

Baumeister, R. F., & Vohs, K. D. (2001). Narcissism as addiction to esteem. *Psychological Inquiry, 12,* 206–210.

Baumrind, D. (1971). Current patterns of parental authority. *Developmental Psychology Monographs, 4,* 1–102.

Baumrind, D. (1996). The discipline controversy revisited. *Family Relations: Journal of Applied Family and Child Studies, 45,* 405–414.

Beane, J. A. (1994). Cluttered terrain: The schools' interest in the self. In T. M.

Brinthaupt & R. P. Lipka (Eds.), *Changing the self: Philosophies, techniques, and experiences* (pp. 69–89). Albany: State University of New York Press.

Bechtold, J. (2006). Technology and the self: Approaching the transmodern. In P. C. Vitz & S. M. Felch (Eds.), *The self: Beyond the postmodern crisis* (pp. 183–202). Wilmington, DE: ISI Books.

Becker, A. E. (1995). *Body, self, and society.* Philadelphia: University of Pennsylvania Press.

Beeghly, M., Carlson, V., & Cicchetti, D. (1986, April). *Child maltreatment and the self: The emergence of internal state language in low SES 30-month olds.* Paper presented at the International Conference on Infant Studies, Beverly Hills, CA.

Bell, B., Lawton, R., & Dittmar, H. (2007). The impact of thin models in music videos on adolescent girls' body dissatisfaction. *Body Image, 4,* 137–145.

Bellmore, A. D., & Cillessen, A. H. (2006). Reciprocal influences of victimization, perceived social preference, and self-concept in adolescence. *Self and Identity, 3,* 209–229.

Bem, S. (1985). Androgeny and gender schema theory. In T. B. Sonderegger (Ed.), *Nebraska Symposium on Motivation* (Vol. 32, pp. 180–226). Lincoln: University of Nebraska Press.

Benson, H. (1975). *The relaxation response.* New York: Morrow.

Benson, H. (1984). *Beyond the relaxation response.* New York: Times Books.

Berry, J. W. (1969). On cross-cultural comparability. *International Journal of Psychology, 4,* 119–128.

Berry, J. W. (1980). Acculturation as varieties of adaptation. In A. M. Padilla (Ed.), *Acculturation: Theory, models and some new findings* (pp. 9–25). Boulder, CO: Westview Press.

Berry, J. W. (2005). Acculturation. In W. Friedlmeier, P. Chakkarath, & B. Schwartz (Eds.), *Culture and human development* (pp. 291–302). New York: Psychology Press.

Bertenthal, B. L., & Fischer, K. W. (1978). Development of self-recognition in the infant. *Developmental Psychology, 14,* 44–50.

Bjorklund, D. F. (2007). *Why youth is not wasted on the young: Immaturity in human development.* Oxford, UK: Blackwell.

Blaine, B., & Crocker, J. (1993). Self-esteem and self-serving biases in reactions to positive and negative events: An integrative review. In R. F. Baumeister (Ed.), *Self-esteem: The puzzle of low self-regard* (pp. 55–85). Hillsdale, NJ: Erlbaum.

Bleiberg, E. (1984). Narcissistic disorders in children. *Bulletin of the Menniger Clinic, 48,* 501–517.

Bleiberg, E. (1994). Normal and pathological narcissism in adolescence. *American Journal of Psychotherapy, 48,* 29–51.

Blond, A., Whitaker, A., Lorenz, J., Nieto, M., & Pinto-Martin, J. (2008). Weight concerns in male low birth weight adolescents: Relation to body mass index, self-esteem, and depression. *Journal of Developmental and Behavioral Pediatrics, 29,* 166–172.

Blos, P. (1962). *On adolescence.* New York: Free Press.

Boekaerts, M., & Roder, I. (1999). Stress, coping, and adjustment in children with a chronic disease: A review of the literature. *Disability and Rehabilitation Multidisciplinary Journal, 21,* 311–337.

Bolognini, M., Plancheral, B., Bettschart, W., & Halfon, O. (1996). Self-esteem and mental health in early adolescence: Development and gender differences, *Journal of Adolescence, 19,* 233–245.

Bornstein, M. H., Tamis-LeMonda, C. S., Tal, J., Ludeman, P., Toda, S., & Rahn, C. W. (1992). Maternal responsiveness to infants in three societies: The United States, France, and Japan. *Child Development, 63,* 808–821.

Bowlby, J. (1973). *Attachment and loss: Vol. 2. Separation.* New York: Basic Books.

Bowlby, J. (1979). *The making and breaking of affectional bonds.* London: Tavistock.

Bowlby, J. (1988). *A secure base.* New York: Basic Books.

Boyes, A., Fletcher, G., & Latner, J. (2007). Male and female body image and dieting in the context of intimate relationships. *Journal of Family Psychology, 21,* 764–768.

Brake, D. L. (2010). *Getting in the game: Title IX and the women's sports revolution.* New York: New York University Press.

Bretherton, I. (1990). Open communication and internal working models: Their role in the development of attachment relationships. In R. A. Thompson (Ed.), *Nebraska Symposium on Motivation: Vol. 36. Socio-emotional development* (pp. 59–113). Lincoln: University of Nebraska Press.

Bretherton, I. (1991). Pouring new wine into old bottles: The social self as internal working model. In M. R. Gunnar & L. A. Sroufe (Eds.), *Minnesota Symposium on Child Psychology: Vol. 23. Self-processes and development* (pp. 1–41). Hillsdale, NJ: Erlbaum.

Bretherton, I. (1993). From dialogue to internal working models: The co-construction of self in relationships. In C. A. Nelson (Ed.), *Minnesota Symposium on Child Psychology: Vol. 26. Memory and affect* (pp. 237–263). Hillsdale, NJ: Erlbaum.

Bretherton, I., & Beeghly, M. (1982). Talking about internal states: The acquisition of an explicit theory of mind. *Developmental Psychology, 18,* 529–548.

Bretherton, I., & Munholland, K. A. (2008). Internal working models in attachment relationships: Elaborating a central construct. In J. Cassidy & P. R. Shaver (Eds.), *Handbook of attachment: Theory, research, and clinical applications* (2nd ed., pp. 102–130). New York: Guilford Press.

Bridges, L. J., Connell, J. P., & Belsky, J. (1988). Similarities and differences in infant–mother and infant–father interaction in the strange situation: A component process analysis. *Developmental Psychology, 24,* 92–100.

Briere, J. (1989). *Therapy for adults molested as children.* New York: Springer.

Briere, J. (1992). *Child abuse trauma: Theory and treatment of the lasting effects.* Newbury Park, CA: Sage.

Brim, O. B. (1976). Life span development of a theory of oneself: Implications for child development. In H. W. Reese (Ed.), *Advances in child development and behavior* (Vol. 11, pp. 82–103). New York: Academic Press.

Brown, B. B. (1990). Peer groups and peer cultures. In S. S. Feldman & G. Elliot (Eds.), *At the threshold: The developing adolescent* (pp. 171–196). Cambridge, MA: Harvard University Press.

Brown, R. (2008). American and Japanese beliefs about self-esteem. *Asian Journal of Social Psychology, 11,* 293–299.

Brown, R. P., & Zeigler-Hill, V. (2004). Narcissism and the non-equivalence of self-esteem measures: A matter of dominance? *Journal of Research in Personality, 38,* 585–592.

Bruner, J. (1990). *Acts of meaning.* Cambridge, MA: Harvard University Press.

Buchmann, M. (1989). *The script of life in modern society: Entry into adulthood in a changing world.* Chicago: Chicago University Press.

Bukowski, W. M., Schwartzman, A., Santo, J., Bagwell, C., & Adams, R. (2009). Reactivity and distortions in the self: Narcissism, types of aggression, and the functioning of the hypothalamic–pituitary–adrenal axis during early adolescence. *Development and Psychopathology, 21,* 1249–1262.

Bushman, B. J., & Baumeister, R. F. (1998). Threatened egotism, narcissism, self-esteem, and direct and displaced aggression: Does self love or self-hate lead to violence? *Journal of Personality and Social Psychology, 75,* 219–229.

Buss, A. H. (1980). *Self-consciousness and social anxiety.* San Francisco: Freeman.

California Task Force to Promote Self-Esteem and Personal and Social Responsibility. (1990). *Toward a state of self-esteem.* Sacramento: California State Department of Education.

Campbell, J. D., Trapnell, P. D., Heine, S., Katz, I. M., Lavallee, L. F., & Lehman, D. R. (1996). Self-concept clarity: Measurement, personality correlates, and cultural boundaries. *Journal of Personality and Social Psychology, 70,* 141–156.

Campbell, W. K., & Buffardi, L. E. (2008). The lure of the noisy ego: Narcissism as a social trap. In H. A. Wayment & J. J. Bauer (Eds.), *Transcending self-interest.* Washington, DC: American Psychological Association.

Campbell, W. K., Foster, J., & Brunell, A. (2004). Running from shame or reveling in pride? Narcissism and the regulation of self-conscious emotions. *Psychological Inquiry, 15,* 150–153.

Campbell, W. K., Goodie, A. S., & Foster, J. D. (2004). Narcissism, confidence, and risk attitude. *Journal of Behavioral Decision Making, 17,* 297–311.

Campbell, W. K., & Green, J. D. (2008). Narcissism and interpersonal self-regulation. In J. V. Wood, A. Tesser, & J. G. Holmes (Eds.), *The self in social relationships* (pp. 73–94). New York: Psychology Press.

Campos, J. J., & Sternberg, C. (1980). Perception, appraisal, and emotion: The onset of social referencing. In M. Lamb & L. Sherrod (Eds.), *Infant social cognition* (pp. 273–314). Hillsdale, NJ: Erlbaum.

Carlson, K. S., & Gjerde, P. F. (2009). Preschool personality antecedents of narcissism in adolescence and young adulthood: A 20-year longitudinal study. *Journal of Research in Personality, 43,* 570–578.

Carlson, V., Cicchetti, D., Barnett, D., & Braunwald, K. (1989). Finding order in disorganization. In D. Cicchetti & V. Carlson (Eds.), *Child maltreatment: Theory and research on the causes and consequences of child abuse and neglect* (pp. 494–528). New York: Cambridge University Press.

Carlson, V. J., & Harwood, R. L. (2003). Attachment, culture, and the caregiving system: The cultural patterning of everyday experience among Anglo and Puerto Rican mother–infant pairs. *Infant Mental Health Journal, 24,* 53–73.

Carnegie Council on Adolesccent Development (1989). *Turning points: Preparing American youth for the 21st century.* Washington, DC: Author.

Carroll, J. J., & Steward, M. S. (1984). The role of cognitive development in children's understandings of their own feelings. *Child Development, 55,* 1486–1492.

Case, R. (1985). *Intellectual development: Birth to adulthood.* New York: Academic Press.

Case, R. (1991). Stages in the development of the young child's first sense of self. *Developmental Review, 11,* 210–230.

Case, R. (1992). *The mind's staircase.* Hillsdale, NJ: Erlbaum.

Cassidy, J., & Kobak, R. R. (1988). Avoidance and its relationship to other defensive processes. In J. Belsky & T. Nezworski (Eds.), *Clinical implications of attachment* (pp. 300–326). Hillsdale, NJ: Erlbaum.

Chandler, C. (1981). *The effects of parenting techniques on the development of motivational orientation in children.* Unpublished doctoral dissertation, University of Denver, Denver, CO.

Chandler, M. J., Lalonde, C. E., Sokol, B. W., & Hallett, D. (2003). Personal persistence, identity development, and suicide: A study of native and non-native North American adolescents. *Monographs of the Society for Research in Child Development, 68,* (2, Series No. 273).

Chao, R. K. (1996). Chinese and European American mothers' views about the role of parenting in children's school success. *Journal of Cross-Cultural Psychology, 27,* 403–423.

Chao, R. K. (2000). Cultural explanations for the role of parenting in the school success of Asian American children. In R. Taylor & M. Wang (Eds.), *Resilience across contexts: Family, work, culture, and community* (pp. 333–363). Mahwah, NJ: Erlbaum.

Chen, A., & Ennis, C. D. (2009). Motivation and achievement in physical education. In K. R. Wentzel & A. Wigfield (Eds.), *Handbook of motivation at school* (pp. 553–576). New York: Routledge (Taylor & Francis Group).

Cheung, M., Gilbert, P., & Irons, C. (2004). An exploration of shame, social rank and rumination in relation to depression. *Personality and Individual Differences, 36,* 1143–1153.

Chodorow, N. (1989). *Feminism and psychoanalytic theory.* New Haven, CT: Yale University Press.

Cicchetti, D. (1989). How research on child maltreatment has informed the study of child development: Perspectives from developmental psychology. In D. Cicchetti & V. Carlson (Eds.), *Child maltreatment: Theory and research on the causes and consequences of child abuse and neglect* (pp. 309–350). New York: Cambridge University Press.

Cicchetti, D. (2004). An odyssey of discovery: Lessons learned through three decades of research on child maltreatment. *American Psychologist, 59,* 728–741.

Cicchetti, D., & Rogosch, F. A. (1996). Equfinality and multifinality in developmental psychopathology. *Development and Psychopathology, 8,* 597–600.

Cicchetti, D., & Toth, S. (2006). Developmental psychopathology and preventive intervention. In W. Damon & R. M. Lerner (Eds.), & K. A. Renninger & I. E.

Sigel (Vol. Eds.) *Handbook of child psychology: Vol. 4. Child psychology in practice* (6th ed., pp. 497–547). New York: Wiley.

Clark, L., & Tiggemann, M. (2008). Sociocultural and individual psychological predictors of body image in young girls: A prospective study. *Developmental Psychology, 44,* 1124–1134.

Clay, D., Vignoles, V., & Dittmar, H. (2005). Body image and self-esteem among adolescent girls: Testing the influence of sociocultural factors. *Journal of Research on Adolescence, 15,* 451–477.

Connell, J. P. (1981). *A model of the relationships among children's self-related cognitions, affects and academic achievement.* Unpublished doctoral dissertation, University of Denver, Denver, CO.

Connell, J. P., & Wellborn, J. G. (1991). Competence, autonomy, and relatedness: A motivational analysis of self-system processes. In M. R. Gunnar & L. A. Sroufe (Eds.), *Minnesota Symposium on Child Psychology: Vol. 23. Self-processes and development* (pp. 125–166). Hillsdale, NJ: Erlbaum.

Cook-Cottone, C., & Phelps, L. (2006). Adolescent eating disorders. Children's needs III: Development, prevention, and intervention (pp. 977–988). Washington, DC: National Association of School Psychologists.

Cooley, C. H. (1902). *Human nature and the social order.* New York: Schribners.

Cooper, C. R. (2011). *Bridging multiple worlds: Cultures, youth identities, and pathways to college.* New York: Oxford University Press.

Cooper, C. R., Grotevant, H. D., & Condon, S. M. (1983). Individuality and connectedness both foster adolescent identity formation and role taking skills. In H. D. Grotevant & C. R. Cooper (Eds.), *Adolescent development in the family: New directions for child development* (pp. 43–59). San Francisco: Jossey-Bass.

Cooper, C. R., Jackson, J. F., Azmitia, M., Lopez, E., & Dunbar, N. (1995). Bridging students' multiple worlds: African American and Latino youth in academic outreach programs. In R. F. Macias & R. G. Garcia-Ramos (Eds.), *Changing schools for changing students: An anthology of research on language minorities* (pp. 211–234). Santa Barbara: University of California Linguistic Minority Research Institute.

Coster, W. J., Gersten, M. S., Beeghly, M., & Cicchetti, D. (1989). Communicative functioning in maltreated toddlers. *Developmental Psychology, 25,* 1020–1029.

Cote, J. E. (1996). Identity: A multidimensional analysis. In G. R. Adams, R. Montemayor, & T. P. Gulotta (Eds.), *Psychosocial development in adolescence: Advances in adolescent development* (pp. 130–180). Thousand Oaks, CA: Sage.

Cote, J. E. (2009). Identity formation and self-development in adolescence. In R. M. Lerner & L. Steinberg (Eds.), *Handbook of adolescent psychology* (3rd ed., Vol. 1, pp. 266–304). New York: Wiley.

Covington, M. (1984). The self-worth theory of achievement motivation: Findings and implications. *Elementary School Journal, 85,* 5–20.

Covington, M. (2006). How can optimal self-esteem be facilitated in children and adolescents by parents and teachers? In M. H. Kernis (Ed.), *Self-esteem: Issues and answers* (pp. 244–250). New York: Psychology Press.

Covington, M. (2009). Self-worth theory: Retrospection and prospects. In K. R.

Wentzel & A. Wigfield (Eds.), *Handbook of motivation at school* (pp. 141–170). New York: Routledge (Taylor & Francis Group).

Cozzarelli, C., Hoekstra, S., & Bylsma, W. (2000). General versus specific mental models of attachment: Are they associated with different outcomes? *Personality and Social Psychology Bulletin, 26,* 605–618.

Crawford, T. N., Cohen, P., & Brook, J. S. (2001). Dramatic-erratic personality disorder symptoms: II. Developmental pathways from early adolescence to adulthood. *Journal of Personality Disorders, 15,* 336–350.

Crittenden, P. M. (1994). Peering into the black box: An exploratory treatise on the development of self in your children. In D. Cicchetti & S. L. Toth (Eds.), *Rochester Symposium on Developmental Psychopathology: Vol. 6. Disorder and dysfunctions of the self* (pp. 79–148). Rochester, NY: University of Rochester Press.

Crittenden, P. M., & Ainsworth, M. D. S. (1989). Child maltreatment and attachment theory. In D. Cicchetti & V. Carlson (Eds.), *Child maltreatment: Theory and research on the causes and consequences of child abuse and neglect* (pp. 432–463). New York: Cambridge University Press.

Crocker, J. (2006a). Having and pursuing self-esteem: Costs and benefits? In M. H. Kernis (Ed.), *Self-esteem: Issues and answers* (pp. 274–280). New York: Psychology Press.

Crocker, J. (2006b). What is optimal self-esteem? In M. H. Kernis (Ed.), *Self-esteem: Issues and answers* (pp. 119–124). New York: Psychology Press.

Crocker, J., & Park, L. E. (2004). The costly pursuit of self-esteem. *Psychological Bulletin, 130,* 392–414.

Crocker, J., & Wolfe, C. T. (2001). Contingencies of self-worth. *Psychological Review, 108,* 593–623.

Crocker, P. R. E., & Ellsworth, J. P. (1990). Perceptions of competence in physical education students. *Canadian Journal of Sports Science, 15,* 262–266.

Cross, S. E., & Gore, J. S. (2003). Cultural models of the self. In M. R. Leary & J. P. Tangney (Eds.), *Handbook of self and identity* (pp. 536–566). New York: Guilford Press.

Cross, S. E., & Markus, H. R. (1999). The cultural constitution of personality. In L. Pervin & O. John (Eds.), *Handbook of personality and research* (2nd ed., pp. 378–396). New York: Guilford Press.

Cushman, P. (1995). *Constructing the self, constructing America: A cultural history of psychotherapy.* New York: Addison Wesley.

Dahl, R. E. (2004). Adolescent brain development: A period of vulnerabilities and opportunities. In R. E. Dahl & L. P. Spear (Eds.), *Adolescent brain development: Vulnerabilities and opportunities* (pp. 1–22). New York: New York Academy of Sciences.

D'Amico, A., Carmeci, F., & Cardaci, M. (2006). The self-concept beliefs: Self-referential and comparative frames of reference. In A. P. Prescott (Ed.), *The concept of self in education, family and sports* (pp. 179–189). Hauppauge, NY: Nova Science.

Damon, W. (1995). *Greater expectations: Overcoming the culture of indulgence in America's homes and schools.* New York: Free Press.

Damon, W., & Hart, D. (1988). *Self-understanding in childhood and adolescence.* New York: Cambridge University Press.

Danis, B., & Harter, S. (1996). *Self-perceptions of anorectic and bulimic female college students.* Unpublished manuscript, University of Denver, Denver, CO.

Davison, T., & McCabe, M. (2006). Adolescent body image and psychological functioning. *Journal of Social Psychology, 146,* 15–30.

Dawson, T. L., Fischer, K. W., & Stein, Z. (2006). Reconsidering qualitative and quantitative research approaches: A cognitive developmental perspective. *New Ideas in Psychology, 24,* 229–239.

Deci, E. L. (1975). *Intrinsic motivation.* New York: Plenum Press.

Deci, E. L., & Ryan, R. M. (1985). *Intrinsic motivation and self-determination in human Behavior.* New York: Plenum.

Deci, E. L., & Ryan, R. M. (1991). A motivational approach to self: Integration in personality. In R. Diensbier (Ed.), *Nebraska Symposium on Motivation: Vol. 38. Perspectives on motivation* (pp. 237–288). Lincoln: University of Nebraska Press.

Deci, E. L., & Ryan, R. M. (2000). The "what" and the "why" of goal pursuits: Human needs and the self-determination of behavior. *Psychological Inquiry, 11,* 227–268.

DeKlyen, M., & Greenberg, M. T. (2008). Attachment and psychopathology in childhood. In J. Cassidy & P. R. Shaver (Eds.), *Handbook of attachment: Theory, research, and clinical applications* (2nd ed., pp. 1637–1665). New York: Guilford Press.

Denmark, F., Klara, M., & Baron, E. (2008). Bullying and hazing: A form of campus harassment. In M. A. Paludi (Ed.), *Understanding and preventing campus violence* (pp. 27–40). Westport, CT: Praeger Greenwood Group.

Dennison, S., & Stewart, A. (2006). Facing rejection: New relationships, broken relationships, shame, and stalking. *International Journal of Offender Therapy and Comparative Criminology, 50,* 324–337.

De Rubeis, S., & Hollenstein, T. (2009). Individual differences in shame and depressive symptoms during early adolescence. *Personality and Individual Differences, 46,* 477–482.

Devos, T. (2006). Implicit bicultural identity among Mexican American and Asian American college students. *Cultural Diversity and Ethnic Minority Psychology, 12,* 381–402.

Dickstein, E. (1977). Self and self-esteem: Theoretical foundations and their implications for research, *Human Development, 20,* 129–140.

Diener, E., & Diener, M. (2009). Cross-cultural correlates of life satisfaction and self-esteem. In E. Diener (Ed.), *The collective works of Ed Diener* (pp. 71–91). New York: Springer Science and Business Media.

Dohnt, H., & Tiggemann, M. (2006). The contribution of peer and media influences to the development of body satisfaction and self-esteem in young girls: A prospective study. *Developmental Psychology, 42,* 929–936.

Donaldson, S. K., & Westerman, M. A. (1986). Development of children's understanding of ambivalence and causal theories of emotion. *Developmental Psychology, 22,* 655–662.

Dost, A., & Yagmurlu, B. (2008). Are constructiveness and destructiveness essential features of guilt and shame feelings respectively? *Journal for the Theory of Social Behavior, 38,* 109–129.

DuBois, D. L., Burk-Braxton, C., Swenson, L. P., Tevendale, H. D., Lockerd, E. M., & Moran, B. L. (2002). Getting by with a little help from self and others: Self-esteem and social support as resources during early adolescence. *Developmental Psychology, 18,* 822–839.

DuBois, D. L., & Flay, B. R. (2004). The healthy pursuit of self-esteem: Comment on an alternative to the Crocker and Park (2004) formulation. *Psychological Bulletin, 130,* 415–420.

DuBois, D. L., & Tevendale, H. D. (1999). Self-esteem in childhood and adolescence: Vaccine or epiphemenon? *Applied and Preventitive Psychology, 8,* 103–117.

Duncan, M., Al-Nakeeb, Y., Jones, M., & Nevill, A. (2007). Body image, adiposity, and physical activity in British children. *Advances in Psychology Research, 50,* 99–113.

Duncan, M., Al-Nakeeb, Y., & Woodfield, L. (2008). Relationships between body esteem, objectively measured physical activity, and anthropometry in children. In M. P. Simmons & L. A. Foster (Eds.), *Sport and exercise psychology research advances* (pp. 1–8). Hauppauge, NY: Nova Biomedical Books.

Dunn, J. (1988). *The beginnings of social understanding.* Cambridge, MA: Harvard University Press.

Dunn, J., Brown, J., & Beardsall, L. (1991). Family talk about feeling states and children's later understanding of others' emotions. *Developmental Psychology, 27,* 445–448.

Dunning, D. (2003). The relation of self to social perception. In M. R. Leary & J. P. Tangney (Eds.), *Handbook of self and identity* (pp. 421–444). New York: Guilford Press.

Dweck, C. S. (1986). Motivational processes affecting learning. *American Psychologist, 41,* 1040–1048.

Dweck, C. S. (1999). *Self-theories: Their role in motivation, personality, and development.* Philadelphia: Psychology Press.

Dweck, C. S., & Grant, H. (2008). Self-theories, goals, and meaning. In J. Y. Shah & W. L. Gardner (Eds.). *Handbook of motivation science* (pp. 405–416). New York: Guilford Press.

Dweck, C. S., & Leggett, E. L. (1988). A social-cognitive approach to motivation and personality. *Psychological Review, 95,* 256–273.

Dweck, C. S., & Master, A. (2009). Self-theories and motivation: Students' beliefs about intelligence. In K. R. Wentzel & A. Wigfield (Eds.), *Handbook of motivation at school* (pp. 123–140). New York: Routledge (Taylor & Francis Group).

Eccles, J. S., & Blumenfeld, P. (1985). Classroom experiences and student gender: Are there differences and do they matter. In L. C. Wilkinson & C. B. Marrett (Eds.), *Gender influences in classroom interaction* (pp. 79–114). Orlando, FL: Academic Press.

Eccles, J. S., & Midgley, C. (1989). Stage/environment fit: Developmentally appropriate classrooms for early adolescents. In R. Ames & C. Ames (Eds.), *Research on motivation in education* (Vol. 3, pp. 139–181). San Diego, CA: Academic Press.

Eccles, J. S., Midgley, C., & Adler, T. (1984). Grade-related changes in the school environment: Effects on achievement motivation. In J. G. Nicholls (Ed.), *The development of achievement motivation* (pp. 283–331). Greenwich, CT: JAI Press.

Eccles, J. S., & Roeser, R. W. (2009). Schools, academic motivation, and stage-environment fit. In R. M. Lerner & L. Steinberg (Eds.), *The handbook of adolescent psychology: Vol. I. Individual bases of adolescent development.* (3rd ed., pp. 404–434). New York: Wiley.

Eccles, J. S., Wigfield, A., & Schiefele, U. (1998). Motivation to succeed. In W. Damon (Series Ed.) & N. Eisenberg (Vol. Ed.), *Handbook of child psychology: Vol. 3. Social, emotional, and personality development* (5th ed., pp. 1017–1096). New York: Wiley.

Edelstein, R. S., & Shaver, P. R. (2007). A cross-cultural examination of lexical studies of self-conscious emotions. In J. L. Tracy, R. W. Robins, & J. P. Tangney (Eds.), *The self-conscious emotions: Theory and research* (pp. 194–208). New York: Guilford Press.

Eichenbaum, L., & Orbach, S. (1983). *Understanding women: A feminist psycho-analytic approach.* New York: Basic Books.

Eid, M., & Diener, E. (2001). Norms for experiencing emotions in different cultures: Inter- and intra-national differences. *Journal of Personality and Social Psychology, 81,* 869-885.

Eisenberg, A. (1985). Learning to describe past experiences in conversation. *Discourse Processes, 8,* 177–204.

Eisenberg, M., Neumark-Sztainer, D., Haines, J., & Wall, M. (2006). Weight-teasing and emotional well-being in adolescents: Longitudinal findings from Project EAT. *Journal of Adolescent Health, 38,* 675–683.

Elison, J., & Dansie, E. J. (in press). Humiliation. In B. B. Brown & M. Prinstein (Eds.), *Encyclopedia of adolescence.* New York: Academic Press.

Elison, J., & Harter, S. (2007). Humiliation: Causes, correlates, and consequences. In J. L. Tracy, R. W. Robins, & J. P. Tangney (Eds.), *The self-conscious emotions: Theory and research* (pp. 310–329). New York: Guilford Press.

Elkind, D. (1967). Egocentrism in adolescence. *Child Development, 38,* 1025–1034.

English, T., & Chen, S. (2007). Culture and self-concept stability: Consistency across and within contexts among Asian Americans and European Americans. *Journal of Personality and Social Psychology, 93,* 478–490.

Epstein, S. (1973). The self-concept revisited or a theory of a theory. *American Psychologist, 28,* 405–416.

Epstein, S. (1981). The unity principle versus the reality and pleasure principles, or the tale of the scorpion and the frog. In M. D. Lynch, A. A. Norem-Hebeisen, & K. Gergen (Eds.), *Self-concept: Advances in theory and research* (pp. 82–110). Cambridge, MA: Ballinger.

Epstein, S. (1991). Cognitive-experiential self theory: Implications for developmental psychology. In M. R. Gunnar & L. A. Sroufe (Eds.), *Minnesota Symposium on Child Psychology: Vol. 23. Self-processes and development (pp. 111–137). Hillsdale, NJ: Erlbaum.*

Erikson, E. H. (1959). Identity and the life cycle. *Psychological Issues, 1,* 1–171.

Erikson, E. H. (1963). *Childhood and society* (2nd ed.). New York: Norton.

Erikson, E. H. (1968). *Identity, youth, and crisis.* New York: Norton.

Erkolahti, R., Ilonen, T., & Saarijarvi, S. (2003). Self-image of adolescents with diabetes mellitus type I and rheumatoid arthritis. *Nordic Journal of Psychiatry, 57,* 309–312.

Erlbaum, B. (2002). The self-concept of students with learning disabilities: A meta-analysis of comparisons across different placements. *Learning Disabilities Research and Practice, 17,* 216–226.

Exline, J. J. (2008). Taming the wild ego: The challenge of humility. In H. A. Wayment & J. J. Bauer (Eds.), *Transcending self-interest: Psychological explorations of the quiet ego* (pp. 53–62). Washington, DC: American Psychological Association.

Faber, M., & Kruger, H. S. (2005). Dietary intake, perceptions regarding body weight, and attitudes toward weight control of normal weight, overweight, and obese black females in a rural village in South Africa. *Ethnicity and Disease, 15,* 238–245.

Faludi, S. (1999). *Stiffed: The betrayal of the American man.* New York: Morrow.

Farrant, K., & Reese, E. (2000). Maternal style and children's participation in reminiscing: Stepping stones in children's autobiographical memory development. *Journal of Cognition and Development, 1,* 193–225.

Fasig, L. (2000). Toddler's understanding of ownership: Implications for self-concept development. *Social Development, 9,* 370–382.

Feiring, C., Taska, L., & Lewis, M. (2002). Adjustment following sexual abuse discovery: The role of shame and attributional style. *Developmental Psychology, 38,* 79–92.

Ferguson, T. J., Brugman, D., White, J., & Eyre, H. (2007). Shame and guilt as morally warranted experiences. In J. L. Tracy, R. W. Robins, & J. P. Tangney (Eds.), *The self-conscious emotions: Theory and research* (pp. 330–348). New York: Guilford Press.

Ferguson, T. J., & Eyre, H. (2000). Engendering gender differences in shame and guilt: Stereotypes, socialization, and situation pressures. In A. H. Fischer (Ed.), *Gender and emotion: Social psychological perspectives* (pp. 254–276). New York: Cambridge University Press.

Fernald, A., & Morikawa, H. (1993). Common themes and cultural variation in Japanese and American mothers' speech to infants. *Child Development, 64,* 637–656.

Fessler, D. M. T. (2007). From appeasement to conformity: Evolutionary and cultural perspectives on shame, competition, and cooperation. In J. L. Tracy, R. W. Robins, & J. P. Tangney (Eds.), *The self-conscious emotions: Theory and research* (pp. 174–193). New York: Guilford Press.

Fischer, K. W. (1980). A theory of cognitive development: The control and construction of hierarchies of skills. *Psychological Review, 87,* 477–531.

Fischer, K. W., & Ayoub, C. (1994). Affective splitting and dissociation in normal and maltreated children: Developmental pathways for self in relationships. In D. Cicchetti & S. Toth (Eds.), *Rochester Symposium on Developmental Psychopathology: Vol. 5. Disorders and dysfunctions of the self* (pp. 149–222). Rochester, NY: University of Rochester Press.

Fischer, K. W., & Bidell, T. R. (2006). Dynamic development of action and thought. In W. Damon & R. M. Lerner (Eds.) & R. M. Lerner (Vol. Ed.), *Handbook of child psychology: Vol. 1. Theoretical models of human development* (6th ed., pp. 313–399). New York: Wiley.

Fischer, K. W., & Canfield, R. (1986). The ambiguity of stage and structure in behavior: Person and environment in the development of psychological structure. In I. Levin (Ed.), *Stage and structure: Reopening the debate* (pp. 246–267). New York: Plenum.

Fischer, K. W., Hand, H., Watson, M., Van Parys, M., & Tucker, J. (1984). Putting the child into socialization: The development of social categories in preschool children. In L. Katz (Ed.), *Current topics in early childhood education* (Vol. 5, pp. 27–72). Norwood, NJ: Ablex.

Fischer, K. W., Shaver, P., & Carnochan, P. (1990). How emotions develop and how they organize development. *Cognition and Emotion, 4,* 81–127.

Fiske, A. P., & Fiske, S. T. (2007). Social relationships in our species and culture. In S. Kitayama & D. Cohen (Eds.), *Handbook of cultural psychology.* New York: Guilford Press.

Fivush, R., & Buckner, J. P. (2003). Creating gender and identity through autobiographical narratives. In R. Fivush & C. A. Haden (Eds.), *Autobiographical memory and the construction of a narrative self* (pp. 149–168). Mahwah, NJ: Erlbaum.

Fivush, R., & Haden, C. A. (Eds.). (2003). *Autobiographical memory and the construction of a narrative self.* Mahwah, NJ: Erlbaum.

Fivush, R., & Hamond, N. R. (1990). Autobiographical memory across the preschool years: Toward reconceptualizing childhood amnesia. In R. Fivush & J. A. Hudson (Eds.), *Knowing and remembering in young children* (pp. 223–248). New York: Cambridge University Press.

Fivush, R., & Hudson, J. A. (Eds.). (1990). *Knowing and remembering in young children.* New York: Cambridge University Press.

Flavell, J. H. (1985). *Cognitive development* (2nd ed.). Englewood Cliffs, NJ: Prentice-Hall.

Forbes, G., Adams-Curtis L., Rade, B., & Jaberg, P. (2001). Body dissatisfaction in women and men. The role of gender-typing and self-esteem. *Sex Roles, 44,* 461–484.

Forehand, R., & Long, N. (1995). *Parenting the strong-willed child: The clinically proven five-week program for parents of two- to six-year-olds.* Lincolnwood, IL: Contemporary Books.

Foster, J. D., Campbell, W. K., & Twenge, J. M. (2003). Individual differences in narcissism: Inflated self-views across the lifespan and around the world. *Journal of Research in Personality, 37,* 469–486.

Foster, J. D., Shrira, I., & Campbell, W. K. (2006). Theoretical models of narcissism, sexuality, and relationship commitment. *Journal of Social and Personality Relationships, 23,* 367–386.

Fottland, H. (2000). Childhood cancer and the interplay between illness, self-evaluation, and academic experiences. *Scandinavian Journal of Educational Research, 44,* 253–273.

Fox, K., Page, A., Armstrong, N., & Kirby, B. (1994). Dietary restraint and self-perceptions in early adolescence. *Personality and Individual Differences, 17,* 87–96.

Fox, M. (2002). The self-esteem of children with physical disabilities: A review of research. *Journal of Research in Special Educational Needs, 2,* 24–32.

Frankenberger, K. D. (2000). Adolescent egocentrism: A comparison among adolescents and adults. *Journal of Adolescence, 23,* 343–354.

Freud, A. (1965). *Normality and pathology in childhood.* New York: International Universities Press.

Freud, S. (1914). On narcissism: An introduction. *The standard edition of the complete psychological works of Sigmund Freud* (Vol. 14, 67–102). London: Hogarth Press.

Freud, S. (1952). *A general introduction to psychoanalysis.* New York: Washington Square Press.

Frey, K. S., & Ruble, D. N. (1990). Strategies for comparative evaluation: Maintaining a sense of competence across the life span. In R. J. Sternberg & J. Kolligian, Jr. (Eds.), *Competence considered* (pp. 167–189). New Haven, CT: Yale University Press.

Freyer, K. (1996). *The impact of team sports on the adolescent female.* Unpublished doctoral dissertation, University of Denver, Denver, CO.

Friedman, R., & Liu, W. (2009). Bicultural in management: Leveraging the benefits of intrapersonal diversity. In R. S. Wyer, C. Chiu, & Y. Hong (Eds.), *Understanding culture: Theory, research, and application.* New York: Psychology Press.

Frost, L. (2003). Doing bodies differently? Gender, youth, appearance, and damage. *Journal of Youth Studies, 6,* 53–70.

Garbarino, J. (1999). *Lost boys: Why our sons turn violent and how we can save them.* New York: Free Press.

Gardner, W., Gabriel, S., & Lee, A.Y. (1999). "I" value freedom but "we" value relationships: Self-conscious priming mirrors cultural differences in judgment. *Psychological Science, 10,* 321–326.

Garner, D. M., & Garfinkel, P. E. (1980). Sociocultural factors in the development of anorexia. *Psychological Medicine, 10,* 647–656.

Geller, J., Srikameswaran, S., Cockell, S. J., & Zaitsoff, S. L. (2000). The assessment of shape and weight-based self-esteem in adolescents. *International Journal of Eating Disorders, 28,* 339–345.

Geller, J., Zaitsoff, S., & Srikameswaran, S. (2002). Beyond shape and weight: Exploring the relationship between non-body determinants of self-esteem and eating disorder symptoms in adolescent females. *International Journal of Eating Disorders, 32,* 344–351.

Gergen, K. J. (1968). Personal consistency and the presentation of self. In C. Gordon & J. Gergen (Eds.), *The self in social interaction* (pp. 299–308). New York: Wiley.

Gergen, K. J. (1977). The social construction of self-knowledge. In T. Mischel (Ed.), *The self: Psychological and philosophical issues* (pp. 139–169). Totowa, NJ: Erlbaum.

Gergen, K. J. (1991). *The saturated self.* New York: Basic Books.

Gergen, K. J. (1996). Technology and the self: From the essential to the sublime. In D. Grodin & T. R. Lindloff (Eds.), *Constructing the self in a mediated world* (pp. 156–178). Thousand Oaks, CA: Sage.

Gergen, K. J. (1998). *The self: Death by technology.* Charlottesville: University of Virginia Press.

Gervis, M., & Dunn, N. (2004). The emotional abuse of elite child athletes by their coaches. *Child Abuse Review, 13,* 215–223.

Gilbert, P. (1997). The evolution of social attractiveness and its role in shame, humiliation, guilt and therapy. *British Journal of Medical Psychology, 70,* 113–147.

Gilligan, C. (1982). *In a different voice: Psychological theory and women's development.* Cambridge, MA: Harvard University Press.

Gilligan, C. (1993). Joining the resistance: Psychology, politics, girls, and women. In L. Weis & M. Fine (Eds.), *Beyond silenced voices* (pp. 143–168). Albany: SUNY University of New York Press.

Gilligan, C., Lyons, N., & Hanmer, T. J. (1989). *Making connections.* Cambridge, MA: Harvard University Press.

Gilovich, T., Epley, N., & Hanko, K. (2005). Shallow thoughts about the self: The automatic components of self-assessment. In M. D. Alicke, D. Dunning, & J. Krueger (Eds.), *The self in social judgment* (pp. 67–84). New York: Psychology Press.

Giner-Sorolla, R., Castano, E., Espinosa, P., & Brown, R. (2008). Shame expressions reduce the recipient's insult from outgroup reparations. *Journal of Experimental Social Psychology, 44,* 519–526.

Gleason, J., Alexander, A., & Somers, C. (2000). Late adolescents' reactions to three types of childhood teasing: Relations with self-esteem and body image. *Social Behavior and Personality, 28,* 471–480.

Glick, M., & Zigler, E. (1985). Self-image: A cognitive-developmental approach. In R. Leahy (Ed.), *The development of self* (pp. 1–54). New York: Academic Press.

Gnepp, J., McKee, E., & Domanic, J. A. (1987). Children's use of situational information to infer emotion: Understanding emotionally equivocal situations. *Developmental Psychology, 23,* 114–123.

Goetz, J., & Keltner, D. (2007). Shifting meanings of self-conscious emotions across cultures: A social-functioning approach. In J. L. Tracy, R. W. Robins, & J. P. Tangney (Eds.), *The self-conscious emotions: Theory and research* (pp. 153–173). New York: Guilford Press.

Goldman, B. M. (2006). Making diamonds out of coal: The role of authenticity in healthy (optimal) self-esteem and psychological functioning. In M. H. Kernis (Ed.), *Self-esteem: Issues and answers* (pp. 132–139). New York: Psychology Press.

Goldman, B. M., & Kernis, M. H. (2002). The role of authenticity in healthy psychological functioning and subjective well-being. *Annals of the American Psychotherapy Association, 5,* 18–20.

Gordon, M. M. (1964). *Assimilation in American life: The role of race, religion, and national origins.* New York: Oxford University Press.

Gordon, C. (1968). Self-conceptions: Configurations of content. In C. Gordon & K. J. Gergen (Eds.), *The self in social interaction* (pp. 115–136). New York: Wiley.

Graham, S. (1988). Children's developing understanding of the motivational role of affect: An attributional analysis. *Cognitive Development, 3,* 71–88.

Gralinsky, J., Fesbach, N. D., Powell, C., & Derrington, T. (1993, April). *Self-understanding: Meaning and measurement of maltreated children's sense of self.* Paper presented at the meeting of the Society for Research in Child Development, New Orleans, LA.

Granlese, J., & Joseph, S. (1993). Factor analysis of the Self-Perception Profile for Children. *Personality and Individual Differences, 15,* 343–345.

Grant, H., & Dweck, C. (2001). Cross-cultural response to failure: Considering outcome attributions with different goals. In F. Salili & C. Chiu (Eds.), *Student motivation: The culture and context of learning* (pp. 203–219). Dordrecht, Netherlands: Kluwer Academic.

Greene, M., & Way, N. (2005). Self-esteem trajectories among ethnic minority adolescents: A growth curve analysis of the patterns and predictors of change. *Journal of Research on Adolescence, 15,* 151–178.

Greenwald, A. G. (1980). The totalitarian ego: Fabrication and revision of personal history. *American Psychologist, 7,* 603–618.

Griffin, N., Chassin, L., & Young, R. D. (1981). Measurement of global self-concept versus multiple role-specific self-concepts in adolescents. *Adolescence, 16,* 49–56.

Griffin, S. (1992). Structural analysis of the development of their inner world: A neo-structural analysis of the development of intrapersonal intelligence. In R. Case (Ed.), *The mind's staircase* (pp. 189–206). Hillsdale, NJ: Erlbaum.

Grotevant, H. D., & Cooper, C. R. (Eds.). (1983). *Adolescent development in the family: New directions for child development.* San Francisco: Jossey-Bass.

Grum, D., Lebaric, N., & Kolenc, J. (2004). Relation between self-concept, motivation for education and academic achievement: A Slovenian case. *Studia Psychologica, 46,* 105–126.

Guay, F., Marsh, H., & Boivin, M. (2003). Academic self-concept and academic achievement: Developmental perspectives on their causal ordering. *Journal of Educational Psychology, 95,* 124–136.

Guzman, M. (1983). *The effects of competence and anxiety level on problem-solving performance and preference for challenge.* Unpublished master's thesis, University of Denver, Denver, CO.

Guzman, M. (1986). *Acculturation of Mexican-American adolescents.* Unpublished doctoral dissertation, University of Denver, Denver, CO.

Haden, C. A. (2003). Joint encoding and joint reminiscing: Implications for young children's understanding and remembering of personal experiences. In R. Fivush & C. A. Haden (Eds.), *Autobiographical memory and the construction of a narrative self* (pp. 49–70). Mahwah, NJ: Erlbaum.

Haltiwanger, J. (1989, April). *Behavioral referents of presented self-esteem in young children.* Paper presented at the meeting of the Society for Research in Child Development, Kansas City, MO.

Hamamura, T., Heine, S., & Paulhus, D. (2008). Cultural differences in response styles: The role of dialectical thinking. *Personality and Individual Differences, 44,* 932–942.

Haney, P., & Durlak, J. A. (1998). Changing self-esteem in children and adolescents: A meta-analytic review. *Journal of Clinical Child Psychology, 27,* 423–433.

Hanh, T. N. (1987). *Interbeing: Fourteen guidelines for engaged Buddhism*. Berkeley, CA: Parallax Press.

Hanh, T. N. (1995). *Living Buddha, living Christ*. New York: Riverhead Books.

Hanh, T. N. (1999). *Going home: Jesus and Buddha as brothers*. New York: Riverhead Books.

Hansford, B. C., & Hattie, J. A. (1982). The relationship between self and achievement/performance measures. *Review of Educational Research, 52,* 123–142.

Hardin, E., Leong, F., & Bhagwat, A. (2004). Factor structure of the self-construal scale revisited: Implications for the multi-dimensionality of self-construal. *Journal of Cross-Cultural Psychology, 35,* 327–345.

Hargreaves, D., & Tiggemann, M. (2002). The effects of television on mood and body dissatisfaction: The role of appearance-schema activation. *Journal of Social and Clinical Psychology, 21,* 287–308.

Harris, P. L. (2003). What children know about the situations that provoke emotion. In M. Lewis & C. Saarni (Eds.), *The socialization of affect* (pp. 162–185). New York: Plenum Press.

Harris, P. L. (2008). Children's understanding of emotion. In M. Lewis, J. M. Haviland-Jones, & L. F. Barrett (Eds.), *Handbook of emotions* (3rd ed., pp. 320–343). New York: Guilford Press.

Harris, P. L., Olthof, T., Meerum Terwogt, M., & Hardman, C. E. (1987). Children's knowledge of the situations that provoke emotion. *International Journal of Behavioral Development, 10,* 319–343.

Harris-Britt, A., Valrie, C., Kurtz-Costes, B., & Rowley, S. (2007). Perceived racial discrimination and self-esteem in African American youth: Racial socialization as a protective factor. *Journal of Research on Adolescence, 17,* 669–682.

Harrison, K. (2001). Ourselves, our bodies: Thin-ideal media, self-discrepancies, and eating disorder symptomatology. *Journal of Social and Clinical Psychology, 20,* 289–323.

Hart, D. (1988). The adolescent self-concept in social context. In D. K. Lapsley & F. C. Power (Eds.), *Self, ego, and identity* (pp. 71–90). New York: Springer-Verlag.

Hart, D., & Matsuba, M. K. (2007). The development of pride and moral life. In J. L. Tracy, R. W. Robins, & J. P. Tangney (Eds.), *The self-conscious emotions: Theory and research* (pp. 114–133). New York: Guilford Press.

Harter, S. (1981). A new self-report scale of intrinsic versus extrinsic orientation in the classroom: Motivational and information components. *Developmental Psychology, 17,* 300–312.

Harter, S. (1982). The perceived competence scale for children. *Child Development, 53,* 87–97.

Harter, S. (1983). Developmental perspectives on the self-system. In P. Mussen & E. M. Hetherington (Eds.), *Handbook of child psychology: Vol. 4. Socialization, personality, and social development* (4th ed., pp. 275–385). New York: Wiley.

Harter, S. (1985). *The self-perception profile for children*. Unpublished manual, University of Denver, Denver, CO.

Harter, S. (1986). Processes underlying the construction, maintenance, and enhancement of the self-concept in children. In J. Suls, & A. G. Greenwald (Eds.), *Psychological perspectives on the self* (Vol. 3, pp. 137–181). Hillsdale, NJ: Erlbaum.

Harter, S. (1990). Adolescent self and identity development. In S. S. Feldman & G. R. Elliott (Eds.), *At the threshold: The developing adolescent* (pp. 352–387). Cambridge, MA: Harvard University Press.

Harter, S. (1992). The relationship between perceived competence, affect, and motivational orientation within the classroom: Processes and patterns of change. In A. K. Boggiano & T. Pittman (Eds.), *Achievement and motivation: A social-developmental perspective* (pp. 43–69). Cambridge, UK: Cambridge University Press.

Harter, S. (1993). Causes and consequences of low self-esteem in children and adolescence. In R. F. Baumeister (Ed.), *Self-esteem: The puzzle of low self-regard* (pp. 87–116). New York: Plenum.

Harter, S. (1996). Teacher and classmate influences on scholastic motivation, self-esteem, and choice. In K. Wentzel & J. Juvonen (Eds.), *Social motivation: Understanding children's school adjustment* (pp. 11–42). Cambridge, UK: Cambridge University Press.

Harter, S. (1997). The personal self in social context: Barriers to authenticity. In R. Ashmore & L. Jussim (Eds.), *Self and identity: Fundamental issues* (pp. 81–105). New York: Oxford University Press.

Harter, S. (1998). The effects of child abuse on the self-system In B. B. Rossman & M. S. Rosenberg (Eds.), *Multiple victimization of children: Conceptual, developmental, research, and treatment issues*. New York: Haworth Press.

Harter, S. (1999). *The construction of the self*. New York: Guilford Press.

Harter, S. (2000). Is self-esteem only skin-deep? The inextricable link between physical appearance and self-esteem among American youth. *Reclaiming children and youth. 9*, 135–138.

Harter, S. (2006a). The self. In W. Damon & R. Lerner (Eds.) & N. Eisenberg (Vol. Ed.), *Handbook of child psychology: Vol. 3, Social, emotional, and personality development* (6th ed., pp. 505–570). New York: Wiley.

Harter, S. (2006b). Self-processes and developmental psychopathology. In D. Cicchetti & D. Cohen (Eds.), *Handbook of developmental psychopathology* (2nd ed., pp. 370–415). New York: Wiley.

Harter, S. (2011). The challenge of framing a problem: What is your burning question? In C. F. Conrad & R. C. Serlin (Eds.), *The SAGE handbook for research in education: Engaging ideas and enriching theory* (pp. 131–148). Thousands Oaks, CA: SAGE.

Harter, S. (2012). Emerging self-processes during childhood and adolescence. In M. Leary & J. P. Tangney (Ed.), *Handbook of self and identity* (2nd ed., pp. 680–715). New York: Guilford Press.

Harter, S., Bresnick, S., Bouchey, H. A., & Whitesell, N. R. (1997). The development of multiple role-related selves during adolescence. *Development and Psychopathology, 9*, 835–854.

Harter, S., & Buddin, B. (1987). Children's understanding of the simultaneity of two emotions: A five-stage developmental acquisition sequence. *Developmental Psychology, 23*, 388–399.

Harter, S. & Buddin, B. (2011). *The effects of parental modeling and support for adolescents' level of voice.* Unpublished manuscript, University of Denver, Denver, CO.

Harter, S., & Connell, J. P. (1984). A comparison of alternative models of the relationship between academic achievement and perceptions of competence, control, and motivational orientation. In J. Nichols (Ed.), *The development of achievement-related cognitions and behaviors* (pp. 64–82). Greenwich, CT: JAI Press.

Harter, S., & Freyer, K. (2012). *The psychological benefits of sports participation for high school athletes.* Unpublished manuscript, University of Denver, Denver, CO.

Harter, S., & Jackson, B. K. (1992). Trait versus non-trait conceptualizations of intrinsic and extrinsic motivational orientation. *Motivation and Emotion, 16,* 209–230.

Harter, S., Kiang, L., Whitesell, N. R., & Anderson, A. V. (2003, April). *A prototype approach to the emotion of humiliation in college students.* Poster session presented at the biannual meeting of the Society of Research in Child Development, Tampa, FL.

Harter, S., Low, S., & Whitesell, N. R. (2003). What have we learned from Columbine: The impact of the self-system on suicidal and violent ideation among adolescents. *Journal of Youth Violence, 2,* 3–26.

Harter, S., & Marold, D. (1993). The directionality of the link between self-esteem and affect: Beyond causal modeling. In D. Cicchetti & S. L. Toth (Eds.), *Rochester Symposium on Developmental Psychopathology: Vol. 5. Disorders and dysfunctions of the self* (pp. 333–379). Rochester, NY: University of Rochester Press.

Harter, S., Marold, D. B., Whitesell, N. R., & Cobbs, G. (1996). A model of the effects of parent and peer support on adolescent false self behavior. *Child Development, 67,* 360–374.

Harter, S., & McCarley, K. (2004, April). *Self-esteem versus narcissism in the prediction of violent ideation among adolescents.* Poster session presented at the annual American Psychiatric Association convention, Honolulu, HI.

Harter, S., & Monsour, A. (1992). Developmental analysis of conflict caused by opposing attributes in the adolescent self-portrait. *Developmental Psychology, 28,* 251–260.

Harter, S., Nowakowsi, M., & Marold, D. B. (1988). *The Dimensions of Depression Profile.* Unpublished manual, University of Denver, Denver, CO.

Harter, S., & Pike, R. (1984). The pictorial scale of perceived competence and social acceptance for young children. *Child Development, 55,* 1969–1982.

Harter, S., Rienks, S., & McCarley, K. (2006, March). *Do young adolescents detect gender bias in the classroom?* Poster presented at the Society for Research on Adolescence, San Francisco, CA.

Harter, S., Stocker, C., & Robinson, N. S. (1996). The perceived directionality of the link between approval and self-worth: The liabilities of a looking glass self orientation among young adolescents. *Journal of Research on Adolescence, 6,* 285–308.

Harter, S., Waters, P., & Whitesell, N. R. (1997). False self behavior and lack of voice among adolescent males and females. *Educational Psychologist, 32,* 153–173.

Harter, S., Waters, P., & Whitesell, N. R. (1998). Relational self-worth: Differences in perceived worth as a person across interpersonal contexts among adolescents. *Child Development, 69,* 756–766.

Harter, S., Waters, P., Whitesell, N. R., & Kastelic, D. (1998). Predictors of level of voice among high school females and males: Relational context, support, and gender orientation. *Developmental Psychology, 34,* 1–10.

Harter, S., Waters, P. L., Whitesell, N. R., Kofkin, J., & Jordan, J. (1997). Autonomy and connectedness as dimensions of relationship styles in men and women. *Journal of Social and Personal Relationships, 14,* 147–164.

Harter, S., & Whitesell, N. R. (1989). Developmental changes in children's understanding of single, multiple and blended emotion concepts. In C. Saarni & P. L. Harris (Eds.), *Children's understanding of emotion* (pp. 835–854). Cambridge, UK: Cambridge University Press.

Harter, S., & Whitesell, N. R. (2003). Beyond the debate: Why some adolescents report stable self-worth over time and situation, whereas others report changes in self-worth. *Journal of Personality, 71,* 1027–1058.

Harter, S., Whitesell, N. R., & Junkin, L. (1998). Similarities and differences in domain-specific and global self-evaluations of learning-disabled, behaviorally-disordered, and normally achieving adolescents. *American Educational Research Journal, 35,* 653–680.

Harter, S., Whitesell, N. R., & Kowalski, P. (1992). Individual differences in the effects of educational transitions on young adolescents' perceptions of competence and motivational orientation. *American Educational Research Journal, 29,* 777–808.

Hartling, L. M., & Luchetta, T. (1999). Humiliation: Assess the impact of derision, degradation, and debasement. *Journal of Primary Prevention, 19,* 259–278.

Hastings, M., Northman, L., & Tangney, J. P. (2000). Shame, guilt, and suicide. In T. Joiner & M. D. Rudd (Eds.) *Suicide science: Expanding the boundaries* (pp. 67–79). New York: Kluwer Academic/Plenum.

Hatfield, E., & Sprecher, S. (1986). *Mirror, mirror. … The importance of appearance in everyday life.* New York: State University of New York Press.

Hayne, H., & MacDonald, S. (2003). The socialization of autobiographical memory in children and adults: The roles of culture and gender. In R. Fivush & C. A. Haden (Eds.), *Autobiographical memory and the construction of a narrative self* (pp. 99–120). Mahwah, NJ: Erlbaum.

Heine, S. J. (2001). Self as cultural product: An examination of East Asian and North American selves. *Journal of Personality, 69,* 881–906.

Heine, S. J. (2003). An exploration of cultural variation in self-enhancing and self-improving motivations. In R. A. Diensbier (Series Ed.) & V. Murphy-Berman & J. J. Berman (Vol. Eds.), *Nebraska Symposium on Motivation: Vol. 49. Cross-cultural differences in perspectives on the self* (pp. 101–128). Lincoln: University of Nebraska Press.

Heine, S. J. (2007). Culture and motivation: What motivates people to act in the ways that they do? In S. Kitayama & D. Cohen (Eds.), *Handbook of cultural psychology* (pp. 714–733). New York: Guilford Press.

Heine, S. J., & Hamamura, T. (2007). In search of East Asian self-enhancement. *Personality and Social Psychology Review, 11,* 4–27.

Heine, S. J., Kitayama, S., Lehman, D. R., Takata, T., Ide, E., Leung, C., et al. (2001). Divergent consequences of success and failure in North America and Japan: An investigation of self-improving motivations and malleable selves. *Journal of Personality and Social Psychology, 81,* 599–615.

Heine, S. J., Lehman, D. R., Markus, H. R., & Kitayama, S. (1999). Is there a universal need for positive self-regard? *Psychological Review, 106,* 766–794.

Hendry, L. B., & Kloep, M. (2011). Lifestyles in emerging adulthood: Who needs stages anyway? In J. J. Arnett, M. Kloep, L. B. Hendry, & J. L. Tanner (Eds.), *Debating emerging adulthood: Stage or process?* (pp. 77–106). New York: Oxford University Press.

Herman, J. (1992). *Trauma and recovery.* New York: Basic Books

Higgins, E. T (1991). Development of self-regulatory and self-evaluative processes: Costs, benefits, and tradeoffs. In M. R. Gunnar & L. A. Sroufe (Eds.), *Minnesota Symposium on Child Psychology: Vol. 23. Self-processes and development* (pp. 125 166). Hillsdale, NJ: Erlbaum.

Higgins, E. T., & Bargh, J. A. (1987). Social cognition and social perception. *Annual Review of Psychology, 38,* 369–425.

Hill, J. P., & Holmbeck, G. N. (1986). Attachment and autonomy during adolescence. In G. J. Whitehurst (Ed.), *Annals of child development* (Vol. 3, pp. 145–189). Greenwich, CT: JAI Press.

Hines, S., & Groves, D. L. (1989). Sports competition and its influence on self esteem development. *Adolescence, 24,* 861–869.

Hobza, C., Walker, K., Yakushko, O., & Peugh, J. (2007). What about men? Social comparison and the effects of media images on body- and self-esteem. *Psychology of Men and Masculinity, 8,* 161–172.

Hodges, B., Regehr, G., & Martin, D. (2001). Difficulties in recognizing one's own incompetence: Novice physicians who are unskilled and unaware of it. *Academic Medicine, 76,* 87–89.

Hoffman, L., Stewart, S., Warren, D., & Meek, L. (2009). Toward a sustainable myth of self: An existential response to the postmodern crisis. *Journal of Humanistic Psychology, 49,* 135–173.

Hoffman, M. L. (2008). Empathy and prosocial behavior. In M. Lewis, J. M. Haviland-Jones, & L. F. Barrett (Eds.), *Handbook of emotions* (3rd ed., pp. 440–455). New York: Guilford Press.

Hofstede, G. (1980). *Culture's consequences: International differences in work-related values.* London: Sage..

Hong, Y., I., G., Chiu, C., Morris, M., & Menon, T. (2001). Cultural identity and dynamic construction of the self: Collective duties and individual rights in Chinese and American cultures. *Social Cognition, 19,* 251–268.

Hong, Y., Morris, M. W., Chiu, C., & Benet-Martinez, V. (2000). Multicultural minds: A dynamic constructivist approach to culture and cognition. *American Psychologist, 55,* 709–720.

Hong, Y., Wan, C., No, S., & Chiu, C. (2007). Multicultural identities. In S. Kitayama & D. Cohen (Eds.), *Handbook of cultural psychology* (pp. 323–345). New York: Guilford Press.

Hoorens, V. (1993). Self-enhancement and superiority biases in social comparison. *European Review of Social Psychology, 4,* 113–139.

Horney, K. (1950). *Neurosis and human growth.* New York: Norton.

Howe, M. L. (2003). Memories from the cradle. *Current Directions in Psychological Science, 12,* 62–65.

Howe, M. L., & Courage, M. L. (1993). On resolving the enigma of infantile amnesia. *Psychological Bulletin, 113,* 305–326.

Hudson, J. A. (1990). Constructive processes in children's autobiographical memory. *Developmental Psychology, 26,* 180–187.

Hyun, K. (2001). Is an independent self a requisite for Asian immigrants' psychological well-being in the U.S.? The case of Korean Americans. *Journal of Human Behavior in the Social Environment, 3,* 179–200.

Ip, K., & Jarry, J. L. (2008). Invstment in body image for self-definition results in greater vulnerability to the think media that does investment in appearance management. *Body Image, 5,* 59–69.

Jackson, M. A. (2000). Distinguishing shame and humiliation. *Dissertation Abstracts International, 61*(4), 2272.

Jacobs, J., Lanza, S., Osgood, D., Eccles, J., & Wigfield, A. (2002). Changes in children's self-competence and values: Gender and domain differences across grades one throughTwelve. *Child Development, 73,* 509–527.

James, W. (1890). *Principles of psychology.* Chicago: Encyclopedia Britannica.

James, W. (1892). *Psychology: The briefer course.* New York: Holt.

Jia, Y., Way, N., Ling, G., Yoshikawa, H., Chen, X., Hughes, D., et al. (2009). The influence of student perception of school climate on socioemotional and academic adjustment: A comparison of Chinese and American adolescents. *Child Development, 80,* 1514–1540.

Joffe, N. G., & Sandler, J. (1967). Some conceptual problems involved in the consideration of disorders of narcissism. *Journal of Child Psychotherapy, 2,* 56–66.

Jones, D., & Crawford, J. (2005). Adolescent boys and body image: Weight and muscularity concerns as dual pathways to body dissatisfaction. *Journal of Youth and Adolescence, 34,* 629–636.

Jordan, J. V. (1991). The relational self: A new perspective for understanding women's development. In J. Strauss & G. Goethals (Eds.), *The self: Interdisciplinary approaches* (pp. 136–149). New York: Springer-Verlag.

Jung, C. G. (1928). *Two essays on analytical psychology.* New York: Dodd, Mead.

Jung, J., & Lee, S. (2006). Cross-cultural comparisons of appearance self-schemas, body image, self-esteem, and dieting behavior between Korean and U.S. women. *Family and Consumer Science Research Journal, 34,* 350–365.

Jung, J., & Lennon, S. (2003). Body image, appearance self-schema, and media images. *Family and Consumer Sciences Research Journal, 32,* 27–51.

Juvonen, J., Le, V. N., Kaganoff, T., Augustine, C., & Constant, L. (2004). *Focus on the wonder years: Challenges facing the American middle school.* Santa Monica, CA: Rand Corporation.

Kagan, J. (1984). *The nature of the child.* New York: Basic Books.

Kagan, J., & Lamb, S. (Eds). (1987). *The emergence of morality in young children.* Chicago: University of Chicago Press.

Kagitcibasi, C. (2005). Autonomy and relatedness in cultural context. *Journal of Cross-Cultural Psychology, 36,* 403–422.

Kanagawa, C., Cross, S. E., & Markus, H. R. (2001). "Who am I?" The cultural psychology of the conceptual self. *Personality and Social Psychology Bulletin,* *27,* 90–103.

Kang, S., Shaver, P., Sue, S., Min, K., & Jing, H. (2003). Culture-specific patterns in the prediction of life satisfaction: Roles of emotion, relationship quality, and self-esteem. *Personality and Social Psychology Bulletin, 29,* 1596–1608.

Kaplan, A., & Maehr, M. L. (2007). The contributions and prospects of goal orientation theory. *Educational Psychology Review, 19,* 91–110.

Karcher, M. J., & Fischer, K. W. (2004'. A developmental sequence of skills in adolescents' intergroup understanding. *Applied Development Psychology, 25,* 259–282.

Kashima, E. S., & Kashima, Y. (1998). Culture and language: The case of cultural dimensions and personal pronouns. *Journal of Cross-Cultural Psychology, 29,* 461–486.

Kashima, Y., Kashima, E., Farsides, T., Kim, U., Strack, F., & Werth, L. (2004). Culture and context-sensitive self: The amount and meaning of context-sensitivity of phenomenal self differ across cultures. *Self and Identity, 3,* 125–141.

Keating, D. P. (1990). Adolescent thinking. In S. S. Feldman & G. Elliot (Eds.), *At the threshold: The developing adolescent* (pp. 54–90). Cambridge, MA: Harvard University Press.

Kelly, A. E., Schochet, T., & Landry, C. F. (2004). Risk taking and novelty seeking in adolescence. In R. E. Dahl & L. P. Spear (Eds.), *Adolescent brain development* (pp. 27–32). New York: New York Academy of Sciences.

Kelly, G. A. (1955). *The psychology of personal constructs.* New York: Norton.

Keltner, D., & Beer, J. (2005). Self-conscious emotion and self-regulation. In A. Tesser, J. V. Wood, & D. A. Staple (Eds.), *On building, defending and regulating the self: A psychological perspective* (pp. 197–215). New York: Psychology Press.

Kendall-Tackett, K. A., Williams, L. M., & Finkelhor, D. (1993). Impact of sexual abuse on children: A review and synthesis of recent empirical studies. *Psychological Bulletin, 113,* 164–180.

Kendrick, D. T., & Funder, D. C. (1988). Profiting from controversy: Lessons from the person-situation debate. *American Psychologist, 43,* 23–34.

Kernberg, O. F. (1975). *Borderline conditions and pathological narcissism.* New York: Aronson.

Kernberg, O. F. (1986). Further contributions to the treatment of narcissistic personalities. In A. Morrison (Ed.), *Essential papers on narcissism* (pp. 244–292). New York: New York University Press.

Kernis, M. H., & Goldman, B. M. (2003). Stability and variability in self-concept and self-esteem. In M. R. Leary & J. P. Tangney (Eds.), *Handbook of self and identity* (pp. 106–127). New York: Guilford Press.

Kernis, M. H., & Goldman, B. M. (2006). Assessing stability of self-esteem and contingent self-esteem? In M. H. Kernis (Ed.), *Self-esteem: Issues and answers* (pp. 77–87). New York: Psychology Press.

Kernis, M. H., & Heppner, W. L. (2008). Individual differences in quiet ego functioning: Authenticity, mindfulness, and secure self-esteem. In H. A. Wayment & J. J. Bauer (Eds.), *Transcending self-interest* (pp. 85–94). Washington DC: American Psychological Association.

Kiang, L., & Harter, S. (2006). Sociocultural values of appearance and attachment processes: An integrated model of eating disorder symptomatology. *Eating Behaviors, 7,* 134–151.

Kiang, L., Harter, S., & Whitesell, N. R. (2007). Relational expression of ethnic identity in Chinese Americans. *Journal of Social and Personal Relationships, 24,* 277–296.

Kihlstrom, J. F. (1993). What does the self look like? In T. K. Srull & R. S. Wyer, Jr. (Eds.), *The mental representations of trait and autobiographical knowledge about the self book: Advances in social cognition* (Vol. 17, pp. 2–40). Hillsdale, NJ: Erlbaum.

Kilbourne, J. (1995). *Slim hopes: Advertising and the obsession with thinness* [Video]. (Available from the Media Education Foundation, 28 Center Street, Northampton, MA 01060)

Kilbourne, J. (1999). *Deadly persuasion: Why women must fight the addictive power of advertising.* New York: Free Press.

Kim, H., & Markus, H. R. (1999). Deviance or uniqueness, harmony or conformity? A cultural analysis. *Journal of Personality and Social Psychology, 77,* 785–800.

Kim, J., Kim, M., Kam, K., & Shin, H. (2003). Influence of self-construals on the perception of different self-perception styles in Korea. *Asian Journal of Social Psychology, 6,* 89–101.

Kim, Y., Butzel, J. S., & Ryan, R. M. (1998). *Interdependence and well-being: A function of culture and relatedness needs.* Paper presented at the International Society for the Study of Personal Relationships, Saratoga Springs, NY.

Kitayama, S., Duffy, S., & Uchida, Y. (2007). Self as cultural mode of being. In S. Kitayama & D. Cohen (Eds.), *Handbook of cultural psychology* (pp. 136–174). New York: Guilford Press.

Kitayama, S., & Park, H. (2007). Cultural shaping of self, emotion, and well-being. How does it work? *Social and Personality Compass, 1,* 202–222.

Kitchner, K. S. (1986). The reflective judgment model: Characteristics, evidence, and measurement. In R. A. Mines & K. S. Kitchner (Eds.), *Adult cognitive development: Methods and models* (pp. 76–91). New York: Praeger.

Kitchner, K. S., King, P. M., & DeLuca, S. (2006). Development of reflective judgment in adulthood. In C. Hoare (Ed.), *Handbook of adult development and learning* (pp. 73–98). New York: Oxford University Press.

Klein, D. C. (1991). The humiliation dynamic: An overview. *Journal of Primary Prevention, 12,* 93–121.

Kohut, H. (1977). *The restoration of the self.* New York: International Universities Press.

Kohut, H. (1986). Forms and transformations of narcissism. In A. P. Morrison (Ed.), *Essential papers on narcissism.* New York: New York University Press.

Kornilaki, E. N., & Chloverakis, G. (2004). The situational antecedents of pride and happiness: Developmental and domain differences. *British Journal of Developmental Psychology, 22,* 605–619.

Kowalski, P. S. (1985). *The role of affective experience in early adolescents' network of self-perceptions.* Unpublished doctoral dissertation, University of Denver, Denver, CO.

Kruger, J., & Dunning, D. (1999). Unskilled and unaware of it: How difficulty in recognizing one's own incompetence lead to inflated self-assessments. *Journal of Personality and Social Psychology, 77,* 1121–1134.

Kuhn, D., & Franklin, S. (2006). The second decade: What develops (and how). In W. Damon & R. M. Lerner (Eds.) & D. Kuhn & R. S. Siegler (Vol. Eds.), *Handbook of child psychology: Vol. 2. Cognition, perception, and language)* pp. 953–994). New York: Wiley.

Lagattuta, K. H., & Thompson, R. (2007). The development of self-conscious emotions: Cognitive processes and social influences. In J. L. Tracy, R. W. Robins, & J. P. Tangney (Eds.). *The self-conscious emotions: Theory and research* (pp. 91–113). New York: Guilford Press.

Lancelotta, K. (1994). *The importance of appearance in western culture: The implications of perceiving an association between appearance and popularity in a young adolescent sample.* Unpublished master's thesis, University of Denver, Denver, CO.

Lancelotta, K. (1999). *Sociocultural factors associated with the incidence of disordered eating among college students.* Unpublished doctoral dissertation, University of Denver, Denver, CO.

Lane, P. (1998). *The impact of teaching styles on students' styles and academic outcomes.* Unpublished doctoral dissertation, University of Northern Colorado, Greeley, CO.

Langer, E. (1989). *Mindfulness.* New York: Da Capo Press (Perseus Books Group).

Langer, E. (2009). Mindfulness versus positive evaluation. In S. J. Lopez & C. R. Snyder (Eds.), *Oxford handbook of positive psychology* (2nd ed., pp. 279–294). New York: Oxford University Press.

Langeveld, N., Grootenhuis, M., Voute, P., De Haan, R., & Van den Bos, C. (2004). Quality of life, self-esteem, and worries in young adult survivors of childhood cancer. *Psycho-Oncology, 13,* 867–881.

Lapsley, D. K. (1993). Toward an integrated theory of adolescent ego development: The "new look" at adolescent egocentrism. *American Journal of Orthopsychiatry, 63,* 562–571.

Lapsley, D. K. (2008). Integrative mechanisms and implicit moral reasoning in adolescence. In W. Sinnott-Armstrong (Ed.), *Moral psychology: Vol. 3. The neuroscience of morality: Emotion, brain disorders, and development* (pp. 343–350). Cambridge, MA: MIT Press.

Lapsley, D. K., & Murphy, M. (1985). Another look at the theoretical assumptions of adolescent egocentrism. *Developmental Review, 5,* 201–217.

Lapsley, D. K., & Rice, K. (1988). The "new look" at the imaginary audience and personal fable: Toward a general model of adolescent ego development. In D. K. Lapsley & F. C. Power (Eds.), *Self, ego, and identity: Integrative approaches* (pp. 109–129). New York: Springer-Verlag.

Lapsley, D. K., & Stey, P. C. (in press). Adolescent narcissism. In R. Levesque (Ed.), *Encyclopedia of adolescence.* New York: Springer.

Lawrence, J., Rosenberg, L., & Fauerbach, J. (2007). Comparing the body esteem of pediatric survivors of burn injury with the body esteem of an age-matched comparison group without burns. *Rehabilitation Psychology, 52,* 370–379.

Leahy, R. L. (1985). The costs of development: Clinical implications. In R. L. Leahy (Ed.), *The development of the self* (pp. 267–294). New York: Academic Press.

Leahy, R. L., & Shirk, S. (1985). Social cognition and the development of the self. In R. L. Leahy (Ed.), *The development of the self* (pp. 123–150). New York: Academic Press.

Leary, M. R. (2004). *The curse of the self: Self-awareness, egotism, and the quality of human life.* Oxford, UK: Oxford University Press.

Leary, M. R. (2007). How the self became involved in affective experience. In J. L. Tracy, R. W. Robins, & J. P. Tangney (Eds.), *The self-conscious emotions: Theory and research* (pp. 38–52). New York: Guilford Press.

Leary, M. R. (2008). Functions of the self in interpersonal relationships: What does the self actually do? In J. V. Wood, A. Tesser, & J. G. Holmes (Eds.), *The self in social relationships* (pp. 95–137). New York: Psychology Press.

Leary, M. R., & Baumeister, R. F. (2000). The nature and function of self-esteem sociometr Theory. In M. P. Zanna (Ed.), *Advances in experimental social psychology* (pp. 1–62). San Diego: Academic Press.

Leary, M. R., & Forsyth, D. R. (1987). Attributions of responsibility for collective endeavors. In C. Hendrick (Ed.), *Group processes* (pp. 167–188). Newbury Park, CA: Sage.

Leary, M. R., Koch, E., & Hechenbleikner, N. (2001). Emotional responses to interpersonal rejection. In M. R. Leary (Ed.), *Interpersonal rejection* (pp. 145–166). New York: Oxford University Press.

Leary, M. R., Kowalski, R. M., Smith, L., & Phillips, S. (2003). Teasing, rejection, and violence: Case studies of the school shootings. *Aggressive Behavior, 29,* 202–214.

Leary, M. R., & MacDonald, G. (2003). Individual differences in self-esteem: A review and theoretical integration. In M. R. Leary & J. P. Tangney (Eds.), *Handbook of self and identity* (pp. 401–418). New York: Guilford Press.

Leary, M. R., & Tangney, J. P. (2003). The self as an organizing construct in the behavioral and social sciences. In M. R. Leary & J. P. Tangney (Eds.), *Handbook of self and identity* (pp. 1–14). New York: Guilford Press.

LeBovidge, J., Lavigne, J., Donenberg, G., & Miller, M. (2003). Psychological adjustment of children and adolescents with chronic arthritis: A meta-analytic review. *Journal of Pediatric Psychology, 28,* 29–39.

Lecky, P. (1945). *Self-consistency: A theory of personality.* New York: Island Press.

Leichtman, M. D., Wang, Q., & Pillemer, D. B. (2003). Cultural variations in interdependence and autobiographical memory: Lessons from Korea, China, India, and the United States. In R. Fivush & C. A. Haden (Eds.), *Autobiographical memory and the construction of a narrative self: Developmental and cultural perspectives* (pp. 73–98). Mahwah, NJ: Erlbaum.

Leit, R. A., Gray, J. J., & Pope, H. G. (2002). The media's representation of the ideal male body: A cause for muscle dysmorphia? *International Journal of Eating Disorders, 31,* 334–338.

Lennon, S., Lillethun, A., & Buckland, S. (1999). Attitudes toward social comparison as a function of self-esteem: Idealized appearance and body image. *Family and Consumer, 67,* pp. 311–339.

Lepper, M. R., Corpus, J. H., & Iyengar, S. S. (2005). Intrinsic *and* extrinsic motivation in the classroom. *Journal of Educational Psychology, 97,* 184–196.

Lepper, M. R., & Gilovich, T. J. (1981). The multiple fuctions of reward: A social-developmental perspective. In S. S. Brehm, S. M. Kassin, & F. Gibbons (Eds.), *Developmental Social Psychology* (pp. 243–269). New York: Oxford University Press.

Lepper, M. R., & Greene, D. (1975). Turning play into work: Effects of adult surveillance and extrinsic rewards on children's intrinsic motivation. *Journal of Personality and Social Psychology, 31*, 479–486.

Lepper, M. R., & Henderlong, J. (2000). Turning "play" into "work" and "work" into "play": 25 years of research on intrinsic versus extrinsic motivation. In C. Sansone & J. M. Harackiewicz (Eds.), *Intrinsic and extrinsic motivation: The search for optimal motivation and performance* (pp. 257–307). San Diego, CA: Academic Press.

Lerner, H. G. (1993). *The dance of deception*. New York: HarperCollins.

Levine, M. P., & Harrison, K. (2004). Medig's role ion the perpetuation and prevention of negaqtive body image and disordered eating. In J. K. Thompson (Ed.), *Handbook of eating disorders and obesity* (pp. 695–717). New York: Wiley.

Levinson, D. J. (1978). *Seasons of a man's life*. New York: Knopf.

Lewis, H. B. (1987). *The role of shame in symptom formation*. Hillsdale, NJ: Erlbaum.

Lewis, M. (1992). *Shame: The exposed self*. New York: Free Press.

Lewis, M. (1994). Myself and me. In S. T. Parker, R. W. Mitchell, & M. L. Boccia (Eds.), *Self-awareness in animals and humans: Developmental perspectives* (pp. 20–34). New York: Cambridge University Press.

Lewis, M. (2000). Self-conscious emotions: Embarrassment, pride, shame, and guilt. In M. Lewis & J. Haviland-Jones (Eds.), *Handbook of emotions* (2nd ed., pp. 623–636). New York: Guilford Press.

Lewis, M. (2007). Self-conscious emotional development. In J. L. Tracy, R. W. Robins, & J. P. Tangney (Eds.), *The self-conscious emotions: Theory and research* (pp. 134–149). New York: Guilford Press.

Lewis, M. (2008). Self-conscious emotions: Embarrassment, pride, shame, and guilt. In M. Lewis, J. M. Haviland-Jones, & L. F. Barrett (Eds.), *Handbook of emotions* (3rd ed., pp. 742–756). New York: Guilford Press.

Lewis, M., & Brooks-Gunn, J. (1979). *Social cognition and the acquisition of the self*. New York: Plenum.

Lewis, M., & Haviland-Jones, J. M. (Eds.). (2000). *Handbook of emotions* (2nd ed.). New York: Guilford Press.

Lewis, M., Haviland-Jones, J. M., & Barrett, L. F. (Eds.). (2008). *Handbook of emotions* (3rd ed.). New York: Guilford Press.

Li, H., Zhang, Z., Bhatt, G., & Yum, Y. (2006). Rethinking culture and self-construal: China as a middle land. *Journal of Social Psychology, 146*, 591–610.

Li, J., Wang, L., & Fischer, K. F. (2004). The organization of Chinese shame concepts. *Cognition and Emotion, 18*, 767–797.

Li, J., & Yue, X. (2004). Self in learning among Chinese children. In M. Mascolo & J. Li (Eds.), *Culture and developing selves: Beyond dichotomization*. San Francisco: Jossey-Bass.

Lickel, B., Schmader, T., Curtis, M., Scarnier, M., & Ames, D. R. (2005). Vicarious shame and guilt. *Group Processes and Intergroup Relations, 8*, 145–147.

Lifton, R. J. (1993). *The protean self*. New York: Basic Books.

Linville, P. W. (1987). Self-complexity as a cognitive buffer against stress-related illness and depression. *Journal of Personality and Social Psychology, 52,* 663–676.

Locker, J., & Cropley, M. (2004). Anxiety, depression, and self-esteem in secondary school children: An investigation into the impact of standard assessment tests (SATs) and other important school examinations. *School Psychology International, 25,* 333–345.

Loevinger, J. (1976). *Ego development.* San Francisco: Jossey-Bass.

Lopez, S. J., & Snyder, C. R. (Eds.). *Oxford handbook of positive psychology.* New York: Oxford University Press.

Lowery, S., Kurpius, S., Befort, C., Blanks, E., Sollenberger, S., & Nicpon, M. (2005). Body image, self-esteem, and health-related behaviors among male and female first year college students. *Journal of College Student Development, 46,* 612–623.

Lyons-Roth, K., & Jacobvitz, D. (2008). Attachment disorganization: Genetic factors, parenting contexts, and developmental transformation from infancy to adulthood. In J. Cassidy & P. R. Shaver (Eds.), *Handbook of attachment: Theory, research, and clinical applications* (2nd ed., pp. 666–697). New York: Guilford Press.

Maccoby, E. (1980). *Social development.* New York: Wiley.

Maccoby, E. E. (1990). Gender and relationships: A developmental account. *American Psychologist, 45,* 513–520.

Maccoby, E. E. (1994). Commentary: Gender segregation in childhood. In C. Leaper (Ed.), *Childhood gender segregation: Causes and consequences* (pp. 87–98). San Francisco: Jossey-Bass.

Maccoby, E. E. (1998). *The two sexes: Growing apart and coming together.* Cambridge, MA: Harvard University Press.

Maczewski, M. (2002). Exploring identities through the internet: Youth experience online. *Child and Youth Care Forum, 31,* 111–129.

Maddux, J. E., & Gosselin, J. T. (2003). Self-efficacy. In M. R. Leary & J. P. Tangney (Eds.), *Handbook of self and identity* (pp. 218–238). New York: Guilford Press.

Maeda, K. (1997). *The Self-Perception Profile for Children administered to a Japanese sample.* Unpublished data, Ibaaraki Prefectural University of Health Sciences, Ibarki, Japan.

Mahalik, J., Pierre, M., & Wan, S. (2006). Examining racial identity and masculinity as correlates of self-esteem and psychological distress in black men. *Journal of Multicultural Counseling and Development, 34,* 94–104.

Main, M., & Solomon, J. (1990). Procedures for identifying infants as disorganized/disoriented during the Ainsworth Strange Situation. In M. Greenwald, D. Cicchetti, & M. Cummings (Eds.), *Attachment during the preschool years: Theory, research, and intervention* (pp. 121–160). Chicago: University of Chicago Press.

Makris-Botsaris, E., & Robinson, W. P. (1991). Harter's Self-Perception Profile for Children: A cross-cultural validation in Greece. *Evaluation and Research in Education, 5,* 135–143.

Marcia, J. H. (1980). Identity in adolescence. In J. Adelson (Ed.), *Handbook of adolescent psychology* (pp. 113–128). New York: Wiley.

Marcia, J. H. (1988). Common processes underlying ego identity, cognitive or moral development, and individuation. In D. K. Lapsley & F. C. Power (Eds.), *Self, ego, and identity: Integrative approaches* (pp. 211–266). New York/Berlin: Springer-Verlag.

Markus, H. R. (1977). Self-schemata and processing information about the self. *Journal of Personality and Social Psychology, 35,* 63–78.

Markus, H. R. (1980). The self in thought and memory. In D. M. Wegner & R. R. Vallacher (Eds.), *The self in social psychology* (pp. 42–69). New York: Oxford University Press.

Markus, H. R., & Cross, S. (1990). The interpersonal self. In L. A. Pervin (Ed.), *Handbook of personality: Theory and research* (pp. 576–608). New York: Guilford Press.

Markus, H. R., & Hamedani, M. G. (2007). Sociocultural psychology: The dynamic interdependence among self systems and social systems. In S. Kitayama & D. Cohen (Eds.), *Handbook of cultural psychology* (pp. 3–39). New York: Guilford Press.

Markus, H. R., & Kitayama, S. (1991). Culture and the self: Implications for cognition, emotion, and motivation. *Psychological Review, 98,* 224–253.

Markus, H. R., & Kitayama, S. (2003). Models of agency: Socialcultural diversity in the construction of action. In R. A. Dienstbier (Ed.) & V. Murphy-Berman & J. J. Berman (Vol. Eds.), *Nebraska Symposium on Motivation: Vol. 49. Cross-cultural differences in perspective on the self* (pp. 1–58). Lincoln: University of Nebraska Press.

Markus, H. R., & Nurius, P. (1986). Possible selves. *American Psychologist, 41,* 954–969.

Markus, H. R., Uchida, Y., Omoregie, H., Townsend, S. S., & Kitayama, S. (2006). Going for the gold: Models of agency in Japanese and American contexts. *Psychological Science, 17,* 103–112.

Marsh, H. W., & Craven, R. (2006). Reciprocal effects of self-concept and performance from a multidimensional perspective: Beyond seductive pleasure and unidimensional perspectives. *Perspectives on Psychological Science, 1,* 133–163.

Marsh, H. W., & Hau, K. (2003). Big-fish-little-pond effect on academic self-concept. *American Psychologist, 58,* 364–376.

Marsh, H. W., Trautwein, U., Lüdtke, O., & Köller, O. (2008). Social comparison and big-fish-little-pond effects on self-concept and other self-belief constructs; role of generalized and specific others. *Journal of Educational Psychology, 100,* 510–524.

Marsh, H. W., Trautwein, U., Lüdtke, O., Köller, O., & Baumert, J. (2005). Academic self-concept, interest, grades, and standardized test scores: Reciprocal effects models of causal ordering. *Child Development, 76,* 397–416.

Marshall, S. K., Tilton-Weaver, L. C., & Bosdet, L. (2005). Information management: Considering adolescents' regulation of parental knowledge. *Journal of Adolescence, 28,* 633–647.

Martin, J., & Sugarman, J. (2000). Between the modern and the postmodern: The possibility of self and progressive understanding in psychology. *American Psychologist, 55,* 397–406.

Mascolo, M., & Fischer, K. W. (1995). Developmental transformations in appraisals for pride, shame, and guilt. In J. P. Tangney & K. W. Fischer (Eds.), *Self-conscious emotions: The psychology of shame, guilt, embarrassment, and pride* (pp. 64–113). New York: Guilford Press.

Mascolo, M. F., & Li, J. (Eds.). (2004). *Culture and developing selves: Beyond dichotomization.* San Francisco: Jossey-Bass.

Maslow, A. (1954). *Motivation and personality.* New York: Harper & Row.

Maslow, A. H. (1943). A theory of motivation. *Psychological Review, 50,* 370–396.

Mattaini, M. (2008). Creating a violence-free school climate/culture. In C. Franklin, M. B. Harris, & P. Allen-Meares (Eds.), *The school practitioner's concise companion to preventing violence and conflict* (pp. 27–39). New York: Oxford University Press.

May, R. (1991). *The cry for myth.* New York: Dell.

McAdams, D. P. (2008). Generativity, the redemptive self, and the problem of a noisy ego in American life. In H. A. Wayment & J. J. Bauer (Eds.), *Transcending self-interest: Psychological explorations of the quiet ego* (pp. 235–242). Washington, DC: American Psychological Association.

McCabe, M., Ricciardelli, L. A., & Holt, K. (2005). A longitudinal study to explain strategies to change weight and muscles among normal weight and overweight children. *Appetite, 45,* 225–234.

McCabe, M. P., & Ricciardelli, L.A. (2004). Weight and shape concerns among boys and men. In J. K. Thompson (Ed.), *Handbook of eating disorders and obesity* (pp. 606–634). New York: Wiley.

McCann, I. L., & Pearlman, L. A. (1992). *Psychological trauma and the adult survivor* (pp. 211–259). New York: Brunner/Mazel.

McCarley, K. (2009). *The humiliation experience: Causes, emotional correlates, and behavioral consequences.* Unpublished doctoral dissertation, University of Denver, Denver, CO.

McCarley, K., & Harter, S. (2006, April). *Disentangling high self-esteem from narcissism.* Poster presentation at the Society for Research on Adolescence, San Francisco, CA.

McCoach, D., & Siegle, D. (2003). The structure and function of academic self-concept in gifted and general education students. *Roeper Review, 25,* 61–65.

McCombs, B. (2007). Learning-centered practices: Providing the context for positive learner development, motivation, and achievement. In B. L. McCombs & L. Miller (Eds.), *Learner-centered classroom practices and assessments: Maximizing student motivation, learning, and achievement* (pp. 227–261). Thousand Oaks, CA: Corwin Press.

McCombs, B., & Miller, L. (2008). *The school leader's guide to learner-centered education: From complexity to simplicity.* Thousand Oaks, CA: Corwin Press.

McCrae, R. R. (2001). Trait psychology and culture: Exploring intercultural comparisons. *Journal of Personality, 69,* 819–846.

McGee, J., & DeBernado, C. (1999). The classroom avenger: A behavioral profile of school based shootings. *Forensic Examiner, 8,* 16–18.

McGregor, H., & Elliot, A. (2005). The shame of failure: Examining the link between fear of failure and shame. *Personality and Social Psychology Bulletin, 31,* 218–231.

McVey, G., Davis, R., Tweed, S., & Shaw, B. (2004). Evaluation of a school-based program designed to improve body image satisfaction, global self-esteem, and eating attitudes and behaviors: A replication study. *International Journal of Eating Disorders, 36,* 1–11.

Mead, G. H. (1934). *Mind, self, and society from the standpoint of a social behaviorist.* Chicago: University of Chicago Press.

Meece, J. L., Wigfield, A., & Eccles, J. S. (1990). Predictors of math anxiety and its influence on young adolescents' course enrollment intentions and performance in mathematics. *Journal of Educational Psychology, 82,* 60–70.

Mehta, T. (2005). *Multiple selves in South Asian adolescents.* Unpublished doctoral dissertation, University of Denver, Denver, CO.

Mendelson, M., Mendelson, B., & Andrews, J. (2000). Self-esteem, body esteem, and body mass in late adolescence. *Journal of Applied Developmental Psychology, 21,* 249–266.

Meredith, W. H., Abbott, D. A., & Zheng, F. M. (1991). Self-concept and sociometric outcomes: A comparison of only children and sibling children from urban and rural areas in the Peoples' Republic of China. *Journal of Psychology, 126,* 411–421.

Meredith, W. H., Wang, A., & Zheng, F. M. (1993). Determining constructs of self-perception for children in Chinese cultures. *School Psychology International, 14,* 371–380.

Mezulis, A., Abramson, L., Hyde, J., & Hankin, B. (2004). Is there a universal positivity bias in attributions? A meta analytic review of individual, developmental, and cultural differences in the self-serving attributional bias. *Psychological Bulletin, 130,* 711–747.

Mikulincer, M. (1997). Adult attachment style and information processing: Individual differences in curiosity and cognitive closure. *Journal of Personality and Social Psychology, 72,* 1217–1230.

Mikulincer, M. (1998). Adult attachment style and affect regulation: Strategic variations in self-appraisals. *Journal of Personality and Social Psychology, 75,* 420–435.

Mikulincer, M., & Shaver, P. R. (2007). *Attachment in adulthood: Structure, dynamics, and change.* New York: Guilford Press.

Miller, A. (1990). *Thou shalt not be aware.* New York: Meridan.

Miller, C., & Downey, K. (1999). A meta-analysis of heavyweight and self-esteem. *Personality and Social Psychology Review, 3,* 68–84.

Miller, J. (2003). Culture and agency: Implications for psychological theories of motivation and social development. In R. A. Dienstbier (Series Ed.) & V. Murphy-Berman & J. Berman (Vol. Eds.), *Nebraska Symposium on Motivation: Vol. 49. Cross-cultural differences in perspectives on the self* (pp. 59–100). Lincoln: University of Nebraska Press.

Miller, J. B. (1986). *Toward a new psychology of women* (2nd ed.). Boston: Beacon Press.

Miller, L. (2006). *Beauty up: Exploring contemporary Japanese body aesthetics.* Berkeley: University of California Press.

Miller, P. J., Potts, R., Fung, H., Hoogstra, L., & Mintz, J. (1990). Narrative practices and the social construction of self in childhood. *American Ethnologist, 17,* 292–311.

Miller, P. J., Wang, S., Sandel, T., & Cho, G. E. (2002). Self-esteem as folk theory:

A comparison of European American and Taiwanese mothers' beliefs. *Parenting: Science and Practice, 2,* 209–239.

Miller, R. S. (2007). Is embarrassment a blessing or a curse? In J. L. Tracy, R. W. Robins, & J. P. Tangney (Eds.), *The self-conscious emotions: Theory and research* (pp. 245–262). New York: Guilford Press.

Miller, S. B. (1988). Humiliation and shame: Comparing two affect states as indicators of narcissistic stress. *Bulletin of the Menninger Clinic, 52,* 40–51.

Mills, J., & D'Alfonso, S. (2007). Competition and male body image: Increased drive for muscularity following failure to a female. *Journal of Social and Clinical Psychology, 26,* 505–518.

Mischel, W. (1973). Toward a cognitive social learning reconceptualization of personality. *Psychological Review, 80,* 252–283.

Mischel, W., & Morf, C. C. (2003). The self as a psycho-social dynamic processing system: A meta-perspective on a century of the self in psychology. In M. R. Leary & J. P. Tangney (Eds.), *Handbook of self and identity* (pp. 15–47). New York: Guilford Press.

Misra, G. (2001). Culture and self: Implications for psychological inquiry. *Journal of Indian Psychology, 19,* 1–20.

Miyahara, M., & Pick, J. (2006). Self-esteem of children and adolescents with physical disabilities: Quantitative evidence from a meta-analysis. *Journal of Developmental and Physical Disabilities, 18,* 219–234.

Miyake, K., Chen, S. J., & Campos, J. J. (1985). Infant temperament, mother's mode of interaction, and attachment in Japan: An interim report. *Monographs of the Society for Research in Child Development, 50,* 276–297.

Moneta, G., Schneider, B., & Csikszentmihalyi, M. (2001). A longitudinal study of the self-concept and experiential components of self-worth and affect across adolescence. *Applied Developmental Science, 5,* 125–142.

Montemayor, R., & Eisen, M. (1977). The development of self-conceptions from childhood to adolescence. *Developmental Psychology, 13,* 314–319.

Morelli, G. A., & Rothbaum, F. (2007). Situating the child in context: Attachment relationships and self-regulation in different cultures. In S. Kitayama & D. Cohen (Eds.), *Handbook of cultural psychology* (pp. 500–527). New York: Guilford Press.

Moretti, M. M., & Higgins, E. T. (1990). The development of self-esteem vulnerabilities: Social and cognitive factors in developmental psychopathology. In R. J. Sterberg & J. Kolligian, Jr. (Eds.), *Competence considered* (pp. 286–314). New Haven, CT: Yale University Press.

Morf, C., & Rhodewalt, F. (2001). Unraveling the paradoxes of narcissism: A dynamic self-regulatory processing model. *Psychological Inquiry,12,* 177–196.

Morling, B., & Kitayama, S. (2008). Culture and motivation. In J. Y. Shah & W. L. Gerdner (Eds.), *Handbook of motivational science* (pp. 417–433). New York: Guilford Press.

Morrison, A. (2007). Shame: A major instigator of secrets. In P. Buirski & A. Kottler (Eds.), *New developments in self psychology practice* (pp. 167–179). Lanham, MD: Aronsen.

Mruk, C. J. (2006). Defining self-esteem: An often overlooked issue with crucial implications. In M. H. Kernis (Ed.), *Self-esteem: Issues and answers* (pp. 10–15). New York: Psychology Press.

Mullen, B., & Goethals, G. R. (1990). Social projection, actual consensus, and violence. *British Journal of Social Psychology, 29,* 279–282.

Muramoto, Y. (2003). An indirect self-enhancement in relationship among Japanese. *Journal of Cross-Cultural Psychology, 34,* 552–566.

Myers, D. G. (1982). *The inflated self: Human illusions and the biblical call to hope.* New York: Seabury Press.

Neff, K. D. (2001). Judgments of personal autonomy and interpersonal responsibility in the context of Indian spousal relationships: An examination of young people's reasoning in Mysore, India. *British Journal of Developmental, 19,* 233–257.

Neff, K. D. (2008). Self-compassion: Moving beyond the pitfalls of a separate self-concept. In H. A. Wayment & J. J. Bauer (Eds.), *Transcending self-interest: Psychological explorations of the quiet ego* (pp. 95–106). Washington, DC: American Psychological Association.

Neff, K. D., & Harter, S. (2002). The role of power and authenticity in relationship styles emphasizing autonomy, connectedness, or mutuality among adult couples. *Journal of Social and Personal Relationships, 18,* 835–857.

Negrao, C., Bonanno, G., Noll, J., Putnam, F., & Trickett, P. (2005). Shame, humiliation, and childhood sexual abuse: Distinct contributions and emotional coherence. *Child Maltreatment, 10,* 350–363.

Negy, C., Shreve, T., Jensen, B., & Uddin, N. (2003). Ethnic identity, self-esteem, and ethnocentrism: A study of social identity versus multicultural theory of development. *Cultural Diversity and Ethnic Minority Psychology, 9,* 333–344.

Nelson, K. (1986). *Event knowledge: Structure and function in development.* Hillsdale, NJ: Erlbaum.

Nelson, K. (1989). *Narratives from the crib.* Cambridge, MA: Harvard University Press.

Nelson, K. (1990). Remembering, forgetting, and childhood amnesia. In R. Fivush & J. A. Hudson (Eds.), *Knowing and remembering in young children* (pp. 301–316). New York: Cambridge University Press.

Nelson, K. (1993). Events, narratives, memory: What develops? In C. A. Nelson (Ed.), *Minnesota Symposium on Child Psychology: Vol. 26. Memory and affect* (pp. 1–24). Hillsdale, NJ: Erlbaum.

Nelson, K. (2003). Narrative and self, myth and memory: Emergence of the cultural self. In R. Fivush & C. A. Haden (Eds.), *Autobiographical memory and the construction of a narrative self* (pp. 3–28). Mahwah, NJ: Erlbaum.

Nelson, K., & Fivush, R. (2004). The emergence of autobiographical memory: A socio-cultural developmental theory. *Psychological Review, 111,* 486–511.

Nelson, L. J., Badger, S., & Wu, B. (2004). The influence of culture in emerging adulthood. Perspectives of Chinese college students. *International Journal of Behavioral Development, 28,* 26–36.

Nelson, L. J., & Barry, C. M. (2005). Distinguishing features of emerging adulthood: The role of self-classification as an adult. *Journal of Adolescent Research, 20,* 242–262.

Newcombe, R., & Reese, E. (2004). Evaluations and orientations in mother–child narratives as a function of attachment security: A longitudinal investigation. *International Journal of Behavioral Development, 28,* 230–245.

Nezlek, J., Sorrentino, R., Yasunaga, S., Otsubo, Y., Allen, M., & Kouhara, S. (2008). Cross-cultural differences in reactions to daily events as indicators of cross-cultural differences in self-construction and affect. *Journal of Cross-Cultural Psychology, 39,* 685–702.

Ng, S. H., & Han, S. (2009). The bicultural self and the bicultural brain. In R. S. Wyer, C. Chiu, & Y. Hong (Eds.), *Understanding culture: Theory, research, and application* (pp. 329–342.) New York: Psychology Press.

Nichols, J. G. (1984). Achievement motivation: Concepts of ability, subjective experience, task choice, and performance. *Psychological Review, 91,* 328–346.

Nichter, M. (2000). *Fat talk: What girls and their parents say about dieting.* Cambridge, MA: Harvard University Press.

Niemiec, C. P., Ryan, R. M., & Brown, K. W. (2008). The role of awareness and autonomy in quieting the ego: A self-determination theory perspective. In H. A. Wayment & J. J. Bauer (Eds.), *Transcending self-interest: Psychological explorations of the quiet ego* (pp. 107–116). Washington, DC: American Psychological Association.

Nisbett, R. E., Peng, K., Choi, I., & Norenzayan, A. (2001). Culture and systems of thought: Holistic versus analytic cognition . *Psychological Bulletin, 108,* 291–310.

Nisbett, R. E., & Ross, L. (1980). *Human inference: Strategies and shortcomings of social judgment.* Englewood Cliffs, NJ: Prentice-Hall.

Noam, G. G., & Borst, S. (Eds.). (1994). *Children, youth and suicide: Developmental perspectives.* San Francisco: Jossey-Bass.

Nolen-Hoeksema, S. (2000). The role of rumination in depressive disorders and mixed anxiety/depressive symptoms. *Journal of Abnormal Psychology, 109,* 504–511.

Nolen-Hoeksema, S., & Girus, J. S. (1994). The emergence of gender differences in depression during adolescence. *Psychological Bulletin, 115,* 435–442.

Norman, K. L. (2006). The self at the human/computer interface: A postmodern artifact in a different world. In P. C. Vitz & S. M. Felch (Eds.), *The self: Beyond the postmodern crisis.* Wilmington, DE: ISI Books.

O'Dea, J. (2006). Self-concept, self-esteem, and body weight in adolescent females: A three-year longitudinal study. *Journal of Health Psychology, 11,* 599–611.

Ogden, C. L., Carroll, M. D., & Flegal, K. M. (2008). High body mass index for age among U.S. children and adolescents, 2003–2006. *Journal of the American Medical Association, 299,* 2401–2405.

Olweus, D. (2008). Social problems in school. In A. Slater & G. Bremner (Eds.), *An introduction to developmental psychology* (pp. 437–454). Malden, MA: Blackwell.

Oosterwegel, A., & Oppenheimer, L. (1993). *The self-system: Developmental changes between and within self-concepts.* Hillsdale, NJ: Erlbaum.

Orth, U., Berking, M., & Burkhardt, S. (2006). Self-conscious emotions and depression: Rumination explains why shame but not guilt is maladaptive. *Personality and Social Psychology Bulletin, 32,* 1608–1619.

Owens, K. B. (1995). *Raising your child's inner self-esteem: The authoritative guide from infancy through the teen years.* New York: Plenum.

Oyserman, D., Bybee, D., Terry. K., & Hart-Johnson, T. (2004). Possible selves as roadmaps. *Journal of Research in Personality, 38,* 130–149.

Oyserman, D., Coon, H., & Kemmelmeier, M. (2002). Rethinking individualism and collectivism: Evaluation of theoretical assumptions and meta-analysis. *Psychological Bulletin, 128,* 3–72.

Oyserman, D., Gant, L.,& Ager, J. (1995). A socially contextualized model of African-American identity: Possible selves and school persistence. *Journal of Personality and Social Psychology, 69,* 1216–1232.

Oyserman, D., & Lee, S. W. S. (2008). Does culture influence what and how we think? Effects of priming individualism and collectivism. *Psychological Bulletin, 134,* 311–342.

Oyserman, D., & Sorensen, N. (2009). Understanding cultural syndrome effects on what and how we think: A saturated cognitive model. In R. S. Wyer, C. Chiu, & Y. Hong (Eds.), *Understanding culture: Theory, research, and application* (pp. 25–52). New York: Psychology Press.

Park, L., & Manor, J. (2009). Does self-threat promote social connection? The role of self-esteem and contingencies of self-worth. *Journal of Personality and Social Psychology, 96,* 203–217.

Paulhus, D. L., Harms, P. D., Bruce, M. N., & Lysy, D. C. (2004). The over-claiming technique: Measuring self-enhancement independent of ability. *Journal of Personality and Social Psychology, 84,* 890–904.

Paulhus, D. L., & Martin, C. L. (1988). Functional flexibility: A new conceptualization of interpersonal flexibility. *Journal of Personality and Social Psychology, 55,* 88–101.

Paxton, S., Neumark-Sztainer, D., Hannan, P., & Eisenberg, M. (2006). Body dissatisfaction prospectively predicts depressive mood and low self-esteem in adolescent girls and boys. *Journal of Clinical Child and Adolescent Psychology, 35,* 539–549.

Pedrabissi, L., Santinello, M., & Scarpazza, V. (1988). Contributo all-adattamento itliano del Self-Perception Profile for Children di Susan Harter. *Bollettino di Psycolgia Applicata, 185,* 19–26.

Pekrun, R. (2009). Emotions at school. In K. R. Wentzel & A. Wigfield (Eds.), *Handbook of motivation at school* (pp. 575–604). New York: Routledge (Taylor & Francis Group).

Pekrun, R., Goetz, T., Perry, R. P., Kramer, K., & Hochstadt, M. (2004). Beyond test anxiety: Development and validation of the Test Emotions Questionnaire (TEQ). *Anxiety, Stress, and Coping, 17,* 287–316.

Peterson, K. L., & Roscoe, B. (1991). Imaginary audience behavior in older adolescent females, *Adolescence, 26,* 195–200.

Pfeffer, C. R. (1988). Risk factors associated with youth suicide: A clinical perspective. *Psychiatric Annals, 18,* 652–656.

Phillips, D. (2007). Punking and bullying: Strategies in middle school, high school, and beyond. *Journal of Interpersonal Violence, 22,* 158–178.

Phillips, D. A., & Zimmerman, M. (1990). The developmental course of perceived competence and incompetence among competent children. In R. J. Sternberg & J. Kolligian, Jr. (Eds.), *Competence considered* (pp. 41–66). New Haven, CT: Yale University Press.

Piaget, J. (1932). *The moral judgment of the child.* New York: Harcourt, Brace, & World.

Piaget, J. (1960). *The psychology of intelligence.* Patterson, NJ: Littlefield-Adams.

Pike, K. M., Devlin, M. J., & Loeb, K. (2004). Cognitive-behavioral therapy in the treatment of anorexia, bulimia nervosa, and binge-eating disorder. In J. K. Thompson (Ed.), *Handbook of eating disorders and obesity* (pp. 130–162). New York: Wiley.

Pincus, A. K., & Lukowitsky, M. R. (2010). Pathological narcissism and narcissistic personality disorder. *Annual Review of Clinical Psychology, 6,* 421–446.

Pipp, S. (1990). Sensorimotor and representational internal working models of self, other, and relationship: Mechanisms of connection and separation. In D. Cicchetti & Beeghly (Eds.), *The self in transition: Infancy to childhood* (pp. 243–264). Chicago: University of Chicago Press.

Pollack, W. (1998). *Real boys.* New York: Random House.

Pomerantz, E. V., Ruble, D. N., Frey, K. S., & Greulich, F. (1995). Meeting goals and confronting conflict: Children's changing perceptions of social comparison. *Child Development, 66,* 723–738.

Pronin, E., Lin, D. Y., & Ross, L. (2002). The bias blind spot: Perceptions of bias in self versus others. *Personality and Social Psychology Bulletin, 28,* 369–381.

Pulham, D. (2009). *Humiliation and its relationship to embarrassment and shame.* Unpublished doctoral dissertation, University of Denver, Denver, CO.

Puoane, T., Fourie, J. M., Shapiro, M., Rosling, L., Tsaka, N. C., & Oelofse, A. (2005). Big is beautiful—An exploration with urban black community health workers in a South African township. *South African Journal of Clinical Nutrition, 18,* 6–15.

Putman, F. W. (1993). Dissociation and disturbances of the self. In D. Cicchetti & S. Toth (Eds.), *Rochester Symposium Developmental Psychopathology: Vol. 5. Disorders and dysfunctions of the self* (pp. 251–266). Rochester, NY: University of Rochester Press.

Pyszczynski, T. (2006). What role does self-esteem play in the ills and triumphs of society? In M. H. Kernis (Ed.), *Self-esteem: Issues and answers* (pp. 407–411). New York: Psychology Press.

Raeff, C. (2004). Within-culture complexities: Multifaceted and interrelated autonomy and connectedness characteristics in late adolescent selves. In M. F. Mascolo & J. Li (Eds.), *Culture and developing selves: Beyond dichotomization.* San Francisco: Jossey-Bass.

Raskin, R. N., & Terry, H. (1988). A principal-components analysis of the narcissistic personality inventory and further evidence of its construct validity. *Journal of Personality and Social Psychology, 54,* 890–902.

Read, G., & Morris, J. (2008). Body image disturbance in eating disorders. G. Read (Ed.), In *ABC of eating disorders* (pp. 9–14). Williston, VT: Wiley-Blackwell.

Reese, E. (2002). Social factors in the development of autobiographical memory: The state of the art. *Social Development, 11,* 124–142.

Reissland, N. (1985). The development of concepts of simultaneity in children's understanding of emotions. *Journal of Child Psychology and Psychiatry, 26,* 811–824.

Renick, M. J., & Harter, S. (1989). The impact of social comparisons on the developing self-representations of learning disabled students. *Journal of Educational Psychology, 81,* 631–638.

Rhee, S., Chang, J., & Rhee, J. (2003). Acculturation, communication patterns, and self-esteem among Asian and Caucasian American adolescents. *Adolescence, 38,* 749–768.

Rhee, U. (1993). Self-perceptions of competence and social support in Korean children, *Early Child Development and Care, 85,* 57–66.

Rhodewalt, F. (2006). Possessing and striving for high self-esteem. In M. H. Kernis (Ed.), *Self-esteem: Issues and answers* (pp. 281–287). New York: Psychology Press.

Riddle, M. (1986). *The effects of the transition to seventh grade on students' perceived competence, anxiety, motivational orientation and sense of control.* Unpublished doctoral dissertation, University of Denver, Denver, CO.

Rienks, S., & Harter, S. (2006). *Does classroom gender composition matter in public high schools?* Poster presented at the Society for Research on Adolescence, March 2006, San Francisco, CA.

Rinpoche, S. (1993). *The Tibetan book of the living and dying.* New York: HarperCollins.

Rinpoche, T. (1976). *The myth of freedom.* Berkeley, CA: Shambhalla Books.

Robbins, B., & Parlavecchio, H. (2006). The unwanted exposure of the self: A phenomenological study of embarrassment. *Humanistic Psychologist, 34,* 321–345.

Roberts, T., & Goldenberg, J. L. (2007). Wrestling with nature: An existential perspective on the body and gender in self-conscious emotions. In J. L. Tracy, R. W. Robins, & J. P. Tangney (Eds.), *The self-conscious emotions. Theory and research* (pp. 389–406). New York: Guilford Press.

Roberts, T., & Waters, P. (2004). Self-objectification and that "not so fresh feeling": Feminist therapeutic interventions for healthy female embodiment. *Women and Therapy, 27,* 5–21.

Robins, R. W., & Pals, J. L. (2002). Implicit self-theories in the academic domain: Implications for goal orientation, attributions, affect, and self-esteem change. *Self and Identity, 1,* 313–336.

Rochat, P. (2003). Five levels of self-awareness as they unfold early in life. *Consciousness and Cognition: An International Journal, 12,* 717–731.

Rochat, P. (2009). *Others in mind: Social origins of self-consciousness.* New York: Cambridge University Press.

Rogers, C. R. (1951). *Client-centered therapy.* Boston: Houghton Mifflin.

Rogoff, B. (1990). *Apprenticeship in thinking.* New York: Oxford University Press.

Rosenberg, M. (1979). *Conceiving the self.* New York: Basic Books.

Rosenberg, M. (1986). Self-concept from middle childhood through adolescence. In J. Suls & A. G. Greenwald (Eds.), *Psychological perspective on the self* (Vol. 3, pp. 107–135). Hillsdale, NJ: Erlbaum.

Rosenberg, S. (1988). Self and others: Studies in social personality and autobiography. In L. Berkowitz (Ed.), *Advances in experimental social psychology* (Vol. 21, pp. 56–96). New York: Academic Press.

Ross, L. R., & Spinner, B. (2001). General and specific attachment representations in adulthood: Is there a relationship? *Journal of Social and Personal Relationships, 18,* 747–766.

Rossman, B. B., & Rosenberg, M. S. (Eds.). (1998). *Multiple victimization of children.* New York: Haworth Press.

Rubin, K. H., Bukowski, W. M., & Parker, J. G. (2006). Peer interactions, relationships, and groups. In W. Damon & R. Lerner (Eds.) & N. Eisenberg (Vol. Ed.), *Handbook of child psychology: Vol. 3. Social, emotional, and personality development* (6th ed., pp. 571–649). New York: Wiley.

Rubin, L. (1985). *Just friends: The role of friendship in our lives.* New York: Harper.

Ruble, D. N., & Dweck, C. (1995). Self-conceptions, person conception, and their development. In N. Eisenberg (Vol. Ed.), *Review of personality and social psychology: The interface* (Vol. 15, pp. 109–139). Thousand Oaks, CA: Sage.

Ruble, D. N., & Frey, K. S. (1991). Changing patterns of comparative behavior as skills are acquired: A functional model of self-evaluation. In J. Suls & T. A. Wills (Eds.), *Social comparison: Contemporary theory and research* (pp. 70–112). Hillsdale, NJ: Erlbaum.

Ruble, D. N., Martin, C. L., & Berenbaum, S. A. (2006). Gender development. In W. Damon & R. Lerner (Eds.) & N. Eisenberg (Vol. Ed.), *Handbook of Child Psychology: Vol. 3. Social, emotional, and personality development* (6th ed., pp. 858–932). New York: Wiley.

Rusk, N., & Rothbaum, F. (2010). From stress to learning: Attachment theory meets goal orientation theory. *Review of General Psychology, 14,* 31–43.

Ruthig, J., Haynes, T., Perry, R., & Chipperfield, J. (2007). Academic optimistic bias: Implications for college student performance and well-being. *Social Psychology of Education, 10,* 115–137.

Rutter, M. (1993). *Developing minds: Challenge and continuity across the life span.* New York: HarperCollins.

Ryan, R. M., & Brown, K. W. (2006). What is optimal self-esteem? The cultivation and consequences of contingent vs. true self-esteem as viewed from the self-determination theory perspective. In M. H. Kernis (Ed.), *Self-esteem: Issues and answers* (pp. 120–131). New York: Psychology Press.

Ryan, R. M., Connell, J. P., & Deci, E. L. (1985). A motivational analysis of self-determination and self-regulation in education. In C. Ames & R. E. Ames (Eds.), *Research on motivation in education: The classroom milieu* (pp. 13–51). New York: Academic Press.

Ryan, R. M., & Deci, E. L. (2000). Self-determination theory and the facilitation of intrinsic motivation, social development and well-being. *American Psychologist, 55,* 68–78.

Ryan, R. M., & Deci, E. L. (2009). Promoting self-determined self-engagement. In K. R. Wentzel & A. Wigfield (Eds.), *Handbook of motivation at school* (pp. 171–196). New York: Routledge.

Ryder, A., Alden, L., & Paulhus, D. (2000). Is acculturation unidimensional or bidimensional? A head to head comparison in the prediction of personality, self-identity, and adjustment. *Journal of Personality and Social Psychology, 79,* 49–65.

Saarni, C., Campos, J. J., Camras, L. A., & Witherington, D. (2006). Emotional development: Action, communication, and understanding. In W. Damon & R. Lerner (Eds.) & N. Eisenberg (Vol. Ed.), *Handbook of child psychology: Vol. 3. Social, emotional, and personality development* (6th ed., pp. 226–229). New York: Wiley.

Sadker, M., & Sadker, D. (1994). *Failing at fairness: How America's schools cheat girls.* New York: Scribners.

Sakura, S. (1983). Development of the Japanese version of Harter's Perceived Competence Scale for Children. *Japanese Journal of Educational Psychology, 31,* 245–249.

Sanchez, D., & Kwang, T. (2007). When the relationship becomes her: Revisiting women's body concerns from a relationship contingency perspective. *Psychology of Women Quarterly, 31,* 401–414.

Sarbin, T. R. (1962). A preface to a psychological analysis of the self. *Psychological Review, 59,* 11–22.

Sarnoff, A. C. (1987). *Psychotherapeutic strategies in late latency through early adolescence.* Northvale, NJ: Aronson.

Sarphatie, H. (1993). On shame and humiliation: Some notes on early development and pathology. In H. Groen-Prakken & A. Laden (Eds.), *Dutch annual of psychoanalysis* (Vol. 1, pp. 191–204). Lisse, Netherlands: Swets & Zeitlinger.

Sarwer, D. B., Magee, L., & Crevand, E. E. (2004). Cosmetic surgery and cosmetic medical treatments. In J. K. Thompson (Ed.), *Handbook of eating disorders and obesity* (pp. 421–442). New York: Wiley.

Savacool, J. (2009). *The world has curves.* New York: Rodale Books.

Schlenker, B. R., & Miller, R. S. (1977). Egotism in groups: Self-serving bias or logical information processing. *Journal of Personality and Social Psychology, 35,* 755–764.

Schmader, T., Major, B., & Gramzow, R. (2001). Coping with ethnic stereotypes in the academic domain: Perceived injustice and psychological disengagement. *Journal of Social Issues, 57,* 93–111.

Schneider, W. (1988). Performance prediction in young children: Effects of skill, metacognition and wishful thinking. *Developmental Science, 1,* 291–297.

Schur, E. A., Sanders, M., & Steiner, H. (2000). Body dissatisfaction and dieting in young children. *International Journal of Eating Disorders, 27,* 74–82.

Schwartz, B., Shafermeier, E., & Trommsdorff, G. (2005). Relations between value orientation, child rearing goals, and parenting: A comparison of German and South Korean mothers. In W. Friedlmeier, P. Chakkarath, & B. Schwartz (Eds.), *Culture and human development: The importance of cross-cultural research to the social sciences.* New York: Psychology Press.

Schwartz, P. D., Maynard, A. M., & Uzelac, S. M. (2008). Adolescent egocentrism: A contemporary view. *Adolescence, 43,* 441–448.

Schwartz, S. J. (2001). The evolution of Eriksonian and neo-Eriksonian identity theory and research: A review and integration. *Identity: An International Journal of Theory and Research, 1,* 7–58.

Sedikides, C., & Herbst, K. (2002). How does accountability reduce self-enhancement?: The role of self-focus. *Revue Internationale de Psychologie Sociale, 15,* 113–128.

Sedikides, C., Horton, R. S., & Gregg, A. P. (2007). The why's the limit: Curtailing self-enhancement with explanatory introspection. *Journal of Personality, 75,* 783–824.

Sedikides, C., Wildschut, T., Routledge, C., Arndt, J., & Zhou, X. (2009). Buffering acculturative stress and facilitating cultural adaptation: Nostalgia as a psychological resource. In R. S. Wyer, C. Chiu, & Y. Hong (Eds.), *Understanding culture: Theory, research, and application*. New York: Psychology Press.

Selman, R. L. (1980). *The growth of interpersonal understanding*. New York: Academic Press.

Selman, R. L. (2003). The promotion of social awareness. New York: Russell Sage Foundation.

Serpell, L., Neiderman, M., Roberts, V., & Lask, B. (2007). The Shape- and Weight-Based Self-Esteem Inventory in adolescent girls with eating disorders and adolescent controls. *Psychotherapy Research, 17,* 321–327.

Shapiro, D., Moffett, A., Lieberman, L., & Dummer, G. (2008). Domain-specific ratings of importance and global self-worth of children with visual impairment. *Journal of Visual Impairment and Blindness, 102,* 232–244.

Shapiro, D. H. (1980). *Meditation: Self-regulation and altered states of consciousness*. New York: Aldine.

Shapiro, S. L. (2009). Meditation and positive psychology. In S. J. Lopez & C. R. Snyder (Eds.), *Oxford handbook of positive psychology* (2nd ed., pp. 601–610). New York: Oxford University Press.

Shaver, P. R., & Mikulincer, M. (2011). An attachment perspective on self-protection and self-enhancement. In M. D. Alicke & C. Sedikides (Eds.), *Handbook of self-enhancement and self-protection* (pp. 279–297). New York: Guilford Press.

Shaver, P. R., Wu, S., & Schwartz, J. C. (1992). Cross-cultural similarities and differences in emotion and its representation: A prototype approach. In M. S. Clark (Ed.), *Review of personality and social psychology* (pp. 175–212). Newbury Park, CA. Sage.

Sheler, J. L. (1997, March 31). New science suggests a "grand design" and ways to imagine eternity. *U.S. News and World Report,* 65–66.

Showers, C., & Larson, B. (1999). Looking at body image: The organization of self-knowledge about physical appearance and its relation to disordered eating. *Journal of Personality, 67,* 659–700.

Shulman, S., Feldman, B., Blatt, S. J., Cohen, O., & Mahler, A. (2005). Emerging adulthood: Age-related tasks and underlying self processes. *Journal of Adolescent Research, 20,* 577–603.

Siegler, R. S. (1991). *Children's thinking* (2nd ed.). Englewood Cliffs, NJ: Prentice-Hall.

Silfver, M. (2007). Coping with guilt and shame: A narrative approach. *Journal of Moral Education, 36,* 169–183.

Silfver, M., Helkama, K., Lönnquist, J., & Verkasalo, M. (2008). The relation between value priorities and proneness to guilt, shame, and empathy. *Motivation and Emotion, 32,* 69–80.

Simmons, R. G., & Blyth, D. A. (1987). *Moving into adolescence: The impact of pubertal change and school context*. New York: Aldine.

Singelis, T. M. (1994). The measurement of independent and interdependent self-construals. *Personality and Social Psychology Bulletin, 20,* 580–591.

Skinner, E. A., Kindermann, T. A., Connell, J. P., & Wellborn, J. G. (2009). Engagement and disaffection as organizational constructs in the dynamics of motivational development. In K. R. Wentzel & A. Wigfield (Eds.), *Handbook of motivation at school* (pp. 223–246). New York: Routledge (Taylor & Francis Group).

Smith, M. B. (1994). Selfhood at risk: Postmodern perils and the perils of postmodernism. *American Psychologist, 49,* 405–411.

Smith, R. H., Webster, J. M., Parrott, W. G., & Eyre, H. L. (2002). The role of public exposure in moral and nonmoral shame and guilt. *Journal of Personality and Social Psychology, 83,* 13–18.

Smolak, L., & Murnen, S. K. (2004). A feminist approach to eating disorders. In J. K. Thompson (Ed.), *Handbook of eating disorders and obesity* (pp. 590–605). New York: Wiley.

Smollar, J., & Youniss, J. (1985). Adolescent self-concept development. In R. L. Leahy (Ed.), *The development of self* (pp. 247–266). New York: Academic Press.

Snow, K. (1990). Building memories: The ontogeny of autobiography. In D. Cicchetti & M. Beeghly (Eds.), *The self in transition. Infancy to childhood* (pp. 213–242). Hillsdale, NJ: Erlbaum.

Snyder, H., & Pope, A. (2003). Presenting a different face to the world: Social comparisons and the self-evaluation of children with facial difference. In A. Pope (Ed.), *Inhabitants of the unconscious: The grotesque and the vulgar in everyday life* (pp. 41–60). New York: Haworth Press.

Snyder, M. (1987). *Public appearances, private realities: The psychology of self-monitoring.* New York: Freeman.

Spencer-Rodgers, J., Boucher, H., Mori, S., Wang, L., & Peng, K. (2009). The dialectical self-concept: Contradiction, change, and holism in East Asian cultures. *Personality and Social Psychology Bulletin, 35,* 29–44.

Spencer-Rodgers, J., Peng, K., Wang, L., & Hou, Y. (2004). Dialetical self-esteem and East–West differences in psychological well-being. *Personality and Social Psychology Bulletin, 30,* 1416–1432.

Sroufe, L. A. (1990). An organizational perspective on the self. In D. Cicchetti & M. Beeghley (Eds.), *The self in transition: Infancy to childhood* (pp. 281–308). Chicago: University of Chicago Press.

Sroufe, L. A., & Fleeson, J. (1986). Attachment and the construction of relationships. In W. Hartup & Z. Rubin (Eds.), *Relationships and development* (pp. 51–71). New York: Cambridge University Press.

Statman, D. (2000). Humiliation, dignity and self-respect. *Philosophical Psychology, 13,* 523–540.

Steele, C. M. (1988). The psychology of self-affirmation: Sustaining the integrity of the self. In L. Berkowitz (Ed.), *Advances in experimental social psychology* (Vol. 21, pp. 261–302). San Diego, CA: Academic Press.

Steinberg, L. (1990). Interdependency in the family, autonomy, conflict, and harmony in the parent–adolescent relationship. In S. Feldman & G. Elliot (Eds.), *At the threshold: The developing adolescent* (pp. 255–276). Cambridge, MA: Harvard University Press.

Steinberg, L. (2004). Risk taking in adolescence: What changes, and why? In R. E. Dahl & L.P. Spear (Eds.), *Adolescent brain development* (pp. 51–58). New York: New York Academy of Sciences.

Steinberg, L., & Silverberg, S. B. (1986). The vicissitudes of autonomy in early adolescence. *Child Development, 57,* 841–851.

Stern, D. (1985). *The interpersonal world of the infant.* New York: Basic Books.

Stevenson, H. W., & Stigler, J. W. (1992). *The learning gap.* New York: Simon & Schuster.

Stewart, T. M., & Williamson, D. A. (2004). Assessment of body image disturbances. In J. K. Thompson (Ed.), *Handbook of eating disorders and obesity*
(pp. 495–514). New York: Wiley.

Stigler, J. W., Smith, S., & Mao, L. (1985). The self-perception of competence by
Chinese Children. *Child Development, 56,* 1259–1270.

Stipek, D. (1995). The development of pride and shame in toddlers. In J. P. Tangney
& K. W. Fischer (Eds.), *Self-conscious emotions: The psychology of shame,
guilt, embarrassment, and pride* (pp. 237–252). New York: Guilford Press.

Stipek, D. (1998). Differences between Americans and Chinese in the circumstances
evoking pride, shame, and guilt. *Journal of Cross-Cultural Psychology, 29,*
616–629.

Stipek, D., Recchia, S., & McClintic, S. (1992). Self-evaluation in young children.
Monographs of the Society for Research in Child Development, 57, 1–84.

Strelan, P., Mehaffey, S., & Tiggemann, M. (2003). Self-objectification and esteem
in young women: The mediating role of reasons for exercise. *Sex Roles, 48,*
89–95.

Stryker, S. (1987). Identity theory: Developments and extensions. In K. Yardley &
T. Honess (Eds.), *Self and identity* (pp. 212–232). New York: Wiley.

Suh, E. (2002). Culture, identity consistency, and subjective well-being. *Journal of
Personality and Social Psychology, 83,* 1378–1391.

Sullivan, H. S. (1953). *The interpersonal theory of psychiatry.* New York: Norton.

Suls, J., & Sanders, G. (1982). Self-evaluation via social comparison: A developmental analysis. In L. Wheeler (Ed.), *Review of personality and social psychology* (Vol. 3, pp. 33–66). Beverly Hills, CA: Sage.

Suzuki, L., Davis, H., & Greenfield, P. (2008). Self-enhancement and self-effacement in reaction to praise and criticism: The case of multi-ethnic youth. *Ethos,
36,* 78–97.

Swann, W. B., Jr. (1996). *Self-traps: The elusive question for high self-esteem.* New
York: Freeman.

Swann, W. B.,Jr., Chang-Schneider, C., & Angulo, S. (2008). Self-verification in
relationships as an adaptive process. In J. V. Wood, A. Tesser, & J. G. Holmes
(Eds.), *The self in social relationships* (pp. 49–72). New York: Psychology
Press.

Swann, W. B., Jr., Chang-Schneider, C., & McClarty, K. L. (2007). Do people's
self-views matter? *American Psychologist, 62,* 84–94.

Swartz, T. T., & O'Brien, K. B. (2009). Intergenerational support during the transition to adulthood. In A. Furlong (Ed.), *Handbook of youth and young adulthood* (pp. 3–13).

Tafarodi, R., Lo, C., Yamaguchi, S., Lee, W., & Katsura, H. (2004). The inner self
in three countries. *Journal of Cross-Cultural Psychology, 35,* 97–117.

Tamm, M., & Prellwitz, M. (2001). "If I had a friend in a wheelchair": Children's
thoughts on disabilities. *Child Care, Health, and Development, 27,* 223–
240.

Tangney, J. P. (1995). Shame and guilt in interpersonal relationships. In J. P. Tangney & K. W. Fischer (Eds.), *Self-conscious emotions: The psychology of
shame, guilt, embarrassment, and pride* (pp. 114–139). New York: Guilford
Press.

Tangney, J. P. (2003). Self-relevant emotions. In M. R. Leary & J. P. Tangney (Eds.), *Handbook of self and identity* (pp. 384–400). New York: Guilford Press.

Tangney, J. P. (2009). Humility. In S. J. Lopez & C. R. Snyder (Eds.), *Oxford handbook of positive psychology* (2nd ed., pp. 483–490). New York: Oxford University Press.

Tangney, J. P. & Dearing, R. L. (2002). *Shame and guilt.* New York: Guilford Press.

Tangney, J. P., & Fischer, K. F. (Eds). (1995). *Self-conscious emotions: The psychology of shame, guilt, embarrassment, and pride.* New York: Guilford Press.

Tangney, J. P., Stuewig, J., & Mashek, D. J. (2007). What's moral about the self-conscious emotions? In J. L. Tracy, R. W. Robins, & J. P. Tangney (Eds.), *The self-conscious emotions. Theory and research* (pp. 21–37). New York: Guilford Press.

Tangney, J. P., Wagner, P. E., Fletcher, C., & Gramzow, R. (1992). Shamed into anger? The relation of shame and guilt to anger and self-reported aggression. *Journal of Personality and Social Psychology, 62,* 669–675.

Tanner, J. L. (2006). Recentering during emerging adulthood. In J. J. Arnett & J. L. Tanner (Eds.), *Emerging adults in America: Coming of age in the 21st century* (pp. 193–217). Washington, DC: American Psychological Association.

Taylor, S. E., & Brown, J. D. (1988). Illusion and well-being: A social-psychological perspective on mental health. *Psychological Bulletin, 103,* 193–210.

Teleporos, G., & McCabe, M. (2001). The impact of physical disability on body self-esteem. *Sexuality and Disability, 19,* 293–308.

Teroni, F., & Deonna, J. (2008). Differentiating shame from guilt. *Consciousness and Cognition: An International Journal, 17,* 725–740.

Terr, L. (1991). Childhood traumas: An outline and overview. *American Journal of Psychiatry, 148,* 10–20.

Tesser, A. (1988). Toward a self-evaluation maintenance model of social behavior. In L. Berkowitz (Ed.), *Advances in experimental social psychology* (Vol. 21, pp. 181–227). New York: Academic Press.

Tessler, M. (1991). *Making memories together: The influence of mother–child joint encoding on the development of autobiographical memory style.* Unpublished doctoral dissertation, City University of New York Graduate Center, New York.

Thomaes, S., Bushman, B. J., De Castro, B. O., & Stegge, H. (2009). What makes narcissists bloom? A framework for research on the etiology and development of narcissism. *Development and Psychopathology, 21,* 1233–1247.

Thomaes, S., Bushman, B. J., Stegge, H., & Olthof, T. (2008). Trumping shame by blasts of noise: Narcissism, self-esteem, shame, and aggression in young adolescents. *Child Development, 79,* 1792–1801.

Thompson, J., Shroff, H., Herbozo, S., Cafi, G., Rodriguez, J., & Rodriguez, M. (2007). Relations among multiple peer influences, body dissatisfaction, eating disturbances, and self-esteem: A comparison of average weight, at risk of overweight, and overweight adolescent girls. *Journal of Pediatric Psychology, 32,* 24–29.

Thompson, R. A. (2006). The development of the person: Social understanding, relationships, conscience, self. In W. Damon & R. Lerner (Eds.) & N.

Eisenberg (Vol. Ed.), *Handbook of child psychology: Vol. 3. Social, emotional, and personality development* (6th ed., pp. 24–98). New York: Wiley.

Tice, D. M., & Gailliot, M. (2006). How self-esteem relates to the ills and triumphs of society. In M. H. Kernis (Ed.), *Self-esteem: Issues and answers.* New York: Psychology Press.

Tiggemann, M. (2001). The impact of adolescent girls' life concerns and leisure activities on body satisfaction, disordered eating, and self-esteem. *Journal of Genetic Psychology, 162,* 133–142.

Tiggemann, M. (2005). Body dissatisfaction and adolescent self-esteem. Prospective findings. *Body Image, 2,* 129–135.

Tiggemann, M., & Lynch, J. (2001). Body image across the life-span in adult women: The role of self-objectification. *Developmental Psychology, 17,* 243–253.

Tiggemann, M., Martins, Y., & Churchett, L. (2008). Beyond muscles: Unexplored parts of men's body image. *Journal of Health Psychology, 13,* 1163–1172.

Toth, S. L., Cicchetti, D., Macfie, J., Maughan, A., & Vanmeenen, K. (2000). Narrative representations of caregivers and self in male pre-schoolers. *Attachment and Human Development, 2,* 271–305.

Tracy, J. L., & Robins, R. (2008). The nonverbal expression of pride: Evidence for cross-cultural recognition. *Journal of Personality and Social Psychology, 94,* 516–530.

Tracy, J. L., Robins, R., & Lagattuta, K. H. (2005). Can children recognize the pride expression? *Emotion, 5,* 251–257.

Tracy, J. L., & Robins, R. W. (2004). Putting the self into self-conscious emotions: A theoretical model. *Psychological Inquiry, 15,* 103–125.

Tracy, J. L., & Robins, R. W. (2006). Appraisal antecedents of shame and guilt: Support for a theoretical model. *Personality and Social Psychology Bulletin, 32,* 1339–1351.

Tracy, J. L., & Robins, R. W. (2007a). Emerging insights in the nature and function of pride. *Current Directions in Psychological Science, 16,* 147–150.

Tracy, J. L., & Robins, R. W. (2007b). The prototypical pride expression: Development of a nonverbal behavior coding system. *Emotion, 7,* 789–801.

Tracy, J. L., Robins, R. W., & Tangney, J. P. (Eds.). (2007). *The self-conscious emotions: Theory and research.* New York: Guilford Press.

Trent, L. M., Russell, G., & Cooney, G. (1994). Assessment of self-concept in early adolescence. *Australian Journal of Psychology, 46,* 21–28.

Triandis, H. C. (1989). *Individualism and collectivism.* Boulder, CO: Westview Press.

Triandis, H. C. (2009). Ecological determinants of cultural variation. In R. S. Wyer, C. Chiu, & Y. Hong (Eds.), *Understanding culture: Theory, research, and application* (pp. 189–210). New York: Psychology Press.

Triandis, H. C., McCusker, C., & Hui, C. H. (1990). Multi-method probes of individualism and collectivism. *Journal of Personality and Social Psychology, 59,* 1006–1020.

Trommsdorff, G., & Kornadt, H. J. (2003). Parent–child relations in cross-cultural perspective. In L. Kuczynski (Ed.), *Handbook of dynamics in parent–child relaions* (pp. 271–306). London: Sage.

Trzesniewski, K. H., Kinal, M. P., & Donnellan, M. B. (2010). Self-enhancement and self-protection in a developmental context. In M. D. Alicke & C. Sedikides (Eds.), *Handbook of self-enhancement and self-protection* (pp. 341–357). New York: Guilford Press.

Tsai, J., Ying, Y., & Lee, P. (2001). Cultural predictors of self-esteem: A study of Chinese American female and male young adults. *Cultural Diversity and Ethnic Minority Psychology, 7,* 284–297.

Tsui, A. S., Nifadkar, S. S., & Ou, A.Y. (2009). Nagging problems and modest solutions in cross-cultural research. In R. S. Wyer, C. Chiu, & Y. Hong (Eds.), *Understanding culture: Theory, research, and application* (pp. 163–186). New York: Psychology Press.

Tulku, T. (1978). *Skillful means.* Berkeley, CA: Dharma.

Turiel, E. (2004). Commentary: Beyond individualism and collectivism—A problem or progress? In M. E. Mascola & J. Lin (Eds.), *Culture and developing selves: Beyond dichotomization.* San Francisco: Jossey-Bass.

Turiel, E., & Walnryb, C. (1994). Social reasoning and the varieties of social experiences in cultural contexts. In H. W. Reese (Ed.), *Advances in child and behavior* (Vol. 45, pp. 289–326).

Turkle, S. (1995). *Life on the screen: Identity in the age of the internet.* New York: Simon & Schuster.

Turkle, S. (2005). *The second self: Computers and the human spirit.* Cambridge, MA: MIT Press.

Twenge, J., & Crocker, J. (2002). Race and self-esteem: Meta-analysis comparing Whites, Blacks, Hispanics, Asians, and American Indians and comment of Gray-Little and Hafdahl (2000). *Psychological Bulletin, 128,* 371–408.

Twenge, J. M., Konrath, S., Foster, J. D., Campbell, W. R. & Bushman, B. J. (2008). Egos inflating over time: A cross-temporal meta-analysis of the narcissistic personality inventory. *Journal of Personality, 76,* 875–901.

Valkenburg, P., Schouten, A., & Peter, J. (2005). Adolescents' identity experiments on the internet. *New Media and Society, 7,* 383–402.

Vallacher, R. B. (1980). An introduction to self-theory. In D. M. Wegner & R. R. Vallacher (Eds.), *The self in social psychology* (pp. 3–30). New York: Oxford University Press.

van der Kolk, B. A. (1987). *Psychological trauma.* Washington, DC: American Psychiatric Association Press.

Van Dongen-Melman, J. E. W. M., Koot, H. M., & Verhulst, F. C. (1993). Cross-cultural validation of Harter's Self-Perception Profile for Children in a Dutch sample. *Educational and Psychological Measurement, 53,* 739–753.

Vartanian, L., & Shaprow, J. (2008). Effects of weight stigma on exercise motivation and behavior: A preliminary investigation among college-aged females. *Journal of Health Psychology, 13,* 131–138.

Vartanian, L. R. (2000). Revisiting the imaginary audience and personal fable constructs of adolescent egocentrism: A conceptual review. *Adolescence, 35,* 639–661.

Verplanken, B., & Velsvik, F. (2008). Habitual negative body image thinking as a psychological risk factor in adolescents. *Body Image, 5,* 133–140.

Vitz, P. (2006). Introduction: From the modern and postmodern selves to the transmodern self. In P. C. Vitz & S. M. Felch (Eds.), *The self: Beyond the postmodern crisis.* Wilmington, DE: ISI Books.

Walsh, R., & Shapiro, S. L. (2006). The meeting of meditative disciplines and western psychology: A mutually enriching dialogue. *American Psychologist, 61,* 227–239.

Walter, J., & Burnaford, S. (2006). Developmental changes in adolescents' guilt and shame: The role of family climate and gender. *North American Journal of Psychology, 8,* 321–338.

Wang, Q., & Leichtman, M. D. (2000). Same beginnings, different stories: A comparison of American and Chinese children's narratives. *Child Development, 71,* 1329–1346.

Wang, Q., & Ross, M. (2007). Culture and memory. In S. Kitayama & D. Cohen (Eds.), *Handbook of cultural psychology* (pp. 645–667). New York: Guilford Press.

Wang, Y., & Ollendick, T. (2001). A cross-cultural and developmental analysis of self-esteem in Chinese and western children. *Clinical Child and Family Psychology Review, 4,* 253–271.

Waterman, A. S. (1992). Identity as an aspect of optimal functioning. In G. R. Adams, T. P. Gulotta, & R. Montemayor (Eds.), *Adolescent identity formation* (pp. 314–339). Newbury Park, CA: Sage.

Waters, T. (2011). *Taiwanese adolescents' construction of multiple selves across relational contexts.* Unpublished data. Colorado College, Colorado Springs, CO.

Watkins, D., Mortazavi, S., & Trofimova, I. (2000). Independent and interdependent conceptions of self: An investigation of age, gender, and culture differences in importance and satisfaction ratings. *Cross-Cultural Research: The Journal of Comparative Social Science, 34,* 113–134.

Watkins, D., & Regmi, M. (1999). Self-concepts of mountain children of Nepal. *Journal of Genetic Psychology, 160,* 429–435.

Watson, M. (1990). Aspects of self-development as reflected in children's role playing. In D. Cicchetti & M. Beeghly (Eds.), *The self in transition: Infancy to childhood* (pp. 123–144). Hillsdale, NJ: Erlbaum.

Watson, M., & Fischer, K. F. (1993). Structural change in children's understanding of family roles and divorce. In R. R. Cocking & K. A. Renninger (Eds.), *The development and meaning of psychological distance* (pp. 123–144). Hillsdale, NJ: Erlbaum.

Wayment, H. A., & Bauer, J. J. (2008). *Transcending self-interest: Psychological explorations of the quiet ego.* Washington, DC: American Psychological Association.

Weber, R. J. (2000). *The created self.* New York: Norton.

Weiner, B. (1986). *An attributional theory of motivation and emotions.* New York: Springer.

Weiner, B. (2007). Examining emotional diversity in the classroom: An attribution theorist considers the moral emotions. In P. A. Schutz & R. Pekrun (Eds.), *Emotions in education* (pp. 73–88). San Diego, CA: Academic Press.

Wertheim, E. H., Paxton, S. J., & Blaney, S. (2004). Risk factors for the development of body image disturbances. In J. K. Thompson (Ed.), *Handbook of eating disorders and obesity* (pp. 463–494). New York: Wiley.

Westen, D. (1993). The impact of sexual abuse on self structure. In D. Cicchetti & S. Toth (Eds.), *Rochester Symposium Developmental Psychopathology:*

Vol. 5. Disorders and dysfunctions of the self (pp. 223–250). Rochester, NY: University of Rochester Press.

White, K., Speisman, J., & Costos, D. (1983). Young adults and their parents: Individuation to mutuality. In H. D. Grotevant & C. R. Cooper (Eds.), *New directions for child development: Adolescent development in the family* (pp. 61–76). San Francisco: Jossey-Bass.

Williams, J., & Curie, C. (2000). Self-esteem and physical development in early adolescence: Pubertal timing and body image. *Journal of Early Adolescence, 20,* 129–149.

Williams, K., & Nida, S. (2009). Is ostracism worse than bullying? In M. J. Harris (Ed.), *Bullying, rejection, and peer victimization: A social cognitive neuroscience perspective* (pp. 279–296). New York: Springer.

Williams, L., & Desteno, D. (2008). Pride and perseverance: The motivational role of pride. *Journal of Personality and Social Psychology, 94,* 1007–1017.

Williams, L., Ricciardelli, L. A., McCabe, M. P., Waqa, G. G., & Bavadra, K. (2006). Body image attitudes among indigenous Fijian and European Australian adolescent girls. *Body Image, 3,* 275–287.

Wink, P. (1991). Two faces of narcissism. *Journal of Personality and Social Psychology, 61,* 590–597.

Winnicott, D. W. (1958). *From paediatrics to psychoanalysis.* London: Hogart Press.

Winnicott, D. W. (1965). *The maturational processes and the facilitating environment.* New York: International Universities Press.

Wirtz, D., & Chiu, C. (2008). Perspectives on the self in the east and the west: Searching for the quiet ego. In H. A. Wayment & J. J. Bauer (Eds.), *Transcending self-interest: Psychological explorations of the quiet ego* (pp. 149–158). Washington, DC: American Psychological Association.

Wolf, D. P. (1990). Being of several minds: Voices and versions of the self in early childhood. In D. Cicchetti & M. Beegley (Eds.), *The self in transition: Infancy to childhood* (pp. 183–212). Chicago: University of Chicago Press.

Wolf-Bloom, M. S. (1998). *Using media literacy training to prevent body dissatisfaction and subsequent eating problems in adolescent girls.* Unpublished doctoral dissertation, University of Cincinnati, Cincinnati, OH.

Wolfe, D. (1989). *Child abuse.* Newbury Park, CA: Sage.

Wong, Y., & Tsai, J. (2007). Cultural models of shame and guilt. In J. L. Tracy, R. W. Robins, & J. P. Tangney (Eds.), *The self-conscious emotions: Theory and research* (pp. 209–223). New York: Guilford Press.

Wood, A. M., Linley, P. A., Maltby, J., Baliousis, M., & Joseph, S. (2008). The authentic personality: A theoretical and empirical conceptualization and the development of the authenticity scale. *Journal of Counseling Psychology, 55,* 385–399.

Wrench, J., & Knapp, J. (2008). The effects of body image perceptions and sociocommunicative orientations on self-esteem, depression, and involvement in the gay community. *Journal of Homosexuality, 55,* 471–503.

Wylie, R. C. (1979). *The self-concept: Theory and research on selected topics* (Vol. 2). Lincoln: University of Nebraska Press.

Wylie, R. C. (1989). *Measures of self-concept.* Lincoln: University of Nebraska Press.

Yang, K. (2003). Beyond Maslow's culture-bound linear theory: A preliminary statement of the double-Y model of basic human needs. In R. A. Diestbier (Series Ed.) & V. Murphy-Berman & J. J. Berman (Vol. Eds.), *Nebraska Symposium on Motivation: Vol. 49. Cross-cultural differences in perspectives on the self* (pp. 175–256). Lincoln: University of Nebraska-Press.

Yang, R., & Blodgett, B. (2000). Effects of race and adolescent decision-making on status attainment and self-esteem. *Journal of Ethnic and Cultural Diversity in Social Work, 9,* 135–153.

Zeleke, S. (2004). Self-concepts of students with learning disabilities and their normally-achieving peers: A review. *European Journal of Special Needs Education, 19,* 145–170.

Zumpf, C. (1986). *The effect of a segregated program for the gifted on their perception of competence, social support, and motivational orientation.* Unpublished doctoral dissertation, University of Denver, Denver, CO.

Index

427